SO-EKM-316

Essentials of Paramedic Care
Canadian Edition
Volume 1

WORKBOOK

Robert S. Porter, M.A., NREMT-P
Ronald Bowles, B.Ed., M.Ed. Technology, EMA II
Manager, Instructional Design, Paramedic Academy, Justice Institute of British Columbia

Bryan E. Bledsoe, D.O., F.A.C.E.P., EMT-P
Emergency Department Staff Physician
Baylor Medical Center—Ellis County
Waxahachie, Texas
and
Clinical Associate Professor of Emergency Medicine
University of North Texas Health Sciences Center
Fort Worth, Texas

Robert S. Porter, M.A., NREMT-P
Senior Advanced Life Support Educator
Madison County Emergency Medical Services
Canastota, New York
and
Flight Paramedic
AirOne, Onondaga County Sheriff's Department
Syracuse, New York

Richard A. Cherry, M.S., NREMT-P
Clinical Assistant Professor of Emergency Medicine
Assistant Residency Director
SUNY Upstate Medical University
Syracuse, New York

Dwayne E. Clayden, M.E.M., Paramedic
Assistant to the Medical Director
The City of Calgary Emergency Medical Services
Calgary, Alberta

PEARSON
Prentice
Hall

Toronto

Copyright © 2006 Pearson Education Canada, a division of Pearson Canada Inc., Toronto, Ontario.

Pearson Prentice Hall. All rights reserved. This publication is protected by copyright, and permission should be obtained from the publisher prior to any prohibited reproduction, storage in a retrieval system, or transmission in any form or by any means, electronic, mechanical, photocopying, recording, or likewise. For information regarding permission, write to the Permissions Department.

Original edition, entitled *Workbook Essentials of Paramedic Care*, published by Pearson Education, Inc., Upper Saddle River, New Jersey, USA. Copyright © 2003 by Pearson Education, Inc. This edition is authorized for sale only in Canada.

ISBN 0-13-120307-X

Executive Editor: Samantha Scully
Developmental Editor: Pamela Voves
Production Editor: Marisa D'Andrea
Production Coordinator: Patricia Ciardullo

Printed and bound in Canada.

21 22 23 CP 16 15 14

NOTICE ON CARE PROCEDURES

It is the intent of the authors and publishers that this workbook be used as part of a formal paramedic education program taught by a qualified instructor. The care procedures presented here represent accepted competencies and practices in Canada. They are not offered as a standard of care.

Paramedic-level pre-hospital care in Canada is to be performed under the specific paramedic competencies available in each province. These competencies are specific for Primary Care Paramedics (PCP), Advanced Care Paramedics (ACP), and Critical Care Paramedics (CCP). Medically delegated acts can only be performed by a paramedic certified by a licensed medical physician or base hospital physician. It is the reader's responsibility to know and follow local protocols and follow their scope of practice associated to the system to which they belong. Also, it is the reader's responsibility to remain current of emergency care procedures and changes to their scope of practice. The material in this workbook contains the most current information available at the time of publication. However, federal, provincial, and local guidelines concerning clinical practices, including, without limitation, those governing infection control and universal precautions, change rapidly. The reader should note, therefore, that the new regulations may require changes in some procedures.

It is the responsibility of the reader to familiarize himself or herself with the policies and procedures set by national, provincial, and local agencies as well as the institution or agency where the reader is employed. The authors and the publisher of this workbook disclaim any liability, loss, or risk resulting directly or indirectly from the suggested procedures and theory, from any undetected errors, or from the reader's misunderstanding of the text. It is the reader's responsibility to stay informed of any new changes or recommendations made by any national, provincial, or local agency as well as by his or her employing institution or agency.

Contents

Introduction

To the Self-Instructional Workbook
Essentials of Paramedic Care

Welcome to the self-instructional workbook for *Essentials of Paramedic Care*. This workbook is designed to help guide you through an educational program for initial or refresher training that follows the specific paramedic competencies available in each province. The workbook is designed to be used either in conjunction with your instructor or as a self-study guide you use on your own.

This workbook features many different ways to help you learn the material necessary to become a paramedic, including those listed below.

FEATURES

Review of Chapter Objectives

Each chapter of *Essentials of Paramedic Care, Volume 1 and 2,* begins with objectives that identify the important information and principles addressed in the chapter reading. To help you identify and learn this material, each workbook chapter reviews the important content elements addressed by these objectives as presented in the text.

Content Self-Evaluation

Each chapter of *Essentials of Paramedic Care* presents an extensive narrative explanation of the principles of paramedic practice. The workbook chapter (or chapter part) contains between 10 and 90 multiple-choice, true/false, and matching questions to test your reading comprehension of the textbook material and to give you experience taking typical emergency medical service examinations.

Chapter Parts

Several chapters in *Essentials of Paramedic Care* are long and contain a great deal of subject matter. To help you grasp this material more efficiently, the workbook breaks these chapters into parts with their own objectives and content review.

How to Use
The Self-Instructional Workbook

The self-instructional workbook accompanying *Essentials of Paramedic Care, Canadian Edition, Volume 2* may be used as directed by your instructor or independently by you during your course of instruction. The recommendations listed below are intended to guide you in using the workbook independently.

• Examine your course schedule and identify the appropriate text chapter or other assigned reading.

• Read the assigned chapter in the text carefully. Do this in a relaxed environment, free of distractions, and give yourself adequate time to read and digest the material. The information presented in *Essentials of Paramedic Care* is often technically complex and demanding, but it is very important that you comprehend it. Be sure that you read the chapter carefully enough to understand and remember what you have read.

• Carefully read the Review of Chapter Objectives at the beginning of each workbook chapter (or part). This material includes both the objectives listed in *Essentials of Paramedic Care* and narrative descriptions of their content. If you do not understand or remember what is discussed from your reading, refer to the referenced pages and reread them carefully. If you still do not feel comfortable with your understanding of any objective, consider asking your instructor about it.

• Take the Content Self-Evaluation at the end of each workbook chapter (or part), answering each question carefully. Do this in a quiet environment, free from distractions, and allow yourself adequate time to complete the exercise. Correct your self-evaluation by consulting the answers at the back of the workbook, and determine the percentage you have answered correctly (the number you got right divided by the total number of questions). If you have answered most of the questions correctly (85 to 90 percent), review those that you missed by rereading the material on the pages listed in the answer key and be sure you understand which answer is correct and why. If you have more than a few questions wrong, (less than 85 percent correct), look for incorrect answers that are grouped together. This suggests that you did not understand a particular topic in the reading. Reread the text dealing with that topic carefully, and then retest yourself on the questions you got wrong. If incorrect answers are spread throughout the chapter content, reread the chapter and re-take the Content Self-Evaluation to assure that you understand the material. If you don't understand why your answer to a question is incorrect after reviewing the text, consult with your instructor.

• When you have completed *Essentials of Paramedic Care, Canadian Edition Volume 2* and its accompanying workbook, prepare for a course test by reviewing both the text in its entirety and your class notes.

If, during your completion of the workbook exercises, you have any questions that either the textbook or workbook doesn't answer, write them down and ask your instructor about them. Prehospital emergency medicine is a complex and complicated subject, and answers are not always black-and-white. It is also common for different EMS systems to use differing methods of care. The questions you bring up in class, and your instructor's answers to them, will help you expand and complete your knowledge of prehospital emergency medical care.

Guidelines to Better Test-Taking

The knowledge you will gain from reading the textbook, completing the exercises in the workbook, listening in your paramedic class, and participating in your clinical and field experience will prepare you to care for patients who are seriously ill or injured. However, before you can practice these skills, you will have to pass several classroom written exams and your state's certification exam successfully. Your performance on these exams will depend not only on your knowledge but also on your ability to answer test questions correctly. The following guidelines are designed to help your performance on tests and to better demonstrate your knowledge of prehospital emergency care.

1. Relax and be calm during the test.

A test is designed to measure what you have learned and to tell you and your instructor how well you are doing. An exam is not designed to intimidate or punish you. Consider it a challenge, and just try to do your best. Get plenty of sleep prior to the examination. Avoid coffee or other stimulants for a few hours before the exam, and be prepared.

Reread the text chapters, review the objectives in the workbook, and review your class notes. It might be helpful to work with one or two other students and ask each other questions. This type of practice helps everyone better understand the knowledge presented in your course of study.

2. Read the questions carefully.

Read each word of the question and all the answers slowly. Words such as "except" or "not" may change the entire meaning of the question. If you miss such words, you may answer the question incorrectly even though you know the right answer.

EXAMPLE:
The art and science of Emergency Medical Services involves all of the following EXCEPT:
- **A.** sincerity and compassion.
- **B.** respect for human dignity.
- **C.** placing patient care before personal safety.
- **D.** delivery of sophisticated emergency medical care.
- **E.** none of the above

The correct answer is C, unless you miss the "EXCEPT."

3. Read each answer carefully.

Read each and every answer carefully. While the first answer may be absolutely correct, so may the rest, and thus the best answer might be "all of the above."

EXAMPLE:
Indirect medical control is considered to be:
- **A.** treatment protocols.
- **B.** training and education.
- **C.** quality assurance.
- **D.** chart review.
- **E.** all of the above

While answers A, B, C, and D are correct, the best and only acceptable answer is "all of the above," E.

4. Delay answering questions you don't understand and look for clues.

When a question seems confusing or you don't know the answer, note it on your answer sheet and come back to it later. This will ensure that you have time to complete the test. You will also find that other questions in the test may give you hints to answer the one you've skipped over. It will also prevent you from being frustrated with an early question and letting it affect your performance.

5. Answer all questions.

Even if you do not know the right answer, do not leave a question blank. A blank question is always wrong, while a guess might be correct. If you can eliminate some of the answers as wrong, do so. It will increase the chances of a correct guess.

EXAMPLE:

When a paramedic is called by the patient (through the dispatcher) to the scene of a medical emergency, the medical control physician has established a physician/patient relationship.

     A.   True
     B.   False

    A true/false question gives you a 50 percent chance of a correct guess.

The hospital health professional responsible for sorting patients as they arrive at the emergency department is usually the:

     A.   emergency physician.
     B.   ward clerk.
     C.   emergency nurse.
     D.   trauma surgeon.
     E.   both A and C (correct)

    A multiple-choice question with five answers gives a 20 percent chance of a correct guess. If you can eliminate one or more incorrect answers, you increase your odds of a correct guess to 25 percent, 33 percent, and so on. An unanswered question has a 0 percent chance of being correct. Just before turning in your answer sheet, check to be sure that you have not left any items blank.

Essentials of Paramedic Care

Division 1

Introduction to Prehospital Care

Chapter 1

Introduction to Prehospital Care

Part 1: Introduction to Prehospital Care

Review of Chapter Objectives

With each chapter of the Workbook, we identify the objectives and the important elements of the textbook content. Because Chapter 1 is lengthy, it has been divided into parts. You should review items in these parts and refer to the pages listed if any points are not clear.

After reading this part of the chapter, you should be able to:

1. Describe the relationship between the paramedic and the other members of the allied health professions.   p. 6

The paramedic is the highest-level prehospital care provider and leader of the prehospital care team. He or she is a member of the allied health care professions and specifically a member of the ancillary health care professions, which include health care professionals other than physicians and nurses. Paramedics are credentialed or licensed by an appropriate provincial or territorial agency and approved by their system's medical directors.

2. Identify the attributes and characteristics of the paramedic. p. 7

Paramedics must possess the knowledge, skills, and attitudes consistent with the expectations of the public and the profession. This includes recognizing that you are an essential component in the continuum of care and an advocate for the patient. As a paramedic, you must be flexible enough to work within the various types of EMS systems and adjust to the ever-changing emergency environment. You must be a confident leader, accept the challenges of your profession, have excellent judgment, communicate effectively, develop a rapport with a great diversity of patients, and function independently in a very unstructured environment.

3. Explain the elements of paramedic education and practice that support its stature as a profession. p. 8

In 2001, the Paramedic Association of Canada, in conjunction with Human Resources and Development Canada, released the National Occupational Competency Profile (NOCP). The NOCP established a comprehensive framework for standardizing the fragmented paramedic education programs across Canada. It also serves as a reference point for agencies seeking to facilitate the mobility of Canadian paramedics between provinces and territories. Further, you, as a paramedic, and other members of the profession must commit to supporting research both to define and improve skills and care procedures that benefit patients and to identify those that do not. Only through research can the paramedic profession continue to grow and earn respect for the work of its members. Despite its relative youth, the field of emergency medical services enjoys growing public recognition as an important segment of the health care professions. However, this status must not be taken for granted.

4. Define and give examples of the expanded scope of practice for the paramedic.   p. 8

The scope of practice for paramedics has been expanded in many directions. These include critical care transport, primary health care, tactical EMS, industrial medicine, sports medicine, heavy urban search and rescue, and other specialty teams. Critical care transport is a specialization directed at the needs of critically ill or injured patients as they are moved from one care facility to another. During this transport, paramedics often use equipment far more advanced and complex than that found on standard ambulances. Primary care is the movement of the paramedic into more traditional health care roles in such places as emergency departments, outpatient clinics, physicians' offices, urgent care centres, and patients' homes. Tactical EMS members join specialized law enforcement officers on tactical operations including hostage rescue, drug raids, and similar high-risk emergencies. Industrial medicine is the field in which specially trained paramedics provide on-site services including emergency care, safety inspection, and accident prevention in the work place. Sports medicine sets the paramedic as a partner with the athletic trainer while providing emergency care and advising whether an injured player should return to the game or continue competition. Paramedics also serve as part of interdisciplinary heavy urban search and rescue teams that provide search, rescue, medical, and technical expertise in disaster situations.

CONTENT SELF-EVALUATION

Each of the chapters in this Workbook includes a short content review. The questions are designed to test your ability to remember what you read. At the end of this Workbook, you can find the answers to the questions as well as the pages where the topic of each question was discussed in the text. If you answered a question incorrectly or are unsure of the answer, review the pages listed.

Multiple Choice

      1. The modern ambulance is best described as a(n):
        A.   rapid patient transport vehicle.   **D.**   mobile intensive care unit.
        B.   vehicle for horizontal transport.   **E.**   automated care delivery centre.
        C.   mobile emergency room.

      2. The expanding role of the paramedic includes the role of:
        A.   public educator.   **D.**   facilitator of access to care.
        B.   health promoter.   **E.**   all of the above
        C.   injury and illness prevention advocate.

3. The paramedic is held accountable to which of the following?
   A. the public
   B. the system medical director
   C. the employer
   D. his or her peers
   E. all of the above

4. The best way to ensure that you meet the expectations of the public, peers, and the system medical director is to:
   A. know your protocols.
   B. attend all ongoing education sessions.
   C. record everything well on the prehospital care report.
   D. always act in the best interest of the patient.
   E. act confident and in control while you provide care.

5. Which of the following is NOT a characteristic of a professional paramedic?
   A. confident leadership.
   B. excellent judgment.
   C. strong opinions about ethnic groups.
   D. ability to develop a rapport with a wide variety of patients.
   E. ability to function independently.

6. The National Occupational Competency Profile serves as:
   A. a reference point for provincial or territorial bodies seeking to facilitate the mobility of Canadian paramedics.
   B. a curriculum document for national EMS training.
   C. a blueprint for the Canadian National Registry examination.
   D. description of the key traits and characteristics required by those seeking to build a career in pre-hospital care.
   E. all of the above.

7. Which of the following is an example of the expanded scope of practice for paramedics?
   A. critical care transport
   B. primary care
   C. industrial medicine
   D. sports medicine
   E. all of the above

8. A tactical paramedic is likely to provide support to which of the services listed below?
   A. fire service
   B. utility company
   C. search and rescue
   D. law enforcement
   E. all of the above

True/False

9. While required to be licensed, registered, or credentialed, paramedics still may only function as approved by and under the direction of the system's medical director.
   A. True
   B. False

10. For years, paramedic practice was based on anecdotal data and tradition.
   A. True
   B. False

11. Paramedics must be able to function independently in a nonstructured, constantly changing environment.
   A. True
   B. False

_____ 12. Provision of prehospital care in Canada is a local or municipal responsibility.
   A.   True
   B.   False

_____ 13. The National Occupational Competency Profile, developed in 2001, established a comprehensive framework for standardizing the fragmented paramedic education programs across Canada.
   A.   True
   B.   False

_____ 14. A professional code of ethics and etiquette help ensure that the public interest is maintained above personal, corporate or financial considerations..
   A.   True
   B.   False

_____ 15. HUSAR teams, including paramedics, help take primary health care into the community and keep non-urgent patients out of the hospital Emergency Department.
   A.   True
   B.   False

_____ 16. Paramedics may also serve in occupational health roles, including safety officers and inspectors.
   A.   True
   B.   False

_____ 17. Critical Care transport teams transport serious ill or injured patients from the field to the Emergency Department.
   A.   True
   B.   False

_____ 18. The primary goal of sports medicine is to limit the aggravation of injuries at the scene.
   A.   True
   B.   False

Matching

Write the letter of the paramedic role in the space provided next to the functions to which it applies.

Role

   A. Critical Care Transport   D.   Industrial Medicine
   B. Primary Health Care   E.   Sports Medicine
   C. Tactical EMS   F.   Heavy Urban Search and Rescue

Function

_____ 19. function alongside trainers to prevent injury and help injured persons to return to full function as quickly as possible.

_____ 20. manage complicated inter-facility transports, often involving specially equipped ambulances or aircraft.

_____ 21. accompany specially trained law enforcement officers on operations that may involve sophisticated, prolonged, definitive patient care.

_____ 22. serve as integral member of an interdisciplinary team involved in search, rescue, medical, and technical operations in disaster areas.

_____ 23. provide occupational health care and serve as safety officers and inspectors in areas such as construction sites, oil rigs, and other facilities where these specialized skills are required.

_____ **24.** function in the community to provide cost-effective, convenient medical care in the field or home, triage and direct patients with nonemergency problems to proper nonhospital facilities.

Chapter 1

Introduction to Prehospital Care

Part 2: EMS Systems

Review of Chapter Objectives

After reading this part of the chapter, you should be able to:

1. **Describe key historical events that influenced the national development of Emergency Medical Services (EMS) systems. pp. 10-12**

   There is a long history of individuals providing care in the out-of-hospital setting, beginning in ancient times. The cardinal events in the history of EMS include the first organized use of patient transport (and the ambulance) by Jean Larrey, chief surgeon for Napoleon. While simply a horse-drawn cart called an ambulance volante (flying ambulance), it represented the first recognized attempt to bring the injured from the field to medical care. Wars continued to be the impetus to improve out-of-hospital care. The American Civil War, World Wars I and II, and the Korean and Vietnamese conflicts all brought substantial changes to field care and transport. The war in Vietnam saw a greater reduction in mortality associated with immediate care in the field and rapid access to surgery than was the case in any previous conflict. In Canada, integrated EMS systems grew from fragmented operations during the 1960's and 1970's. Early advanced life support programs started up in various regions throughout the 1970's. However, with health care as a provincial and territorial concern, these programs tended to function at local, municipal, or regional levels. Standards varied from province to province. Canadian systems were influenced by the US Department of Transportation, but developed in many different directions.

2. **Define the following terms:**

   EMS systems   p 13
   An emergency medical services system is a comprehensive network of personnel, equipment, and resources established to deliver aid and emergency medical care to the community.

   Licensure   p. 18

Licensure is a process by which a governmental agency grants permission to engage in an occupation based on an applicant's attaining a required competency sufficient to ensure the public's protection.

Certification   p. 18
Certification is a process by which an agency or association grants recognition to an individual who meets its qualifications.

Registration   p. 18
Registration is the listing of your name and essential information within a particular record of a certifying organization.

Profession p. 18
A profession is a vocation requiring advanced education or training in a specialized body of knowledge and/or skills.

Professionalism   p. 24
Professionalism is the conduct or qualities that characterize a practitioner in a particular field or profession.

Ethics   p. 25
Ethics are rules or standards for conduct of a particular group or profession.

Peer review   p. 25
Peer review is a process of evaluation of the quality of conduct or actions performed by members of a group or profession that is undertaken by other members of that group or profession.

Medical direction   p. 14
Medical direction is the guidance of the actions of prehospital care providers by a physician associated with the emergency medical services system. Medical direction may be on-line or off-line medical direction and includes the physician's involvement in and supervision of personnel education, personnel and equipment selection, protocol development, quality improvement, and advocacy for the EMS system and the patient.

Protocols p. 15
Protocols are policies and procedures addressing primarily triage, treatment, transport, and transfer of patients as well as special circumstances and events within the EMS system.

3. Identify national groups important to the development, education, and implementation of EMS as well as the role of provincial or territorial associations, the Paramedic Association of Canada (PAC), and the roles of various EMS standard-setting agencies.   pp. 19 - 20

The Paramedic Association of Canada is Canada's only national EMS organization. Over 14,000 members belonged to PAC in 2005. Membership is drawn from EMS practitioners in most Canadian provinces and territories, as well as the Canadian Armed Forces. Because health care is a provincial and territorial responsibility in Canada, EMS standards are set at the provincial and territorial level. Although federal laws affect such areas of controlled drugs and medical devices, provincial and territorial bodies govern other aspects of EMS operations.

4. Identify the standards (components) of an EMS system.   p. 12

EMS systems should have the following components:
• **Regulation and policy.** Each province or territory must have laws, regulations, policies, and procedures that govern its EMS system.
• **Resources management.** Each province or territory must have central control of health-care resources to ensure that all patients have equal access to emergency care.
• **Human resources and training.** Each province or territory must require that all EMS providers are taught by qualified instructors using a standardized curriculum.
• **Transportation.** Each province or territory must ensure that patients are safely and reliably

transported by ground or air ambulance.

• **Facilities.** Each province or territory must ensure that every seriously ill or injured patient is delivered to an appropriate medical facility in a timely manner.

• **Communications.** Each province or territory must have a system for public access to EMS along with communications among dispatchers, ambulance crews, and hospital personnel.

• **Trauma systems.** Each province or territory should develop a system of specialized care for trauma patients including the designation of trauma centres and systems to ensure that patients arrive at the appropriate facility in a timely manner.

• **Public information and education.** EMS personnel should participate in programs designed to educate the public in injury prevention, emergency recognition, system access, and first aid.

• **Medical direction.** Each EMS system must have a physician medical director responsible for delegating medical practice to prehospital care providers and overseeing patient care.

• **Evaluation.** Each province or territory must have a quality improvement system for continuing evaluation and upgrading of the EMS system.

5. Differentiate among EMS provider levels: emergency medical responder, primary care paramedic, advanced care paramedic, and critical care paramedic.   pp. 18-19

• **Emergency Medical Responder (EMR).** An emergency medical responder may act as a first responder or as an entry-level position in some EMS systems. EMRs are responsible for primary assessment, BLS treatments and interventions, and the provision of safe and prudent care.

• **Primary Care Paramedic (PCP).** Primary care paramedics may be volunteer or career paramedics and may operate in any EMS setting. PCPs perform patient assessment, treat medical conditions and injuries, and perform delegated medical acts, such as the administration of specific medications, semiautomatic defibrillation, and IV maintenance. PCPs display a sound knowledge of anatomy, physiology, and pathophysiology, and demonstrate excellent problem-solving and decision-making skills.

• **Advanced Care Paramedic (ACP).** Advanced care paramedics provide enhanced levels of care, using advanced life support procedures and protocols. ACP builds on the PCP foundation to provide additional levels of assessment and treatment. ACP competencies include advanced techniques, invasive procedures, pharmacological interventions, and delegated medical acts for managing life-threatening conditions involving airway, breathing, and circulation.

• **Critical Care Paramedic (CCP).** The critical care paramedic is the highest level described by the NOCP. CCP extends ACP competencies to include patient assessment, interpret laboratory and radiological data, demonstrate advanced decision-making and differential discrimination skills, and manage patient autonomously and with consultation of medical authorities. The CPP profile includes a wide range of controlled and delegated medical acts, including the use of invasive hemodynamic monitoring devices.

6. Describe what is meant by "citizen involvement in the EMS system."   pp. 15 - 16

Citizen involvement in the EMS system means that average members of the public can recognize a medical or trauma emergency, know how to access the EMS system, and know how to provide basic life support assistance such as hemorrhage control, CPR, and, possibly, early defibrillation prior to the arrival of EMS personnel.

7. Discuss the role of the EMS physician in providing medical direction, prehospital and out-of-hospital care as an extension of the physician, the benefits of both on-line and off-line medical direction, and the process for the development of local policies and protocols.   pp. 14- 15

A paramedic functions only under the supervision and direction of a medical direction physician. That oversight is provided as either on-line medical direction or off-line medical dirrection. Off-line medical direction involves the physician's participation in personnel and equipment selection, training, protocol development, quality improvement, and acting as an EMS and patient advocate within the health profession. On-line medical direction consists of direct radio or phone consultation and oversight of paramedics and other prehospital care providers while they are caring for a patient. The ultimate responsibility for all care offered by the paramedic rests with the medical direction physician.

The medical director is a physician who is legally responsible for all clinical and patient care aspects of an EMS system. Prehospital care provided by the paramedic or other EMS personnel is provided under the license of the medical director, regardless of who his or her employer is.

The benefits of both on-line and off-line medical direction include the medical supervision of the EMS system and prehospital and out-of-hospital patient care. Among these benefits are the opportunity to practice "prehospital medicine" under the license and supervision of the medical director including use of protocols, standing orders, and algorithms developed by the medical director. Additionally, on-line medical direction provides access to direct medical consultation for EMS personnel during the care of the emergency patient.

Protocols are developed by the medical director (in cooperation with expert EMS personnel) to address the assessment and care offered during triage, treatment, transport, and transfer of the patient. The protocols and other system policies are developed to address not only commonly encountered circumstances but also special situations such as intervener physicians, child, spouse, or elderly abuse, DNR orders, patient refusals, and the like. The protocols and policies set the standards for accountability of EMS personnel and ensure uniform, medically approved care for each and every patient.

8. Describe the relationship between a physician on the scene, the paramedic on the scene, and the EMS physician providing on-line medical direction.   pp. 14-15

At the scene of a medical or trauma emergency, the health care professional with the highest training specific to emergency care should be responsible for patient care. When a nonaffiliated physician is at the scene (an intervener physician), the on-line medical direction physician is ultimately responsible for the patient. When on-line medical direction is not available, the paramedic may relinquish patient care responsibility to the intervener physician as long as that individual identifies him- or herself, demonstrates a willingness to assume patient care responsibilities, and agrees to provide the documentation required by the system. If treatment differs from system protocols, the intervener physician must agree to ride with the patient to the hospital.

9. Describe the components of continuous quality improvement and analyze its contribution to system improvement, continuing medical education, and research.   pp. 23-25

Continuous quality improvement (CQI) is an ongoing effort to refine and improve the system to ensure the highest level of service possible. It involves six basic components: identifying system-wide problems, elaborating on the probable causes, listing solutions, outlining a plan of corrective action, providing resources and support to ensure success, and re-evaluating the results and system performance continuously. CQI system review uses positive reinforcement and support to identify and improve patient care. It can identify areas for improvement and ways to allocate resources to make those improvements, frequently through continuing medical education. When questions arise about the benefits of care offered by a system, a CQI program can suggest research projects to investigate the real value of procedures, equipment, and protocols. The real key to effective CQI is the positive and reinforcing nature of its approach to system improvement.

10. Describe the importance, basic principles, process of evaluating and interpreting, and benefits of research.   p. 25-26

Research is essential to ensuring that the equipment and procedures used in the out-of-hospital setting are safe, benefit the patient, and are worth any potential risks of employing them. Research attempts to objectively evaluate the performance of interventions in an unbiased way. Research begins by asking a question (stating a hypothesis), investigating any existing research, designing a study that is unbiased and fairly measures performance, collects and analyzes data, assesses and evaluates results against the hypothesis, and reports the findings. Research is ultimately needed to determine what is in the best interest of the prehospital patient and what is the value of prehospital care in general. Research is essential to the existence of EMS and the profession's evolution.

CONTENT SELF-EVALUATION

Multiple Choice

_____ 1. The date of the earliest recorded medical care procedures is:
A. about 5,000 years ago.
B. about 2,000 years ago.
C. 1497.
D. 1562.
E. 1666.

_____ 2. Which of the following was NOT a component of the Emergency Medical Services Systems Act of 1973?
A. communications
B. system financing
C. training
D. access to care
E. system evaluation

_____ 3. The intervener physician is a physician who is:
A. not affiliated with the system of medical direction.
B. at the scene of an emergency.
C. a trained emergency physician.
D. both A and B.
E. none of the above.

_____ 4. When on-line medical control does not exist and an intervener physician is present, is willing to accept patient care responsibility, performs interventions consistent with the system protocols, and agrees to document the interventions as required by the system, the paramedic should:
A. relinquish patient care responsibilities.
B. retain patient care authority.
C. relinquish patient care responsibilities only if the physician agrees to ride to the hospital.
D. retain patient care responsibilities in cases of physician disagreement.
E. none of the above.

_____ 5. Off-line medical direction includes which of the following?
A. protocols
B. training guidelines
C. personnel selection policies
D. quality assurance
E. all of the above

_____ 6. Which of the following is NOT one of the four "Ts" of emergency care?
A. triage
B. transfer
C. termination of care
D. transport
E. treatment

_____ 7. Which of the following statements is NOT true?
A. the ability to recognize cardiac emergencies can save lives.
B. in Canada, over 75,000 cardiac-related deaths occurred in 1999.
C. most cardiac arrests happen immediately upon onset of symptoms.
D. if bystanders or the patient call in time, many cardiac arrests can be prevented.
E. all of the above.

_____ 8. The dispatch system that provides caller interrogation, predetermined response configurations, and pre-arrival instructions is:
A. system status management.
B. enhanced 911.
C. priority dispatch.
D. caller interrogation.
E. none of the above

9. The goal of dispatch and response in an effective EMS is to have:
   A. BLS units on the scene within 4 minutes.
   B. ALS units on the scene within 8 minutes.
   C. at least 90 percent of all responses within system time limits.
   D. all of the above
   E. none of the above

10. The process by which a province, territory, or other regulatory agency grants permission to engage in a given occupation is:
   A. licensure.   D. reciprocity.
   B. certification.   E. tenure.
   C. registration.

11. Granting someone recognition for meeting the qualifications of another agency is called:
   A. licensure.   D. reciprocity.
   B. certification.   E. tenure.
   C. registration.

12. The Paramedic Association of Canada National Occupational Competency Profile identifies how many levels of paramedic providers?
   A. 1   D. 4
   B. 2   E. 5
   C. 3

13. The paramedic provider responsible for general patient assessment, CPR, hemorrhage control, and spinal immobilization is the:
   A. Emergency Medical Responder.   D. Critical Care Paramedic.
   B. Primary Care Paramedic.   E. all of the above
   C. Advanced Care Paramedic.

14. Standards for training and licensure for paramedics in Canada are established by:
   A. The Canadian Medical Association.
   B. National Association of Prehospital Care Providers.
   C. Paramedic Association of Canada.
   D. Designated regulatory bodies in each province or territory.
   E. None of the above.

15. Fixed-wing aircraft are usually used for patient transports exceeding:
   A. 25 km.   D. 320 km.
   B. 50 km.   E. 500 km.
   C. 200 km.

16. A standard van with a raised roof that is configured as an ambulance is categorized as which type of ambulance?
   A. Type I   D. Type A
   B. Type II   E. Type B
   C. Type III

17. A Primary Trauma Centre is a facility that:
   A. provides initial triage for all trauma situations in a community.
   B. fulfills the role of the major trauma centre.
   C. coordinates specialty services and ensures appropriate patient distribution.
   D. has a 24-hour emergency department.
   E. all of the above.

18. A hospital designated as a receiving facility for the EMS system should have which of the following?
   A. an emergency department
   B. 24-hour emergency physician coverage
   C. surgical facilities and coverage

D. critical and intensive care units

E. all of the above

19. Which of the following is NOT a part of a well-designed disaster plan?
    A. mutual aid agreements among neighboring municipalities, services, and systems
    B. a rigid communications system
    C. frequent disaster plan tests and drills
    D. integration of all system components
    E. a coordinated central management agency

20. A major complaint regarding quality assurance programs is that they tend to:
    A. be one-time efforts.
    B. address only procedural issues.
    C. focus on punitive actions.
    D. not examine protocol issues.
    E. create divisions among care workers on staff.

21. Continuous quality improvement differs from quality assurance in that it:
    A. emphasizes customer satisfaction.
    B. rewards or reinforces good behaviour.
    C. examines billing practices.
    D. evaluates maintenance activities.
    E. all the above

22. Which of the following is NOT one of the standard rules of evidence used to evaluate a proposed change in the EMS system?
    A. There must be a basis for change.
    B. The old procedure must be deemed no longer medically acceptable.
    C. The change must be clinically important.
    D. The change must be affordable, practical, and teachable.
    E. All of the above are standard rules of evidence.

23. Ethics are best defined as:
    A. protocols and policies for conduct.
    B. rules or standards governing the performance of a profession.
    C. legal principles governing potential lawsuits.
    D. the four elements needed to determine negligence.
    E. justifications for actions.

24. The process in which others care in the profession judge the quality of an individual's emergency is known as:
    A. peer review.   **D.** continuous quality review.
    B. post-incident critique.   **E.** standards of care review.
    C. third-party review.

25. Which of the following research questions would NOT inform discussions on EMS funding and system accountability:
    A. What prehospital interventions actually reduce morbidity and mortality?
    B. Where did early EMS systems develop?
    C. Are the benefits of certain field procedures worth the potential risks?
    D. What is the cost-benefit ratio of sophisticated prehospital equipment and procedures?
    E. Is field stabilization possible, or should paramedics begin immediate transport in every case?

True/False

_____ **26.** An Emergency Medical Services system is a network of personnel, equipment, and resources established to deliver aid and emergency care to the community.
- **A.** True
- **B.** False

_____ **27.** Emergency medical responders in Canada may be trained and licensed to provide advanced life support measures such as drug therapy, intubation, and manual defibrillation.
- **A.** True
- **B.** False

_____ **28.** EMS services in Canada, including training, protocols, and operations may vary across provinces and territories, and even across cities and towns.
- **A.** True
- **B.** False

_____ **29.** The intervener physician is a medical director who is legally responsible for all patient care offered by the system he or she oversees.
- **A.** True
- **B.** False

_____ **30.** Standing orders are preauthorized protocols or treatment algorithms that allow a paramedic to perform delegated medical acts only after consultation with online medical control.
- **A.** True
- **B.** False

_____ **31.** Priority dispatching refers to preferentially dispatching resources within a community based on their level of training.
- **A.** True
- **B.** False

_____ **32.** Reciprocity refers to the process by which an agency grants automatic certification or licensure to an individual who has comparable certification or licensure from another agency.
- **A.** True
- **B.** False

_____ **33.** The Emergency Medical Responder level includes the provision of safe and prudent care. In some communities, EMRs may also provide transport.
- **A.** True
- **B.** False

_____ **34.** Multiple trauma patients should be transported to the nearest hospital whenever possible.
- **A.** True
- **B.** False

_____ **35.** Peer review is an essential component of a professional code of ethics.
- **A.** True
- **B.** False

Matching

Write the letter of the appropriate term in the space provided next to the definition to which it applies.

Term

A. Tertiary Trauma Centre
B. Primary Trauma Centre
C. Critical Care Paramedic
D. Advanced Care Paramedic

E. Primary Care Paramedic
F. Certification
G. Reciprocity
H. Licensure

Definition

_____ **36.** smaller, rural medical centre or nursing station that provides initial triage for all trauma situations.

_____ **37.** highest level of paramedic described by the NOCP; includes a wide range of controlled and delegated medical acts, including the use of invasive hemodynamic monitoring devices.

_____ **38.** regional referral centre for seriously injured patients, staffed with a 24-hour trauma response team.

_____ **39.** process by which a regulatory agency grants permission to engage in a given occupation to an applicant who has attained the degree of competency required to ensure the public's protection.

_____ **40.** process by which an agency or association grants recognition and the ability to practice to an individual who has met its qualifications.

_____ **41.** provides enhanced levels of care using advanced techniques, invasive procedures, pharmacological interventions and delegated medical acts.

Chapter 1

Introduction to Prehospital Care

Part 3: Roles and Responsibilities of the Paramedic

Review of Chapter Objectives

After reading this part of the chapter, you should be able to:

1. Describe the attributes of a paramedic as a health care professional.   **pp. 30-34**

The attributes of a paramedic are related to his or her stature as a health care professional and include leadership, integrity, empathy, self-motivation, appearance and personal hygiene, self-confidence, communication, time management, teamwork and diplomacy, respect, and patient advocacy.

As a paramedic, you must demonstrate leadership in order to coordinate and direct other care providers in attending to the patient. You must know the abilities of your team and ask its members to do only what they are able to do. You must demonstrate integrity to earn the respect of your peers and the medical community. You must demonstrate empathy by appreciating the plight of the patient and demonstrating an understanding of his or her situation. You must be both self-confident and self-motivated to employ life-saving procedures in the worst of conditions. You must strive for excellence in knowledge and skills and have and display confidence as you employ patient care skills. Your appearance must demonstrate a respect for both yourself and your patient. Remember that good grooming and personal hygiene both are important in presenting a professional image. You must be able to communicate effectively both orally and in writing to patients, other care providers, and physicians. You must be able to coordinate your efforts and those of others to quickly address the needs of the patient and to fulfill your responsibilities as a paramedic. You must respect others and, through demonstrating that respect, earn respect for yourself. One way of demonstrating that respect is showing a heightened sensitivity to your patient's rights as a person, including the right to confidentiality. You must become a patient advocate, promoting and ensuring that patients receive the care and attention their illness or injury requires. And finally, you must ensure that you maintain the attributes of a professional through careful delivery of your service, including mastering and refreshing skills; following protocols, policies, and procedures; checking your equipment before its use; and operating the ambulance and equipment safely.

2. Describe the benefits of paramedic continuing education and the importance of maintaining one's paramedic license/certification.   p. 35

Continuing education helps you maintain the knowledge you acquired through your initial paramedic education and expands your own personal knowledge and skills. It helps you keep up with changes in prehospital care and is essential to maintaining your certification and ability to practice.

3. List the primary and additional responsibilities of paramedics.   pp. 27-30

The primary responsibilities of the paramedic include:
• **Preparation:** You must be mentally, physically, and emotionally ready to respond to the call; know your protocols, geography, and equipment; and ensure that your vehicle and equipment are all in proper working order.
• **Response:** You must drive responsibly, ensuring a timely, yet safe, response.
• **Scene size-up:** You must assess the scene to determine: the safety of the scene (including identification of any hazards and the need for BSI; the number of ill or injured; the need for any additional resources; and the mechanism of injury or the nature of the illness.
• **Patient assessment:** Once at the patient's side, you must determine whether or not the patient needs cervical immobilization as well as his or her level of consciousness (or responsiveness) and the stability of the airway, breathing, and circulation. You will then assess for specific injury or illness signs through a focused or rapid trauma assessment. You will also evaluate the patient's medical history and perform ongoing assessments.
• **Recognition of injury or illness:** As a result of the scene size-up and patient assessment, you will identify the illness or injury and the patient's priority for care and transport.
• **Patient management:** You will employ appropriate care procedures, guided by protocols, with your patient and, at times, consult with medical direction to further guide your care.
• **Appropriate disposition:** Based upon the results of your assessment, the effects of the care measures you have employed, and your system's protocols, you will determine the disposition of your patient. That disposition may be transport to an appropriate trauma centre or to another specialized hospital, the closest hospital, or an alternative care facility. An additional possible disposition is to treat and release the patient with instructions to seek the advice of a personal physician.
• **Patient transfer:** As the health care system becomes more complex and facilities become more specialized, you may be charged with the safe and efficient transfer of patients from one facility to another.
• **Documentation:** At the conclusion of your patient care, you will be required to document the results of your assessment and care to ensure the continuity of patient care.
• **Return to service:** At the end of your response, you must ensure that you, your crew, and your ambulance are ready to return to service. This includes cleaning and refueling the vehicle, maintaining equipment, and replacing supplies used during the call.
Additional responsibilities include:
• **Community involvement:** You should promote and participate in programs to help the community recognize when EMS is needed, how to access the system, and what to do until the ambulance arrives. Community involvement also includes participation in the development and presentation of programs to improve health—stressing a healthy diet, for example—and to reduce injury—such as promoting seat belt use.
• **Support for primary care:** Modern health care is evolving in ways aimed at ensuring that costly resources are best directed to serve the patient. In support of this aim, you may be responsible for transporting or directing patients with minor injury or illness to alternate facilities like urgent care centres or physicians' offices.
• **Citizen involvement in EMS:** Ordinary citizens can be highly important evaluators of the EMS system, as they are its consumers and can best say what elements of it are important to them. Pay attention to the comments, suggestions, and criticisms of the patients/citizens you contact and pass what you learn along to the appropriate personnel in your system.
• **Personal and professional development:** To maintain and improve your ability to provide prehospital (and out-of-hospital) care, you must participate in professional development. This may

include taking refresher and continuing education courses, engaging in skill maintenance exercises, and other activities.

4. Define the role of the paramedic relative to the safety of the crew, the patient, and the bystanders.   pp. 27-28

You must evaluate information obtained from the dispatcher and gathered during your scene size-up to identify any potential scene hazards. Then you must take action to ensure your safety and the safety of the patient, other crew members and rescue personnel, and bystanders. You must also monitor the scene during your care to ensure that no hazards develop to threaten you, your patient, fellow rescuers, or bystanders.

5. Describe the role of the paramedic in health education activities related to illness and injury prevention.   p. 29-30

As EMS matures, its members will be expected to become more involved in both injury and illness prevention programs for the public. Such programs provide the most effective ways of increasing overall public health and reducing both death and disability from accidents and injuries.

6. Describe examples of professional behaviours in the following areas: pp. 32-34

• **Integrity:** Be honest and trustworthy in your contacts with patients, crew members, and other health care professionals. Doing this is essential to maintaining personal integrity.
• **Empathy:** You can convey empathy by attempting to understand and appreciate a patient's situation. Specifically, you can show empathy by being supportive and reassuring, demonstrating an understanding of the patient's feelings and the feelings of the family, demonstrating respect for others, and having a calm, compassionate, and helpful demeanor.
• **Self-motivation:** Doing your job well without direct supervision represents self-motivation.
• **Appearance and personal hygiene:** A clean, pressed shirt and trousers and well-kept hair demonstrate a good appearance and appropriate personal hygiene.
• **Self-confidence:** Displaying comfort with the application of emergency skills demonstrates self-confidence.
• **Communications:** In emergency medical services, it is essential to communicate quickly, concisely, accurately, and effectively.
• **Time management:** An emergency scene is often a chaotic place. It is imperative that you be able to organize and direct your actions and those of others quickly and efficiently to ensure that your patient receives appropriate emergency care and transport to definitive care as rapidly as possible.
• **Teamwork and diplomacy:** The emergency response is a team event, and the paramedic, as team leader, must direct many individuals to work together in the patient's best interest.
• **Respect:** Respect is demonstrated by showing regard and consideration for patients, care providers, and others. Listening to these people and indicating that you really hear what they say shows your respect for them and earns you their respect.
• **Patient advocacy:** Ensuring that the needs of your patient remain the first priority of your prehospital emergency care will help you meet your responsibility as patient advocate.
• **Careful delivery of service:** Demonstrate professional behaviour by performing your job to the highest level of excellence, by mastering and maintaining your skills and knowledge, and by conscientiously carrying out equipment checks, driving safely, and following protocols, policies, and procedures.

7. Identify the benefits of paramedics teaching in their community.   pp. 29-30

Teaching in your community places you before your "consumers" before they call for help. This gives you an opportunity to develop a positive public image and explain the workings of the system. It will also help you integrate with the other members of the health care system.

8. Analyze how the paramedic can benefit the health care system by supporting primary care for patients in the out-of-hospital setting.   pp. 28-29

With the increasing costs of health care, it has become necessary to ensure that the patient's needs are best matched to the available resources. This may mean that the paramedic, through assessment and consultation with the medical direction physician, may direct patients to facilities other than the emergency department.

9. Describe how professionalism applies to the paramedic while on and off duty.   p. 31

It is essential that the paramedic display a professional attitude toward his or her patient and the profession as a whole. This applies while both on and off duty since the public often judges a profession by the actions of its members.

CONTENT SELF-EVALUATION

_____ **1.** Prior to responding to a call, you must be:
- **A.** emotionally able to meet the demands of patient care.
- **B.** physically able to meet the demands of patient care.
- **C.** mentally able to meet the demands of patient care.
- **D.** sure the ambulance and equipment are ready for the response.
- **E.** all of the above.

_____ **2.** Prior to responding to a call, you must be familiar with:
- **A.** local EMS protocols.
- **B.** the local communications system.
- **C.** local geography.
- **D.** neighboring EMS agencies.
- **E.** all of the above

_____ **3.** A call involving which of the following is least likely to require additional assistance?
- **A.** a single ill patient
- **B.** reported use of a weapon
- **C.** knowledge of previous violence
- **D.** hazardous materials
- **E.** a rescue situation

_____ **4.** When a patient receives a minor injury and remains on scene after treatment by paramedics, this care is best described as:
- **A.** basic health care.
- **B.** primary health care.
- **C.** treat and release.
- **D.** diversion of care.
- **E.** health maintenance.

_____ **5.** When a patient receives a minor injury and is transported to an alternate care facility like an outpatient clinic, this care is best described as:
- **A.** basic health care.
- **B.** primary heath care.
- **C.** treat and release.
- **D.** diversion of care.
- **E.** health maintenance.

_____ **6.** You are transferring a multiple trauma patient from a local medical centre to a regional trauma centre. You are concerned that the patient will require care beyond your scope of practice. You should:
- **A.** request that the patient remain at the local facility until stable enough to travel.
- **B.** arrange a medical escort that can manage the procedures and equipment you are not licensed to use.
- **C.** refuse to transport the patient until critical care paramedics are available.
- **D.** arrange for the local physician to accompany you .
- **E.** consult with medical direction to obtain permission to perform the procedures that are outside your scope of practice.

_____ **7.** Which of the following items is NOT an essential part of the transfer of a patient between health care facilities?
- **A.** a verbal patient report from the transferring primary care provider
- **B.** a copy of the essential parts of the patient's chart

C. the results of all diagnostic tests
D. a summary of the patient's past medical history
E. a summary of the patient's present medical history

8. Which of the following is a component of returning to service after a call?
   A. refueling the ambulance.
   B. restocking supplies.
   C. stowing equipment.
   D. reviewing the call with the crew.
   E. all of the above.

9. Which of the following is NOT a part of community involvement for the paramedic?
   A. teaching CPR.
   B. transporting patients to alternate care facilities.
   C. conducting EMS demonstrations.
   D. providing prevention programs.
   E. sponsoring programs that help the public recognize when to access EMS.

10. What is the unique benefit of having citizen consumers involved in the development, evaluation, and regulation of the EMS system?
   A. They can help seek out alternative funding.
   B. They provide an outside objective view of the EMS system.
   C. They do not have the prejudices of most EMS providers.
   D. They can provide insight into new care procedures.
   E. all of the above

11. Honesty and trustworthiness are behaviours that indicate your:
   A. leadership.
   B. integrity.
   C. self-confidence.
   D. self-motivation.
   E. diplomacy.

12. Which of the following is NOT a method of displaying empathy?
   A. being supportive and reassuring
   B. demonstrating respect for others
   C. having a calm and helpful demeanor
   D. accepting constructive feedback
   E. understanding a patient's feelings

13. The ability to accurately assess your strengths and limitations and improve any weaknesses helps you develop a sense of:
   A. leadership.
   B. integrity.
   C. self-confidence.
   D. respect.
   E. diplomacy.

14. Showing others deferential regard, consideration, and appreciation are indicators of:
   A. leadership.
   B. integrity.
   C. self-confidence.
   D. respect.
   E. diplomacy.

15. Placing the patient's needs above your own represents which professional attribute?
   A. empathy.
   B. diplomacy.
   C. patient advocacy.
   D. initiative.
   E. self-confidence.

True/False

16. Pathophysiology is the study of the factors that influence the frequency, distribution, and causes of injury, disease, and other health-related events in a population.
   A. True
   B. False

_____ **17.** As a professional, you must put the needs of your patients ahead of your personal safety.
   A.   True
   B.   False

_____ **18.** If your patient requests transport to a facility that is different from the one indicated by your local protocols, you should consult online medical direction for advice.
   A.   True
   B.   False

_____ **19.** "Treat and release" refers to an increasing trend to seek alternative transport destinations and reduce the load on emergency departments.
   A.   True
   B.   False

_____ **20.** The treatment and care of a patient in an interfacility transfer is a shared responsibility of the receiving and accepting physician and the transporting paramedics.
   A.   True
   B.   False

_____ **21.** The role of the paramedic as a professional includes taking an active role in promoting positive health care practices in your community.
   A.   True
   B.   False

_____ **22.** The use of vans to transport non-emergency patients between facilities, disposition of patients to alternate treatment centres, and directing resources into prevention and wellness programs are examples of EMS involvement in cost containment.
   A.   True
   B.   False

_____ **23.** The term profession refers to a generally self-regulating group with a specialized body of knowledge or skills.
   A.   True
   B.   False

_____ **24.** Professionals master their skills and knowledge to the point of mastery so that further refresher courses are unnecessary.
   A.   True
   B.   False

_____ **25.** Your appearance, as well as your behaviour is vital to establishing credibility and instilling confidence.
   A.   True
   B.   False

Matching

Write the letter of the paramedic responsibility in the space provided next to the action to which it applies.

Responsibility

A. Preparation	**E.** Patient transfer
B. Response	**F.** Documentation
C. Patient assessment and management	**G.** Return to service
D. Appropriate disposition	

Action

_____ **26.** Refuel the vehicle.

_____ **27.** Follow local patient care protocols.

_____ **28.** Transport a patient to an outpatient centre.

._____ **29.** Determine the mechanism of injury.

_____ **30.** Record the care you provided.

_____ **31.** Be familiar with local protocols.

_____ **32.** Determine the patient's medical history.

_____ **33.** Categorize the patient's priority for transport.

_____ **34.** Take a report from the sending facility.

_____ **35.** Drive responsibly and safely.

_____ **36.** Deliver a patient to a level II trauma centre.

_____ **37.** Be mentally fit to respond to a call.

_____ **38.** Check crew members for signs of stress.

_____ **39.** Identify the nature of the illness.

_____ **40.** Determine the seriousness of the injury.

Chapter 1

Introduction to Prehospital Care

Part 4: The Well-Being of the Paramedic

Review of Chapter Objectives

After reading this part of the chapter, you should be able to:

1. Discuss the concept of wellness and its benefits, components of wellness, and the role of the paramedic in promoting wellness.   p. 35

Wellness, or personal physical, mental, and emotional well-being, is the result of proper nutrition, basic physical fitness, safe practices to protect you from disease and injury, and the development of effective mechanisms to deal with the stress of the profession. The results of observing practices that promote wellness in your own life are a reduced incidence of work-related injury and illness, a good attitude toward the profession, and a long fruitful career in emergency medical services.

Basic physical fitness is the muscular strength, cardiovascular endurance (aerobic capacity), and flexibility that permit you to perform the tasks associated with prehospital emergency care without risk to the musculoskeletal system.
Good nutrition is the controlled and balanced consumption of carbohydrates, fats, proteins, vitamins, and minerals that meet the body's needs yet is not consumption in excess.
Personal protection from disease includes application of body substance isolation procedures and acquisition of proper immunizations for protection from contagious disease.
Stress and stress management involve the recognition that prehospital emergency care is a stressful profession and that stress management techniques, including critical incident stress management, are essential to a long career in EMS.

General safety considerations include such principles as safe lifting, ensuring a safe environment for EMS operations, safe driving practices, appropriate interpersonal relationships, and the proper dealing with habits and addictions.

The paramedic should, by example, promote basic physical fitness, proper nutrition, the following of safe practices, and the use of appropriate mechanisms to deal with job-related stress. He or she can be a model to peers, patients, and the community in general.

2. Discuss how cardiovascular endurance, weight control, muscle strength, and flexibility contribute to physical fitness. pp. 35-40

Cardiovascular endurance, weight control, muscular strength, and flexibility are all essential to the physical fitness required of the paramedic. Cardiovascular endurance is the measure of the heart's and blood vessels' ability to support physical exercise. Increased cardiovascular endurance improves the body's ability to accommodate the physical stress associated with patient lifting and movement and the carrying of equipment. Weight control is essential to limit cardiovascular and musculoskeletal stresses on the body. Muscular strength is achieved by regular exercise and helps keep the body ready for the stresses of lifting and moving the patient and EMS equipment. Flexibility is the strength and ease of motion through the normal range of motion of the body's major joints. Good flexibility will reduce back pain and the potential for joint and muscle injury during your EMS career.

3. Describe the impact of shift work on circadian rhythms. p. 49

Shift work disturbs the normal biorhythms of the body, called circadian rhythms. Dramatic changes in a person's daily time schedule disturb the normal sleep/awake, appetite, hormonal, and temperature fluctuation cycles of the body and may result in drowsiness and fatigue. To diminish the negative effects of shift work, it is best to maintain a regular 24-hour sleep/awake cycle (sleeping at about the same time), even on days when you do not work.

4. Discuss the contributions that periodic risk assessments and warning sign recognition make to cancer and cardiovascular disease prevention. p. 37

Periodic assessment of your risk for disease is important. Have frequent physical exams and examine your family history to determine the risk for cancer and cardiovascular disease. Know your cholesterol and triglyceride levels and keep them in check. Women past menopause might consider the use of hormonal therapy to reduce the risk of cardiovascular disease and have frequent mammograms and pap smears with advancing age. Males should have periodic prostate exams with advancing age. Also watch for blood in the stool, changes in moles, unexplained weight loss, unexplained chronic fatigue, and unusual lumps.

5. Differentiate proper from improper body mechanics for lifting and moving patients in emergency and non-emergency situations. pp. 38-40

Proper lifting and moving techniques, especially when coupled with good physical fitness and good nutrition, help protect the musculoskeletal system from the high risks for injury associated with prehospital emergency care. Good posture, lifting with the leg muscles, and keeping the back straight, the palms up, and the body close to the object being lifted will reduce the potential for injury. Exhale during a lift, keep your feet apart with one foot ahead of the other, take your time, and ask for help when you think you will need it. These principles will make lifting easier and help keep you from back injury during your years of service.

6. Describe the problems that a paramedic might encounter in a hostile situation and the techniques used to manage the situation. p. 53

Emergency responses occasionally put the caregiver into contact with hostile patients, family members, and bystanders. These individuals may affect your ability to provide care and, at the extreme, threaten you or your patient with physical harm. If there is a significant threat, remove yourself from the scene immediately. Often, however, the hostility of people at the scene can be overcome by appreciating the cultural diversity of those you treat and helping them understand that your reason for being there is to offer help. Treating everyone you attend with dignity and respect will go a long way toward establishing trust in you and in EMS providers in general.

7. Describe the special considerations that should be given to using escorts, dealing with adverse environmental conditions, using lights and siren, proceeding through intersections, and parking at an emergency scene. pp. 53–54

Driving an emergency vehicle provides you with some privileges, but with them come some very important added responsibilities. In general, you must remain especially aware of others on the roadway and remember that they may react unexpectedly to your approach and passage. Also consider the following steps when dealing with these specific situations:

• When following an escort, be aware that some drivers may not realize that you are following from behind and may pull out in front of you.

• Adverse driving conditions (rain, snow, ice, fog) reduce visibility and traction. Give other drivers more time to see you and stop, and respect the increased stopping time and reduced maneuverability of your ambulance in these conditions.

• Lights and sirens are used to alert others of your approach and ask them to yield the right of way. However, some drivers may neither see nor hear them or may react in an unexpected manner. Be alert while using lights and sirens and anticipate the actions of others.

• Intersections pose special problems for emergency vehicles. Driving through a red light or a stop sign is dangerous because other drivers may presume they have the right of way. The situation becomes more complicated and dangerous when multiple emergency vehicles are responding. When proceeding through an intersection, and especially when passing through a red light, slow to almost a stop and keep a good lookout for other vehicles not yielding the right of way.

• Once at the scene, park so as to protect you and your crew, the patient, and other drivers. Place your emergency vehicle between traffic and the crash/care scene and be sure the lights can be seen by all oncoming traffic.

8. Discuss the concept of "due regard for the safety of all others" while operating an emergency vehicle. p. 54

The concept of exercising due regard for the safety of others recognizes that different drivers will react differently to the approach of emergency vehicles. This means that you must maintain an intense lookout for hazards while driving the emergency vehicle. You must anticipate the actions of other drivers on the highway, including those that are unexpected and not in keeping with the right of way given you under the law. Otherwise you may find yourself responsible for injury when your intent was to provide care or, worse, injure yourself.

9. Describe the equipment available in a variety of adverse situations for self-protection, including body substance isolation steps for protection from airborne and bloodborne pathogens. pp. 40-42, 54–56

Equipment available to help protect you from the more common hazards of emergency medical service include helmets, footwear with toe and ankle support, body armor, reflective tape for night visibility, seatbelts, and personal protective equipment used for body substance isolation (gloves, masks, eyewear, respirators, gowns, resuscitation equipment).

Body substance isolation (BSI) practices include the use of personal protective equipment (PPE) to isolate the body from contaminants found in the air and body fluids while caring for a patient. These practices involve using protective latex or plastic gloves to protect yourself when touching a patient if there is reasonable expectation of contact with body fluids, including tears, vomit, saliva, blood, urine, fecal material, cerebrospinal fluid, or any other body fluid or substance. Masks and protective eyewear should be used whenever there is a reasonable expectation that fluid or droplets will be splattered, as is the case with arterial hemorrhage, endotracheal intubation, intensive airway care, childbirths, and the cleaning of contaminated equipment. When a patient has or is suspected of having tuberculosis or another highly contagious airborne disease, use of a special type of mask, either the high-efficiency particulate air (HEPA) or N-95 respirator, offers protection by removing small infectious particles from the air. Gowns are worn to protect clothing and the body from contamination by splashing of body fluids in extreme circumstances (like childbirth). A gown impervious to fluid movement is recommended. When possible, use disposable equipment for patient ventilation and other invasive procedures.

10. Given a scenario in which equipment and supplies have been exposed to body substances, plan for the proper cleaning, disinfection, and disposal of the items.   pp. 42-43

When EMS equipment becomes contaminated (or possibly contaminated), it should be disposed of or properly cleaned and disinfected. Single-use devices, bandaging materials, and other disposable EMS equipment and materials should be placed in a sealed biohazard waste container and disposed of properly. Needles and other sharp contaminated items should be placed in a puncture-proof "sharps" container and disposed of properly. Equipment that has been in contact with a patient or otherwise becomes contaminated should be cleaned with soap and water, disinfected with an appropriate agent (commercial or a bleach solution), or sterilized (by heat, steam, or radiation) as per your service's policies and procedures. Any contaminated cleaning or disinfecting supplies should be disposed of properly.

11. Describe the benefits and methods of smoking cessation.   p. 38

Smoking and the effects of nicotine are well known to be detrimental to respiratory and cardiovascular health and well linked to lung cancer. Smoking cessation programs using replacement therapy (nicotine patches), behaviour modification, aversion therapy, hypnotism, and "cold turkey" approaches represent structured programs of controlled withdrawal from sociocultural, psychological, and physiological dependency on the drug. The result of a successful smoking cessation program is better respiratory and cardiovascular health and a reduced risk of respiratory infection and cancer.

12. Identify and describe the three phases of the stress response, factors that trigger the stress response, and causes of stress in EMS.   pp. 47-50

There are three stages to the human response to stress: alarm, resistance, and exhaustion. Alarm is the initial response, more commonly known as the "fight-or-flight" response. The autonomic nervous system prepares the body to deal with a threat to its well-being by releasing hormones that increase cardiac output (increase heart rate, the strength of contraction, and preload) and blood pressure, induce pupil dilation, increase blood sugar, and relax the respiratory tree. Resistance begins as the body starts to adjust and cope with the stress. During this phase, the blood pressure and pulse rate may return to normal. The final stress response phase is exhaustion. If the exposure to stress is prolonged, the body may become exhausted and lose its ability to resist and adapt to the stressors. The individual becomes more susceptible to physical and psychological ailments.

Stress is a stimulus from the environment that affects the body. Stress can have positive effects (eustress), or it can generate negative effects (distress). Factors that induce the stress response are anything that threatens (or is perceived to threaten) the well-being of the individual. These factors include physical ones, like the threat of violence; emotional ones, like the loss of a loved one; and physiological ones, like physical fatigue or extreme hunger. Each person reacts differently to stressors, bringing his or her previous experiences into the equation.

13. Differentiate between normal or healthy and detrimental physiological and psychological reactions to anxiety and stress.   pp. 50-51

The human stress response is the body's way of dealing with stress, and the outcome is either healthy or unhealthy. Healthy responses result in the individual's quickly adjusting to the stressor and physiologically and psychologically returning to normal. Unhealthy responses result in behavioural and physiologic manifestations like gastrointestinal disturbances, sleep disturbances, headaches, vision problems, fatigue, chest pains, confusion, a reduced attention span, poor concentration, disorientation, memory problems, inappropriate fear, panic, grief, depression, anxiety, and feelings of being overwhelmed, abandoned, or numb to emotion. A person with an unhealthy response may also experience withdrawal from normal social activities, increased use of drugs or alcohol, or inappropriate humor, silence, crying, suspiciousness, or activity levels.

EMS provides an abundant amount of stressors because of the nature of the profession. These stressors include shift work; loud pagers and sounds; poor pay; long hours; periods of boredom followed by short periods of extreme excitement; scene violence; abusive patients; vomit; blood; gory scenes; chaotic scenes; personal fears; frustration; exhaustion; demands of family members, friends, or bystanders; inclement weather; conflicts with co-workers or supervisors; hunger and thirst; and physical demands on the body, like heavy lifting. The personality traits commonly found in EMS members, a strong need to be liked and often unrealistically high self-expectations, also leave these individuals more likely to develop adverse responses to stress.

14. Describe behaviour that is a manifestation of stress in patients and those close to them, and describe how that behaviour relates to paramedic stress.   pp. 50-51

Stress may become evident through almost any unusual behaviour exhibited by the patient, family, or bystanders. It may manifest with hyper- or hypoactivity, withdrawal, suspiciousness, increased smoking, increased alcohol or drug intake, excessive humor or silence, crying spells, or any changes in behaviour, communications, interactions with others, or eating habits. These behaviours can confound the assessment of the patient's mental status and place additional stress on the paramedic.

15. Identify and describe the defense mechanisms and management techniques commonly used to deal with stress, components of critical incident stress management (CISM), and provide example situations in which CISM would be beneficial to paramedics. pp. 50, 51-52

Constructive mechanisms and management techniques used to deal with stress can be divided into two categories—immediate and long term. Immediate coping mechanisms include controlling breathing to reduce adrenaline levels and heart rate, reframing thoughts to encourage or support any needed behaviour on your behalf (like saying to yourself "I can do this!"), and focusing your concentration on the responsibilities at hand (i.e., the needs of the patient), not the stressful problem. For long-term well-being, ensure your physical, mental, and emotional health. Exercise, watch your diet, and work toward supportive and pleasant distractions from the stress, like a non-EMS circle of friends or a vacation away from the job.

Critical incident stress management recognizes that EMS personnel experience events with powerful emotional impacts that may cause acute stress reactions. Such events include the injury or death of an infant, an EMS co-worker, or someone known to EMS personnel; an injury or death of someone due to EMS operations; threats of personal harm; extreme media attention; or prolonged or especially gruesome events. CISM supports EMS personnel by providing pre-incident stress training, on-scene support, advice to command staff during large incidents, follow-up services, and special debriefings to spouses and families. The major components of CISM include initial discussion, defusing, demobilization, and critical incident stress debriefing services. Initial discussion permits those involved to discuss and air their feelings immediately after the incident. Defusing is a more formal gathering within 2 to 12 hours after an incident in which personnel can vent their feelings at a session monitored by a CISM-trained peer. Demobilization is performed at a staging sector at a large incident to help caregivers transition to everyday life. The critical incident stress debriefing is a formal session, proctored by a mental health provider, 24 to 72 hours after an incident.

16. Given a scenario involving a stressful situation, formulate a strategy to help adapt to the stress.   pp. 47-52

When you are called to a situation that places you under stress, make a conscious decision to deal with it in an appropriate manner. Immediately control your breathing by taking deep breaths and letting the air out slowly through your mouth. Repeat this as needed, and then focus your energy on the essential tasks at hand. Tell yourself "I can do it" or "I can make it through this" and attend to the immediate needs of your patient. Once the immediate stressor is removed, make sure that you take care of yourself physically, emotionally, and mentally. Talk with members of your team about the event, and identify what you have done well and areas in which you can improve. Exercise regularly, eat properly, and take a vacation or a few days off. Examine the situation and your options, decide how best to handle the situation in the long term, and go on with your life. If a situation is extremely stressful, take advantage of your system's CISM services.

17. Describe the stages of the grieving process (Kübler-Ross) and the unique challenges for paramedics in dealing with themselves, adults, children, and other special populations related to their understanding or experience of death and dying.pp. 41–45

The grieving patient is likely to progress through five stages of the grieving process as described by Elisabeth Kübler-Ross. Those stages include anger, denial, bargaining, depression, and acceptance.

A grieving person usually progresses though these stages in order, though he or she may skip around or move back and forth between stages. In the anger stage, the person vents the frustration over the inability to control the situation or control the outcome. Denial represents the inability or refusal to accept the reality of the event or situation. Bargaining is an unrealistic attempt to change or put off the outcome. Depression represents despair over the inevitable and withdrawal into a private world. Acceptance is realization and acceptance of the event or the patient's fate.

Even though paramedics are exposed to death and dying, they don't necessarily handle these events better than other people. All people tend to move through the same stages of the grieving process, although age and the patient's special circumstances may alter the presentation of those stages. Children may not recognize the significance and finality of the event or may fear that death may soon happen to themselves or others. Adults react differently, usually experiencing a "paralyzing" feeling followed by intense grief for weeks. The intensity gradually subsides with later peaks of feeling associated with anniversaries, birthdays, and the like. The elderly usually are concerned about the effects of their death on others and their loss of independence.

18. Given photos of various motor-vehicle collisions, assess scene safety and propose ways to make the scene safer.   pp. 53-54

The scene of an emergency is inherently dangerous, especially when it involves an auto crash. The roadway becomes a hazard as oncoming traffic may collide with your ambulance, personnel on the scene, and the wrecked auto(s). The crash produces broken glass, jagged metal, and spilled fluids that may be slippery, hot, caustic (battery acid), or flammable. If the patient involved in the crash is hostile, he or she may pose a threat to care providers as may the patient's friends and family members or other bystanders. The incident may also affect utility poles, breaking their wires to create electrical hazards. The paramedic must use caution when approaching the scene and carefully rule out hazards. If any exist, you must eliminate them or not approach the scene. Do not attempt to correct a scene hazard unless you are specifically and properly trained and equipped to handle it. Place your vehicle to caution oncoming traffic and create a barrier between you and that traffic. At all scenes with jagged metal and broken glass, wear protective clothing, including gloves, boots, helmet, and a protective coat (turnout gear). If need be, "blind" the occupants of a stopped vehicle with a spotlight until you are sure it is safe to enter the scene. If there is any possibility of blood or body fluid exposure, observe body substance isolation procedures.

CONTENT SELF-EVALUATION

1. All of the following are benefits of physical fitness EXCEPT:
   - A. decreased resting heart rate.
   - B. decreased resting blood pressure.
   - C. increased anxiety levels.
   - D. enhanced quality of life.
   - E. increased resistance to disease.

2. The basic elements of physical fitness include all of the following EXCEPT:
   - A. disease resistance.
   - B. muscular strength.
   - C. flexibility.
   - D. cardiovascular endurance.
   - E. aerobic capacity.

3. Exercise performed against stable resistance, where muscles are exercised in a motionless manner, is called:

	A.	isometric.	D.	isotonic.
	B.	polymeric.	E.	polytonic.
	C.	aerobic.		

_____ **4.** The target heart rate for a 50-year-old female with a resting heart rate of 65 is:
   - **A.** 103.
   - **B.** 139.
   - **C.** 152.
   - **D.** 170.
   - **E.** 220.

_____ **5.** Flexibility is obtained by:
   - **A.** isometric exercise.
   - **B.** isotonic exercise.
   - **C.** stretching.
   - **D.** bouncing at the end of a range-of-motion exercise.
   - **E.** weight lifting.

_____ **6.** Which of the following is NOT a major food group?
   - **A.** grains and breads
   - **B.** dairy products
   - **C.** fruits
   - **D.** meat and fish
   - **E.** simple sugars

_____ **7.** A proper and healthy diet minimizes intake of which of the following?
   - **A.** carbohydrates
   - **B.** vitamins
   - **C.** salt
   - **D.** protein
   - **E.** grains

_____ **8.** Which of the following does NOT increase your risk for cancer?
   - **A.** prolonged, chronic, and unprotected sun exposure
   - **B.** consumption of charcoal-grilled foods
   - **C.** eating broccoli
   - **D.** being a postmenopausal woman
   - **E.** elevated cholesterol levels

_____ **9.** Which of the following can reduce the risk of back injury?
   - **A.** doing abdominal crunches
   - **B.** stopping smoking
   - **C.** following good nutritional practices
   - **D.** getting adequate rest
   - **E.** all of the above

_____ **10.** Which of the following is NOT part of proper lifting?
   - **A.** positioning the load as close to the body as possible
   - **B.** locking your back in a slightly extended position
   - **C.** reaching while twisting to distribute weight
   - **D.** bending your knees
   - **E.** keeping your palms up

_____ **11.** Which of the following infectious diseases is NOT transmitted via airborne pathogens?
   - **A.** hepatitis C
   - **B.** pertussis
   - **C.** tuberculosis
   - **D.** varicella
   - **E.** rubella

_____ **12.** Which of the following items of personal protective equipment is/are recommended when suctioning a patient?
   - **A.** gloves
   - **B.** eyewear and mask
   - **C.** gown
   - **D.** both A and B
   - **E.** A, B, and C

13. Which of the following items of personal protective equipment is/are recommended when assisting a mother with childbirth?

    A. gloves
    D. both A and B
    B. eyewear and mask
    E. A, B, and C
    C. gown

14. HEPA and N-95 respirators are intended to protect against:

    A. HIV/AIDS.
    D. hepatitis C.
    B. tuberculosis or SARS.
    E. bacterial meningitis.
    C. hepatitis B.

15. Proper handwashing requires:

    A. removing rings.
    B. lathering hands vigorously.
    C. scrubbing vigorously for at least 15 seconds.
    D. scrubbing under fingernails and in creases of the knuckles.
    E. all of the above

16. Which of the following is a recommended immunization for the paramedic?

    A. tetanus/diphtheria
    D. TB
    B. SARS
    E. all of the above
    C. hepatitis C

17. Used needles are to be disposed by:

    A. placing them in a properly labeled puncture-proof container.
    B. recapping them and placing them in a biohazard bag.
    C. returning them to the pharmacy for disposal.
    D. driving them deeply into the ground.
    E. breaking them and taping them together with the tips covered.

18. Sterilization uses which of the following to kill pathogens?

    A. bleach
    D. pressurized steam
    B. radiation
    E. all of the above except A
    C. disinfectant soap

19. Which of the following represent the standard progression through the stages of grieving?

    A. anger, denial, bargaining, acceptance, depression
    B. denial, bargaining, anger, depression, acceptance
    C. denial, anger, bargaining, depression, acceptance
    D. anger, denial, bargaining, depression, acceptance
    E. depression, anger, denial, bargaining, acceptance

20. A grieving patient who is withdrawing from friends and family and is unwilling to communicate with others is most likely in which stage of loss?

    A. denial
    D. bargaining
    B. anger
    E. acceptance
    C. depression

21. At which age are children most likely to feel that death is a temporary absence from which the deceased person will return?

    A. newborn to age 3
    D. ages 9 to 12
    B. ages 3 to 6
    E. ages 12 to 18
    C. ages 6 to 9

22. The type of stress that has positive effects is:

    A. distress.
    D. eustress.
    B. halcion.
    E. gravitas.
    C. stimulation.

23. Which of the following is NOT a typical stressor for people working in emergency medical services?

A.	shift work	D.	limited responsibilities
B.	violent people	E.	thirst
C.	waiting for calls		

24. The human response to stress progresses through three stages, in this order:
    A. resistance, alarm, exhaustion.   D. resistance, exhaustion, alarm.
    B. alarm, resistance, exhaustion.   E. exhaustion, alarm, resistance.
    C. alarm, exhaustion, resistance.

25. The physiological phenomena that occur at approximately 24-hour intervals and regulate body temperature, sleepiness, and appetite are called:
    A. estrorhythms.   D. fatigue/rest cycles.
    B. circadian rhythms.   E. solar epochs.
    C. lunar tidals.

26. When you work a regular night shift, a technique that may help you maintain the appropriate awake/sleep cycle is:
    A. sleeping during one "anchor time" for both on- and off-duty days.
    B. eating well before going to bed.
    C. sleeping during the day after you work a night shift and at night when off duty.
    D. sleeping in a warm place during the day.
    E. taking short naps rather than long sleep.

27. Which of the following is a warning sign of stress?
    A. withdrawal   D. aching muscles and joints
    B. feeling of being abandoned   E. all of the above
    C. difficulty making decisions

28. Which of the following is NOT a healthy behaviour for dealing with or reducing stress?
    A. controlled breathing
    B. remaining distant from co-workers
    C. reframing
    D. creating a non-EMS circle of friends
    E. taking a vacation

29. An example of an event that is likely to be stressful for an EMS provider is:
    A. serious injury to a child.
    B. the death of a co-worker.
    C. an EMS operation causing a civilian death.
    D. a disaster.
    E. all of the above

30. A short, informal debriefing held within hours of a critical event is:
    A. defusing.   D. critical incident stress management.
    B. demobilization.   E. arbitration.
    C. critical incident stress debriefing.

31. The establishment and staffing of a transition point between a large-scale critical incident and going back to regular duty is:
    A. defusing.   D. critical incident stress management.
    B. demobilization.   E. arbitration.
    C. critical incident stress debriefing.

32. The formal, structured, planned intervention provided by a CISM team, including a mental health professional, is:
    A. defusing.   D. critical incident stress management.
    B. demobilization.   E. arbitration.
    C. critical incident stress debriefing.

33. Which of the following is a hazard commonly associated with auto crashes?
- **A.** downed power lines
- **B.** spilled hazardous chemicals
- **C.** moving traffic
- **D.** adverse weather conditions
- **E.** all of the above

34. When driving an ambulance, a paramedic must:
- **A.** ignore highway regulations as necessary to reach the patient.
- **B.** practice due regard for the safety of others.
- **C.** never exceed speed limits.
- **D.** always use an escort vehicle.
- **E.** none of the above

35. When approaching a roadway incident involving a patient who appears to be slumped over the steering wheel, you should:
- **A.** park behind the vehicle and remain alert as you approach the patient.
- **B.** park in front of the patient's vehicle, on the same side of the street.
- **C.** park in front of the patient's vehicle, on the opposite side of the street.
- **D.** park even with the patient's vehicle, on the opposite side of the street.
- **E.** park a block away and wait for police to arrive.

True/False

36. Isotonic exercise is active and involves working muscles through their range of motion.
- **A.** True
- **B.** False

37. In general, a balanced diet consists of 30 percent fat, 30 percent protein, and 40 percent carbohydrates.
- **A.** True
- **B.** False

38. Exercise helps prevent cardiovascular disease but has no preventative effect for cancer.
- **A.** True
- **B.** False

39. When lifting, always exhale. Do not hold your breath.
- **A.** True
- **B.** False

40. Because a person carrying a contagious disease may present without signs, you must consider the blood and body fluids of every patient you treat as infectious.
- **A.** True
- **B.** False

41. Because paramedics experience death more often than the general population, they experience less stress and are better able to cope with it.
- **A.** True
- **B.** False

42. When informed of the death of a loved one, some family members may explode in anger, throw things, and scream.
- **A.** True
- **B.** False

43. When informing the family of the death of a member, use the words "dead" or "died" rather than less definitive ones such as "moved on" or "has gone to a better place."
- **A.** True
- **B.** False

44. Stress related disease is unavoidable given the many demands of the EMS profession.
   A. True
   B. False

45. When responding with an escort vehicle to a roadway incident, you should travel as close together as possible.
   A. True
   B. False

Matching

Body Substance Isolation Procedures

Write the letter or letters of the appropriate personal protective equipment necessary for each of the following procedures in the space provided.

Term

    A. gloves
    B. mask and eyewear
    C. HEPA or N-95 respirator
    D. gown

Procedure

46. Suctioning

47. Childbirth

48. Endotracheal intubation

49. Patient with suspected TB

50. Serious arterial blood loss

Chapter 1

Introduction to Prehospital Care

Part 5: Illness and Injury Prevention

Review of Chapter Objectives

After reading this part of the chapter, you should be able to:

1. Describe the incidence, morbidity and mortality, and the human, environmental, and socioeconomic impact of unintentional and allegedly unintentional injuries.   pp. 54-56

Injuries remain one of Canada's most important health problems. According to the Alberta Centre for Injury Control and Research, injury is the leading cause of death in Canadians under 45. Head injuries are a serious problem, with over 34,000 admissions per year. Twice as many men as women experience head injuries. Helmet use dramatically lowers both the risk of head injury (85%) and brain injury (88%). Motor vehicle collisions are a leading cause of injury and death for Albertans under 30. Firearms account for more than 1300 deaths in Canada annually. Other causes of traumatic injury include pedestrian injuries, falls, and suicide.

2. Identify health hazards and potential crime areas within the community.   pp. 59-60

Health hazards are plentiful in a community. Homes are frequent sites of injuries to children from burns, falls, and firearm discharges. Geriatric patients also frequently fall in their homes. The home setting is also a place where paramedics are likely to encounter infants of low birth weight, patients discharged early from health care facilities, and patients having problems with medication noncompliance—all groups that are at greater likelihood for needing emergency care. Recreational and workplace injuries are also common in communities. Bars and areas with previous records of high crime rates should also be considered as potential crime areas.

3. Identify local municipal and community resources available for physical, socioeconomic crises.   pp. 56-57, 61

Establish a list of community resources in your locality that are available to assist patients in crisis. Such sites might include prenatal clinics, urgent care centres, and social services organizations that can offer food, shelter, clothing, and mental health counseling or services or referral to clinics or other forms of health care service.

4. List the general and specific environmental parameters that should be inspected to assess a patient's need for preventative information and direction.   pp. 59-60

Factors that should be considered when assessing the need for injury/illness prevention include the availability of prenatal care; level of public compliance with use of proper vehicular restraints for infants and children; awareness of proper firearm control measures; awareness of the dangers of drinking and driving; the home environments of geriatric patients (who are susceptible to falls); awareness of the need for patients to comply with directions for using medications; and local hospital/health organization policies involving the early discharge of patients with illness or injury. By surveying your community in these areas, you may identify parameters in which public education and direction may be beneficial in preventing illness and injury.

5. Identify the role of EMS in local municipal and community prevention programs.   pp. 56-61

The EMS provider can promote prevention by becoming an advocate of injury prevention. This may include teaching CPR and first aid courses for the public, teaching and supporting prevention programs, and being a role model and example by following safe practices (including BSI and ensuring scene safety) him- or herself.

6. Identify the injury and illness prevention programs that promote safety for all age populations.   pp. 59-62

Childhood and flu immunization programs; prenatal, well baby, and elder-care clinics; defensive driving programs; workplace safety courses; and health clinics sponsored by hospitals or health care organizations are just some examples of injury and illness prevention programs available to people across a range of ages in the community.

7. Identify patient situations in which the paramedic can intervene in a preventative manner.   pp. 59-62

The paramedic can intervene at the scene of an illness or injury and take advantage of a teachable moment. In a nonjudgmental, nonthreatening way, the paramedic may identify behaviours that would prevent illness or injury—for example, wearing protective equipment like seat belts in a car or helmets when biking—and instruct the patient in their use. The paramedic may also identify community risks like improperly enclosed swimming pools, which are common sites of children drowning, or poorly designed railway crossings, which are likely sites of train-vs.-auto collisions.

8. Document primary and secondary injury prevention data. pp. 61-62

Frequently, prehospital care reports contain or can be designed to collect information about the patient behaviour regarding safe practices. Information on seatbelt use, airbag deployment, medication compliance, and the like may be helpful in identifying areas in which programs promoting safe practices could reduce illness and injury. The patient care report may also identify mechanisms that frequently result in injury and suggest areas in which preventative practices or safety equipment may help reduce mortality and morbidity.

CONTENT SELF-EVALUATION

1. Wearing a helmet reduces the risk of head and brain injury by approximately:
   - **A.** an insignificant amount.
   - **B.** 30%.
   - **C.** 50%.
   - **D.** 85%.
   - **E.** 99%.

2. One of the leading causes of injury-related deaths for Canadian seniors aged 65 and over is:

    A. firearms.
    D. pedestrian struck incidents.
    B. abuse or assault.
    E. motor vehicle incidents.
    C. falls.

3. A systematic method to collect, analyze, and interpret information about injury data is a(n):

    A. injury risk program.
    D. secondary prevention program.
    B. injury surveillance program.
    E. risk data analysis.
    C. epidemiological intervention.

4. Medical care after an injury that helps prevent further problems is known as a(n):

    A. injury risk program.
    D. tertiary prevention.
    B. primary prevention.
    E. epidemiological intervention
    C. secondary prevention.

5. The primary goal of EMS provider commitment to injury prevention is to:

    A. protect themselves from harm.
    D. increase awareness of injury risks.
    B. protect their patients from harm.
    E. decrease long term disability.
    C. protect their co-workers from harm.

6. You respond to an industrial situation involving hazardous materials. You should:

    A. call law enforcement to establish a secure perimeter.
    B. stay back from the scene and call for local hazmat teams.
    C. establish a Command Post, then approach the scene cautiously.
    D. identify the hazardous materials, then notify the appropriate agencies.
    E. all of the above.

7. The number one cause of death in Canadian children is:

    A. congenital defects.
    D. respiratory distress syndrome.
    B. motor vehicle incidents.
    E. trauma.
    C. drowning.

8. Which of the following is an action you should take as an EMS responder to implement injury prevention strategies?

    A. Preserve response team safety.
    D. Know your community resources.
    B. Recognize scene hazards.
    E. all of the above
    C. Engage in on-scene education.

9. The opportunity presented by an emergency call to provide information to patients/bystanders about the future prevention of such an emergency is:

    A. a prevention protocol.
    D. patient/provider prevention.
    B. a teachable moment.
    E. tertiary prevention.
    C. EMS empowerment.

10. Which of the following is a possible community resource for injury or illness prevention?

    A. childhood and flu immunization program
    B. elder-care clinic
    C. workplace safety course
    D. prenatal and well-baby clinic
    E. all of the above

True/False

11. While injuries are often considered to be caused by accident, they are most likely predictable and preventable.

        A. True
        B. False

_____ **12.** Most pedestrian injuries involving children in Canada occur within one block of their home.
        A. True
        B. False

_____ **13.** Intentional injuries account for two thirds of all injury deaths.
        A. True
        B. False

_____ **14.** EMS providers are well distributed throughout the population, are often considered to be champions of the health care consumer, and are high-profile health care role models.
        A. True
        B. False

_____ **15.** EMS managers and supervisors are responsible for ensuring that employees are properly instructed in the fundamentals of primary prevention.
        A. True
        B. False

_____ **16.** Directing traffic is the primary responsibility of the first responding emergency agency at a motor vehicle incident.
        A. True
        B. False

_____ **17.** A paramedic should enter a hazardous scene only when the proper rescue, utility, or hazardous materials teams are not available.
        A. True
        B. False

_____ **18.** Congenital anomalies account for over 60 percent of neonatal deaths.
        A. True
        B. False

_____ **19.** The term *accident* does not accurately reflect the nature of auto collisions.
        A. True
        B. False

_____ **20.** The early release of patients from health care facilities to help control heath care costs is likely to cause an increase in the number of EMS responses.
        A. True
        B. False

Matching

Injury Prevention Terms

Write the letter or letters of the appropriate term following its definition in the space provided.

Term

        A. epidemiology
        B. injury risk
        C. primary prevention
        D. secondary prevention
        E. injury surveillance program

Description

_____ **21.** Medical care after an injury or illness that helps prevent further problems from occurring.

_____ **22.** Ongoing systematic collection, analysis, and interpretation of injury data.

_____ **23.** Keeping an injury or illness from every occurring.

_____ **24.** Study of factors that influence the frequency, distribution, and causes of injury, disease, and other health-related events in a population.

_____ **25.** Situation that puts people in danger of injury.

Chapter 1

Introduction to Prehospital Care

Part 6: Ethics in Advanced Prehospital Care

Review of Chapter Objectives

After reading this part of the chapter, you should be able to:

1.   Define ethics and morals and distinguish between ethical and moral decisions in emergency medical service.   pp. 63-66

Morals are social, religious, or personal standards of right and wrong. Ethics are rules or standards that govern the conduct of a group or profession. Ethics and morals, along with common law, govern how we function in prehospital emergency care.

Ethical decisions regarding patient care involve what the public and peers expect of the paramedic. Moral decisions involve the paramedic's own values of right and wrong.

2.   Identify the premise that should underlie the paramedic's ethical decisions in out-of-hospital care.   p. 65

Ultimately, the decisions made by the paramedic should be guided by the question: What is in the best interest of the patient?

3.   Analyze the relationship between the law and ethics in EMS.   p. 63

In general, the law takes a narrower and more specific look at behaviour and identifies what is wrong in the eyes of society. Ethics takes a more general view of what is right or good behaviour. Laws or the results of following them may be unethical, and the law often does not resolve ethical dilemmas.

4.   Compare and contrast the criteria used in allocating scarce EMS resources.   pp. 71-72

The most common situation regarding allocation of resources that a member of EMS is likely to face is a multiple-casualty incident (MCI). At an MCI, the triage process sorts casualties into priorities for care because patient needs outstrip the available resources. In the civilian environment, the person with the most need for care (excepting those with mortal injuries) receives care first. In the military domain, those with the least serious injuries receive care first to help maintain the fighting force (and win the battle).

5. Identify issues surrounding advance directives in making a prehospital resuscitation decision. pp. 67-68

Advance directives, such as living wills and Do Not Resuscitate orders, are ways that patients can indicate their desire for the type of medical care they wish to receive should they become incapacitated. Such directives often present ethical dilemmas for paramedics because they are trained and expected to do all that is necessary to preserve life. When a paramedic confronts a situation involving an advance directive, he or she must weigh the patient's right to autonomy against what he or she feels is in the patient's medical best interest. Whenever you are presented with an advance directive, ensure that it is valid, current, and conforms to requirements in your province or territory for such documents. When in doubt, resuscitate.

CONTENT SELF-EVALUATION

————   1. Ethical questions ask:
   A. whether something is right or wrong in the eyes of society.
   B. what is right or good.
   C. what are our personal standards and principles of right and wrong.
   D. what the basis of our decision-making process is.
   E. whether our actions are impartial, consistent, and balanced.

————   2. The concept that each person must decide how to behave and that whatever decision the person makes is acceptable is known as:
   A. Ethical relativism.
   B. Ethical pluralism.
   C. Moral integrity.
   D. impartiality.
   E. existential freedom.

————   3. Which of the following statements is most true when dealing with ethical dilemmas?
   A. Reason, logic, and emotion must be equally considered.
   B. The emotional impact of the issue is more important than the logic of the argument.
   C. Neither logical arguments or emotional appeals should be considered.
   D. Ethical questions can only be resolved if the parties share common values and desires.
   E. Reason and logic must be used and emotion must be excluded as much as possible.

————   4. Practitioners experience ethical distress occurs when:
   A. imposition of a practice causes feelings of guilt, concern, or distaste.
   B. there are ethical reasons both for and against a particular action and one option must be selected.
   C. practitioners neglect or fail to meet their moral obligations to their patients.
   D. their code of ethics fails to address a specific issue.
   E. their professional responsibilities conflict with broad humanitarian concerns.

————   5. When faced with an ethical challenge, the best guiding question is which of the following?
   A. How would I like to be treated?
   B. What would the patient want?

C. Which actions will account for the greatest good?
D. What is in the best interest of the patient?
E. What actions can I defend?

6. The term that means "desiring to do good" is:
    A. benevolence.
    B. justice.
    C. beneficence.
    D. autonomy.
    E. euphylanthropnia.

7. The Latin phrase *primum non nocere* means:
    A. "Do the best you can."
    B. "Avoid mistakes."
    C. "Maintain the patient's best interests."
    D. "First, do no harm."
    E. "Treat all patients fairly."

8. Which question best describes the impartiality test for analyzing an ethical situation?
    A. Can you justify this action to others?
    B. Would you want this procedure if you were in the patient's place?
    C. Would you want this procedure performed on you if you were in similar circumstances?
    D. Will you likely be questioned about the need for this procedure later?
    E. none of the above

9. When in doubt about the validity of a DNR order or the patient's desire to be resuscitated, you should:
    A. begin resuscitation immediately.
    B. await arrival of the DNR to verify its validity.
    C. contact medical direction for advice before beginning resuscitation.
    D. not resuscitate.
    E. begin with CPR and delay advanced interventions.

10. When presented with orders from a physician that do not comply with your protocols and that you believe are not in the patient's best interest, you should:
    A. follow the physician's order and report your concerns to the medical director.
    B. ask the physician to repeat or confirm the order.
    C. ask the physician for an explanation of the order.
    D. not follow the physician's order.
    E. do all except A.

True/False

11. Ethics are generally considered social, religious, or personal standards of right and wrong.
    A. True
    B. False

12. Most codes of ethics provide specific guidance for performance of the professional.
    A. True
    B. False

13. Justice refers to the paramedic's obligation to treat all patients fairly, without regard to conditions such as sex, race, ability to pay, or cultural background.
    A. True
    B. False

14. When attempting to resolve an ethical issue, the first step is to state the issue in a universal form.
    A. True
    B. False

_____ **15.** There are no circumstances in which it is appropriate to breach patient confidentiality.
     A. True
     B. False

Matching

Injury Prevention Terms

Write the letter or letters of the appropriate term following its definition in the space provided.

Term

    A. ethical violations
    B. ethical dilemmas
    C. ethical distress
    D. impartiality test
    E. universality test
    F. interpersonal justifiability test

Description

_____ **16.** Asks whether you would want this action performed in all relatively similar circumstances.

_____ **17.** Situation in which reasons both for and against a course of action are present and one must be chosen.

_____ **18.** Asks whether or not you can defend or justify your actions to others.

_____ **19.** Situation where a practitioner neglects of fails to meet their moral obligations to a patient.

_____ **20.** Asks whether you would be willing to undergo this procedure or action if you were in the patient's place.

Chapter 1

Introduction to Prehospital Care

Part 7: Lifting and Moving Patients

Review of Chapter Objectives

After reading this part of the chapter, you should be able to:

1. **Define body mechanics. p. 74**

   Body mechanics refers to the safest and most efficient methods of using your body to gain a mechanical advantage. Practicing and using good body mechanics every day increases your safety and performance, even in the most stressful emergencies.

2. **Discuss the guidelines and safety precautions that need to be followed when lifting a patient. pp. 74-75**

   Principles of good body mechanics include using your legs, not you back to lift; keeping the weight of the object as close to your body as possible; keeping your shoulders, hips, and feet "stacked" and moving as a unit; and reducing the height or distance you need to move an object.

3. **Describe the power lift and the power grip.   p. 75-76**

   The power lift is your best defense against injury, while helping to protect your patient with a safe and stable move. The power lift is particular useful for rescuers who have weak knees or thighs. Key points in using the power lift include placing your feet a comfortable distance apart, turning your feet slightly outwards, and bending at the knees. Tighten the muscles of your back and abdomen and keep your feet flat. Place your hands about 25 cm apart. Use the power grip (see below). As the lift begins, keep your back locked and drive through the heels and arches of your feet. Your upper body should come up before your hips do.

   When using the power grip, your palms and fingers should come in complete contact with the object and all your fingers should be bent at the same angle.

4. **Explain how good posture and physical fitness can contribute to your well-being as an EMS provider.   pp. 77-78**

Posture is an overlooked, but key element in body mechanics. Poor posture includes swayback, where the stomach is too far forward and the buttocks too far back, and the slouch, where the shoulders are rolled forward, putting increased pressure on every region of the spine.

Demonstrate good posture by having your ears, shoulders, and hips in vertical alignment when you stand. Bend your knees slightly and tuck your pelvis slightly forward. When sitting, distribute your weight evenly on both ischia. Your ears, shoulders, and hips should be in vertical alignment, with your feet flat on the floor or crossed at the ankle. If possible, your lower back should contact the chair back.

Maintain a proactive, well-balanced physical fitness program to improve flexibility, cardiovascular conditioning, strength, and good nutrition.

5. Describe the indications for an emergency move.   p. 79

Emergency moves should only be used when there is an immediate danger to the patient, such as fire or the threat of fire, explosion or the threat of explosion, an inability to protect the patient from other hazards at the scene, an inability to gain access to other patients who need life-saving care, or when life-saving care cannot be given because of the patient's location or position.

To use a Shirt Drag, fasten the patient's hands together, then use the shoulders of the patient's shirt to pull the patient toward you. To use a Blanket Drag, fold a blanket into pleats next to the patient. Roll the patient enough to get the blanket under him. Roll from the other side to grasp the folded pleats and pull them underneath the patient. Wrap the blanket around the patient, then grasp the blanket that is under the patient's head and pull him/her towards you. For the shoulder drag, kneel at the patient's head and slip your hands under the patient's armpits from the back. If necessary reach down and grasp the patient's forearms.

6. Describe the indications for assisting in nonemergency moves.   pp. 82-84

Nonemergency moves are generally performed with other rescuers. In general, nonemergency moves should be used when there is no immediate threat to the patient's life. The direct ground lift requires two or three rescuers and is useful when the patient is unable to sit in a chair, or when a stretcher cannot be brought close to the patient. Use the extremity left to move a patient from a chair, or from the floor, to the stretcher. Do not use this lift if the patient has injuries to the arms or legs.

7. Describe additional types of emergency moves, such as the piggyback carry, one-rescuer crutch, one-rescuer cradle carry, and fire fighter's drag.   pp. 81-82

Nonemergency moves include the sheet drag, the piggyback carry, the one-rescuer crutch, the cradle carry, and the fire fighter's drag.

8. Discuss the various devices associated with moving a patient in the out-of-hospital arena. pp. 85-97

The standard stretcher has wheeled legs and a collapsible undercarriage. Portable stretchers are lightweight folding stretchers that are easy to clean. A scoop, or orthopedic stretcher splits into sections that can be fitted around a patient and reconnected. The patient can then be lifted and moved to a standard stretcher. Stair chairs are lightweight, collapsible devices with wheeled legs, a grab bar, and straps to secure the patient. Backboards immobilize or stabilize a patient's entire body. They are used for patients with suspected spine injury who are supine.

9. Describe the principles of loading and securing the stretcher into, and unloading the stretcher from, an ambulance.   pp. 87-88

Use appropriate lifting technique or transferring device to place your patient onto the stretcher. Ensure that the patient is properly positioned for his or her injuries and that all equipment is secured. At the back of the ambulance, lower IV poles and remove any equipment attached to the sides of the stretcher. Communicate with your partner and ensure that everyone knows the procedures for loading. Once in the ambulance transfer from portable to ambulance-based oxygen, monitoring, and resuscitation equipment as necessary.

When you arrive at your destination, change back to portable equipment, move all required supplies and equipment to the stretcher. Again, ensure effective communication with your partner while you unload from the vehicle.

10. Explain the rationale behind properly lifting and moving patients. pp. 74-75

As a paramedic, you may be asked to lift and carry both patients and heavy equipment. If you do it incorrectly, you could cause yourself injury, strain, and life-long pain. With planning, good health, and skill, you can do your job with minimum risk to yourself, your partner, and your patients.

11. Explain the rationale behind an emergency move. p. 79

Your first priority is to maintain a patient's airway, breathing, and circulation. However, if the scene is unstable or poses an immediate threat, you may have to move the patient before assessment and treatment.

CONTENT SELF-EVALUATION

1. The term body mechanics refers to methods of:
   A. exercising to strengthen your back muscles.
   B. positioning the patient for safe extrication.
   C. lifting and transferring patients safely.
   D. determining how a patient may have been injured.
   E. using your body to gain a mechanical advantage.

2. When lifting a heavy load, you should:
   A. lift with your legs, your back, and your shoulders.
   B. lift with your legs and your shoulders.
   C. lift with your legs and back.
   D. lift with your legs and abdomen.
   E. lift with your legs.

3. Keeping your shoulders, hips, and feet in line, then moving or turning as a unit is referred to as:
   A. stacking your posture.
   B. the power posture.
   C. the power lift.
   D. unit mechanics.
   E. maintaining vertical posture.

4. The key to preventing injuries when lifting, carrying ,moving, reaching, pushing, and pulling is:
   A. balance, strength, and attitude.
   B. correct alignment of the spine.
   C. nutrition, cardiovascular endurance, and strength.
   D. keeping your knees slightly bent.
   E. locking your elbows, wrists, and knees.

5. When using the power lift, you should splint your vulnerable lower back area:
   A. by tightening the muscles of your back and abdomen.
   B. to avoid excessive slouch or swayback.
   C. and take a long, deep breath and lift quickly.

D.   by tightening your hamstrings, quadriceps, and abdominal muscles.

E.   all of the above.

6. When standing with good posture, you should:
A.   keep your knees locked and your head high.
B.   bend your knees slightly and keep your ears, shoulders, and hips in vertical alignment.
C.   bend your knees slightly and tuck your pelvis back.
D.   keep your stomach in and your chin forward.
E.   keep your ears, shoulders, and feet in vertical alignment.

7. Emergency moves should only be attempted when:
A.   there is an immediate danger to the patient.
B.   you cannot provide life-saving interventions because of the patient's position.
C.   the patient is blocking access to other patients who require immediately life-saving interventions.
D.   you cannot remove or secure hazards that threaten the patient and other rescuers.
E.   all of the above

8. The greatest danger in using an emergency move is that you may:
A.   become a victim of the same hazards that threaten the patient.
B.   injure yourself as you do not have time to employ safe body mechanics.
C.   aggravate the patient's injuries or condition.
D.   not be able to move the patient by yourself.
E.   become too fatigued to provide adequate care.

9. When positioning a conscious patient with internal bleeding and shock on your stretcher, you should:
A.   elevate the patient's legs.
B.   elevate the patient's head and torso.
C.   position the patient supine.
D.   position the patient semi-prone.
E.   place the patient sitting upright.

10. The orthopedic stretcher is ideal for patients who are:
A.   lying on uneven or rocky terrain.
B.   lying semi-prone on any surface.
C.   are short of breath or have chest pain and must be evacuated down stairs.
D.   are lying supine on a relatively flat surface.
E.   any patient on the ground.

True/False

11. When lifting a heavy object, keep its weight as close you your body as possible.
A.   True
B.   False

12. Whenever possible, you should use a transferring device or equipment rather than perform a lift.
A.   True
B.   False

13. When sitting with good posture, you feet should be flat on the floor or crossed at the knees.
A.   True
B.   False

14. Proper body mechanics will not help if you are not physically fit.
A.   True
B.   False

_____ **15.** The direct ground lift can be used for patients with spinal injuries.
        A. True
        B. False

Matching

Patient Positioning

Write the letter or letters of the appropriate patient position in the space provided beside the description of the patient's condition or injuries below.

Position

    A. supine
    B. semi-prone, on patient's right side
    C. semi-prone, on patient's left side
    D. supine, knees and feet elevated
    E. sitting or semi-sitting

Condition

_____ **16.** conscious patient who is short of breath

_____ **17.** conscious patient with spinal injuries

_____ **18.** unconscious patient with spinal injuries

_____ **19.** conscious patient with shock and no spinal or extremity injuries

_____ **20.** unconscious medical patient

Chapter 2

Medical-Legal Aspects of Prehospital Care

Review of Chapter Objectives

With each chapter of the Workbook, we identify the objectives and the important elements of the text content. You should review these items and refer to the pages listed if any points are not clear.

After reading this chapter, you should be able to:

Introduction to Advanced Prehospital Care

1. Differentiate legal, ethical, and moral responsibilities.   pp. 90-91

A paramedic's legal responsibility to the patient and others is defined by constitutional, legislative, and common law. Failure to meet this responsibility may result in professional, civil, or criminal sanctions. Ethical responsibilities are those actions expected of a paramedic by the health care profession and by the public. Moral responsibilities are personal values of right and wrong and are governed by conscience. Legal, ethical, and moral factors guide an individual in his or her actions as a paramedic.

2. Describe the basic structure of the Canadian legal system and differentiate between civil and criminal law.   pp. 91-93

There are two legal regimes in Canada. Quebec operates under a system based on the French Code Napoleon and has a civil law-common law fused system. The federal government, other provinces, and territories use a system based on English common law. All federal laws must be written in both English and French.

Civil law is non-criminal legal action between individuals for such things as matrimonial, contract, and personal injury disputes. Tort law is a branch of civil law that deals with issues such as negligence, medical malpractice, assault, battery, and defamation. Criminal law addresses actions against society (crimes) such as homicide, rape, and burglary and will fine and/or imprison those found guilty.

3. Differentiate licensure and certification.   p. 96

Certification is the recognition of an individual who has met predetermined qualifications to participate in a certain activity. It may be given by a certifying agency or by a professional college or association. Licensure is a process whereby a governmental agency grants permission to an individual, after meeting certain qualifications, to engage in a particular profession. Each province and territory sets out requirements for certification, licensure, recertification, and relicensure.

4. List reportable problems or conditions and to whom the reports are to be made.   p. 96-97

Each province or territory has laws that require prehospital care providers to report such matters as suspected spousal abuse, child neglect and abuse, and abuse of the elderly. In many jurisdictions, violent crimes, sexual assault, gunshot wounds, and stab wounds must be reported to law enforcement officials. And public health threats such as animal bites and communicable diseases must also be reported to the proper authorities. You must be familiar with the reporting requirements in your jurisdiction.

5. Define:

a.   Abandonment   pp. 108-109
This is the termination of a patient-paramedic relationship while the patient still desires and needs care without the paramedic's providing for the appropriate continuation of care.

b.   Advance directives   pp. 110-111
Documents created to ensure that certain treatment choices are honoured when a patient is unconscious or otherwise unable to express a choice of treatment.

c.   Assault p. 109
Assault is an act that unlawfully places a person in apprehension of immediate bodily harm without his or her consent.

d.   Battery p. 109
This is the unlawful touching of an individual without his or her consent.

e.   Breach of duty   p. 98
Breach of duty is an action or failure to act that violates the standard of care expected of a similarly trained paramedic under similar circumstances.

f.   Confidentiality p. 103
This is the principle of law that prohibits the release of medical or other information about a patient without his or her permission.

g.   Consent (expressed, implied, informed, involuntary)   pp. 104-106
Consent is the granting of permission to treat. Expressed consent occurs when a patient gives verbal, nonverbal, or written communication that he or she wants to receive medical care. Implied consent occurs when you presume the patient would give expressed consent if he or she were able. Informed consent is consent for treatment that is given based on full discourse of information. Involuntary consent is consent to treat a patient given by the authority of a court order.

h.   Do not resuscitate (DNR) orders p. 111
DNR orders are legal documents, usually signed by the patient and his or her physician, that indicates to medical personnel which, if any, life-sustaining measures should be taken when the patient's heart and respiratory functions have ceased..

i.   Duty to act   p. 98
This is the formal contractual or informal legal obligation to provide care.

j.   Emancipated minor   p. 106
This is generally someone under 18 years of age who is married, pregnant, a parent, a member of the armed forces, or financially independent and living away from home. Such a person is often considered legally able to give informed consent.

k.   False imprisonment   p. 109
This is the intentional and unjustifiable detention of a person without consent or other legal authority.

l.   Immunity   pp. 97, 100
This is the exemption from legal liability.

m.   Liability   pp. 91, 98-102
This is the legal responsibility for one's actions. Any deviation from the duty to act or the standard of care exposes the care provider to liability.

n.   Libel   p. 104
This is the act of injuring a person's character, name, or reputation by false statements made in writing or through the mass media with malicious intent or reckless disregard for the falsity of those statements.

o.   Minor   p. 106
Depending on provincial or territorial law, a minor is a person under 18 years of age.

p.   Negligence   pp. 98-101
This is the deviation from accepted standards of care recognized by the law for the protection of others against the unreasonable risk of harm.

q.   Proximate cause   pp. 100
This is the action or inaction of the paramedic that immediately caused or worsened the damage suffered by the patient.

r.   Scope of practice   pp. 95-96
This is the range of duties and skills paramedics are allowed and expected to perform.

s.   Slander p. 104
This is the act of injuring a person's character, name, or reputation by false and malicious statements spoken with malicious intent or reckless disregard for the falsity of those statements.

t.   Standard of care   pp. 98-99
This is the degree of care, skill, and judgment expected under like or similar circumstances from a similarly trained, reasonable paramedic in the same community.

u.   Tort   p. 93
This is a civil wrong committed by one individual against another.

6. Discuss the legal implications of medical direction.   pp. 95, 101-102

Medical direction, both on-line and off-line, helps define the paramedic's scope of practice. Protocols, policies, and procedures as well as medical direction from an on-line physician define what is the acceptable standard of care. The system medical director is responsible for supervising the protocols and continuing education of the paramedic. The on-line medical direction physician is responsible for supervising and directing the paramedic's actions at the scene and during transport. The paramedic is responsible for ensuring that the medical care given to the patient is appropriate and in keeping with the protocols. Any breach of duty or deviation from the standard of care that results in patient injury may result in charges of negligence.

7. Describe the four elements necessary to prove negligence. pp. 98-100

Four elements must exist before negligence can be proven. They include the duty to act, breach of duty, actual damages, and proximate cause. The duty to act is the direct or indirect responsibility to provide the patient with care. Breach of duty is the failure to meet the standard of care associated with the patient's needs. Damages are the actual physical, psychological, or financial harm suffered by the patient. Proximate cause means that the paramedic's action or inaction directly caused or worsened the harm suffered by the patient.

8. Explain liability as it applies to emergency medical services.   pp. 91, 98-102

Liability in EMS is the legal responsibility to provide appropriate assessment, care, and transport of the ill or injured patient. That liability extends to the system medical director and on-line medical direction physician as well as to the paramedic who supervises the actions of others while at the emergency scene. They must ensure that those they supervise follow the standard of care.

9. Discuss immunity, including Good Samaritan statutes and governmental immunity, as it applies to the paramedic.   pp. 97, 100

The Good Samaritan statute may offer some liability protection to someone who assists at the emergency scene if that person acts in good faith, is not grossly negligent, acts within his or her scope of practice, and does not receive payment for his or her services. In some provinces and territories, Good Samaritan statutes have been expanded to include both paid and unpaid EMS providers. In Canada, there is no positive duty to assist; therefore an off-duty paramedic is not legally required to stop and assist. However, once you start to assist, you must continue, stopping only in accordance with acceptable standards.

Governmental immunity is a judicial doctrine that protects the government from liability unless it accepts that liability. However, most jurisdictions have waived these rights, and courts are becoming increasingly likely to strike any remaining immunity down.

10. Explain the necessity and standards for maintaining patient confidentiality that apply to the paramedic. pp. 103-104

The paramedic, through his or her involvement in patient care, learns sensitive information about the patients he or she treats. To encourage patients to continue to divulge this information, paramedics must respect its confidential nature and only divulge it to those with a need to know. Information regarding a patient may be released to those continuing care, in accordance with the patient's consent to release information, as required by law, and as necessary for billing purposes.

11. Differentiate expressed, informed, implied, and involuntary consent and describe the process used to obtain informed or implied consent.   pp. 104-107

Expressed consent is that given in writing, verbally, or non-verbally, while implied consent is assumed consent from a patient who is unable to give expressed consent. Informed consent is the consent for treatment given by a patient when he or she understands the necessity, nature, risks, and alternatives to care. Involuntary consent is the consent given by the authority of court order to treat an individual.

When a patient summons an ambulance, that action suggests that he or she is asking for help and consenting to treatment. However, a paramedic is obligated to explain what he or she is going to do to and for the patient and why he or she is going to do it. The paramedic must also determine if the patient is alert, oriented, and rational enough to make a competent decision to accept or refuse care. If the patient is not able to make a rational decision regarding care, then the paramedic may need to invoke implied consent. If the patient is a minor and the legal parent or guardian cannot be reached, consent is assumed (implied consent).

12. Discuss appropriate patient interaction and documentation techniques regarding refusal of care.   p. 106-107

When a patient refuses care, the paramedic must assure and document the following: the patient was legally able and competent to make the decision; the need for care and potential consequences of refusing care were explained; on-line medical direction was consulted; the patient was directed to see his or her own physician; and the patient was directed to call the ambulance if the symptoms return or get worse. The refusal form should be signed by the patient and a disinterested witness, such as a police officer. If the patient refuses to sign a refusal of treatment form, then have his or her refusal witnessed by a family member or police officer.

13. Identify legal issues involved in the decision not to transport a patient, or to reduce the level of care.   p. 108

A decision not to continue the care of a patient or to relinquish care to a lesser level of provider may expose the paramedic to charges of abandonment or negligence if the patient suffers harm. This is especially true if the paramedic has initiated advanced care procedures like starting an IV or administering a medication.

14. Describe the criteria and the role of the paramedic in selecting hospitals to receive patients. pp. 110

The patient's request to be transported to a particular hospital should be honored unless his or her particular care needs demonstrate otherwise. The decision to transport a patient to a facility other than the one requested must be based upon the patient's care needs, the capabilities of the requested facility, protocols, and interaction with the on-line medical direction physician.

15. Differentiate assault and battery. p. 109

Assault threatens bodily harm, while battery is unauthorized touching. These civil and criminal actions can be avoided by the paramedic's making sure to obtain expressed consent for treatment and to explain what he or she is planning to do for the patient before doing it.

16. Describe the conditions under which the use of force, including restraint, is acceptable. pp. 97, 109

The use of force to restrain a patient may be necessary when the patient is violent or poses a danger to him- or herself or to others. Then only such force and restraint should be used as is required. In conditions where force and restraint are necessary to care for a patient, law enforcement officers should be involved.

17. Explain advance directives and how they impact patient care. pp. 110-113

Advance directives permit the patient to define what care he or she would desire should they become incapacitated. Advance directives include Do Not Resuscitate (DNR) orders, which limit care actions that can be taken should the patient go into cardiac or respiratory arrest. Living wills are legal documents that also prescribe the care a patient may receive, including his or her desire to donate organs and to die at home or elsewhere. Provincial and territorial legislation and local protocols usually define the authority of DNRs, living wills, and other advance directives.

18. Discuss the paramedic's responsibilities relative to resuscitation efforts for patients who are potential organ donors. p. 113

When presented with a patient who is a possible organ donor, it is essential for the paramedic to maintain adequate perfusion of that organ to ensure its viability. Follow local protocols for employing resuscitation procedures including fluid therapy, cardiac compressions, and ventilation. Notify the medical direction physician that you are transporting a possible organ donor.

19. Describe how a paramedic may preserve evidence at a crime or accident scene. p. 113-114

Your responsibility at the crime scene is first to ensure your safety and that of your patient and then to ensure the health of the victim (your patient). If the patient is not obviously dead, initiate resuscitation and care directed at his or her injuries. Limit any movement of articles around the patient and at the scene and, if possible, document what you moved and from what location you moved it. Do not cut through clothing where objects entered the body; remove the clothing without cutting it, or cut around the openings.

20. Describe the importance of providing accurate documentation of an EMS response. pp. 114-115

Documentation establishes what was found and what was done at the emergency scene. It must be completed promptly, thoroughly, objectively, and accurately. At the same time, the confidentiality of the information obtained must be maintained. The documentation will become a part of the patient's medical record and help guide continuing patient care. It will also become a record of what you did at the emergency scene and during transport should your actions ever come into question. It may also become a legal document in a court of law when someone feels they have been injured (damaged) by someone else.

21. Describe what is required to make the patient care report an effective legal document. pp. 114-115

A patient care report must be completed in a timely manner, must be thorough, must be objective, must be accurate, and must ensure patient confidentiality to be an effective legal document.

CONTENT SELF-EVALUATION

1. The term liability best refers to:
   - A. an illegal act.
   - B. legal responsibility.
   - C. an act of negligence.
   - D. civil responsibility.
   - E. responsibility for damages.

2. Ethical responsibilities are best described as:
   - A. requirements of case law.
   - B. requirements of statute law.
   - C. standards of a profession.
   - D. personal feelings of right and wrong.
   - E. legal concepts of right and wrong

3. Moral issues are best described as:
   - A. requirements of case law.
   - B. requirements of statute law.
   - C. standards of a profession.
   - D. personal feelings of right and wrong.
   - E. legal concepts of right and wrong.

4. Criminal law in Canada is set out in:
   - A. The Criminal Code of Canada.
   - B. The Criminal Code of Canada and various provincial and territorial Criminal Codes.
   - C. provincial and territorial legislation.
   - D. The Criminal Code of Canada and Quebec Code Napoleon.
   - E. case law at the territorial, provincial, and federal levels.

5. Criminal law is best described as dealing with:
   - A. wrongs committed against society.
   - B. conflicts between two or more parties.
   - C. contract disputes.
   - D. negligence.
   - E. breaches of faith.

6. Civil law is best described as dealing with:
   - A. wrongs committed against society.
   - B. conflicts between two or more parties.
   - C. contract disputes.
   - D. negligence.
   - E. breaches of faith.

7. In Canada, licensure and certification requirements are set by:
   - A. federal statute.
   - B. provincial bodies.
   - C. the Paramedic Association of Canada.
   - D. local EMS operators.
   - E. the Canadian Medical Association.

8. Which of the following is NOT a common mandatory reporting event?
- **A.** rape
- **B.** spousal abuse
- **C.** child abuse
- **D.** a seizure episode
- **E.** animal bites

9. Which of the following is NOT one of the elements required to prove a charge of negligence against a paramedic?
- **A.** duty to act
- **B.** proximate cause
- **C.** actual damages suffered by the patient
- **D.** payment to the paramedic
- **E.** breach of duty

10. Which of the following is a duty expected of the paramedic?
- **A.** to respond to the scene of an emergency
- **B.** to conform to the expected standard of care
- **C.** to provide care in accordance with the system's protocols
- **D.** to drive, or ensure the emergency vehicle is driven, appropriately
- **E.** maintain supplementary documentation, such as a personal notebook`

11. The degree of care, skill, and judgment that would be expected under like or similar circumstances by a similarly trained, reasonable paramedic is:
- **A.** the duty to act.
- **B.** the scope of practice.
- **C.** the standard of care.
- **D.** a proximate cause.
- **E.** malfeasance.

12. *Res ipsa loquitur* is a legal term that refers to:
- **A.** contributory negligence.
- **B.** immunity from prosecution.
- **C.** a matter that is self-evident.
- **D.** the victim's liability.
- **E.** the reliability of evidence.

13. Which of the following will NOT protect a paramedic from charges of negligence?
- **A.** Good Samaritan statute
- **B.** governmental immunity
- **C.** the statute of limitations
- **D.** contributory negligence
- **E.** acting while off duty

14. Which of the following is NOT an acceptable reason for the release of confidential patient information?
- **A.** Medical providers need it to care for the patient.
- **B.** A judge has signed a court order demanding its release.
- **C.** It is necessary for third party billing.
- **D.** Other paramedics, not on the call, have requested it.
- **E.** The patient has made a written request for its release.

15. The act of injuring an individual's character, name, or reputation by false written statements and with malicious intent is:
- **A.** slander.
- **B.** breach of confidentiality.
- **C.** malfeasance.
- **D.** misfeasance.
- **E.** libel.

16. The act of injuring an individual's character, name, or reputation by false spoken statements and with malicious intent is:
- **A.** slander.
- **B.** breach of confidentiality.
- **C.** malfeasance.
- **D.** misfeasance.
- **E.** libel.

17. The type of consent that is given by the authority of a court is:
- **A.** expressed.
- **B.** implied.
- **C.** involuntary.
- **D.** informed.
- **E.** common.

18. For a patient's consent to be informed, the patient must be told and understand:

    A. the nature of the treatment.   **D.** the risks of refusing the treatment.

    B. the necessity of the treatment.   **E.** all of the above

    C. the risks of the treatment.

19. In most provinces and territories, a minor is considered someone under the age of:

    A. 16.   **D.** 21.

    B. 18.   **E.** 25.

    C. 19.

20. Which of the following is NOT an essential element in accepting a patient's refusal of care?

    A. The patient is conscious, alert, and rational.

    B. The patient is a minor.

    C. The patient is aware of the possible consequences of his or her decision.

    D. The patient has been advised that he or she may call again for help if necessary.

    E. The patient and/or a disinterested witness has signed a release-from-liability form.

21. Ending a patient–care giver relationship without providing the appropriate continuing care and without the patient's approval could be found to be:

    A. battery.   **D.** abandonment.

    B. defamation.   **E.** assault.

    C. nonfeasance.

22. The unlawful act of touching another person without permission is:

    A. assault.   **D.** slander.

    B. abandonment.   **E.** libel.

    C. battery.

23. Do Not Resuscitate orders usually restrict care providers from:

    A. performing CPR in case of cardiac arrest.

    B. performing a "slow code."

    C. performing a "chemical code."

    D. leaving the scene until the coroner arrives.

    E. contacting medical direction.

24. Which of the following statements is NOT true regarding a paramedic's responsibility at the crime scene?

    A. He or she should contact law enforcement officers if they are not on the scene.

    B. He or she should not enter the scene unless it is safe.

    C. His or her primary responsibility is to preserve the evidence at the scene.

    D. He or she should not disturb the scene unless it is necessary for patient care.

    E. He or she should document the movement of any item at the scene.

25. Which of the following is NOT required when documenting a patient care response?

    A. Completing documentation promptly.

    B. Ensuring that documentation is accurate.

    C. Ensuring that documentation is subjective.

    D. Ensuring that patient confidentiality is maintained.

    E. Ensuring that documentation is thorough.

True/False

26. The preliminary inquiry conducted by the plaintiff's attorney into the facts and circumstances surrounding an incident to determine whether a potential law suit has merit is known as the *discovery phase.*

    A. True

    B. False

27. Paramedics may legitimately refuse an order from online medical direction if the ordered procedures are beyond the paramedic's scope of training and is inconsistent with established protocols.
   A.   True
   B.   False

28. Governmental immunity is a likely protection for the paramedic working for a municipality.
   A.   True
   B.   False

29. Because Canadian law does not require an off-duty paramedic to stop at an accident scene, Good Samaritan laws do not apply.
   A.   True
   B.   False

30. The formal contractual or informal legal obligation to provide care is known as a duty to act.
   A.   True
   B.   False

31. The degree of care, skill, and judgment expected under like or similar circumstances from a similarly trained, reasonable paramedic in the same community is known as the scope of practice.
   A.   True
   B.   False

32. Because civil cases involving negligence only require proof of guilt by a "preponderance of evidence," the burden of proving or disproving negligence rests on the defendant in Canada.
   A.   True
   B.   False

33. Contributory negligence is an action or inaction of the paramedic that immediately causes or worsens the damage suffered by another person.
   A.   True
   B.   False

34. In many jurisdictions, a paramedic would be guilty of practicing without a license if, while off duty, he or she performed advanced life support skills outside his or her system of medical direction.
   A.   True
   B.   False

35. The improper release of information may result in a lawsuit against a paramedic for defamation, breach of confidentiality, breach of contract, or invasion of privacy.
   A.   True
   B.   False

36. Before beginning to treat a patient, a paramedic must obtain expressed consent.
   A.   True
   B.   False

37. Once a patient has given consent for treatment, he or she may not withdraw that consent.
   A.   True
   B.   False

38. Ideally, a police officer should respond to the scene of all problem patients and sign the patient care report as a witness or, if the patient poses a threat to the paramedic, accompany the paramedic and patient to the hospital.

A. True
B. False

_____ **39.** The primary factor in selecting a destination hospital is the wishes of the patient.
    A. True
    B. False

_____ **40.** Even if requested to do so by family members, treating a cardiac arrest patient as a "slow code" with only medications means abandoning airway management and defibrillation and amounts to negligence.
    A. True
    B. False

Matching

Write the letter of the appropriate term in the space provided next to the definition to which it applies.

Term

A. scope of practice	**H.** nonfeasance
B. duty to act	**I.** proximate cause
C. breach of duty	**J.** defamation
D. standard of care	**K.** libel
E. malfeasance	**L.** slander
F. misfeasance	**M.** assault
G. reasonable force	**N.** battery

Definition

_____ **41.** action or inaction of the paramedic that immediately caused or worsened the damage suffered by the person

_____ **42.** the act of injuring a person's character, name, or reputation by false or malicious statements spoken with malicious intent or reckless disregard for the falsity of the statements

_____ **43.** a breach of duty by performance of a wrongful or unlawful act

_____ **44.** an action or inaction that violates the standard of care expected from a paramedic

_____ **45.** the act of injuring a person's character, name, or reputation by false statements made in writing or through the mass media with malicious intent or reckless disregard for the falsity of the statements

_____ **46.** a breach of duty by failure to perform a required act or duty

_____ **47.** a formal contractual or informal legal obligation to provide care

_____ **48.** the unlawful touching of another individual without consent

_____ **49.** a breach of duty by performance of a legal act in a manner that is harmful or injurious

_____ **50.** an act that unlawfully places a person in apprehension of immediate bodily harm without consent

Chapter 3

Operations

Part 1: Ambulance Operations

Review of Chapter Objectives

Because Chapter 3 is lengthy, it has been divided into five parts to aid your study. Read the assigned text pages, then progress through the objectives and self-evaluation materials as you would with other chapters. When you feel secure in your grasp of the content, proceed to the next part.

After reading this part of the chapter, you should be able to:

1. Identify current local and provincial and territorial standards that influence ambulance design, equipment requirements, and staffing of ambulances. pp. 120-125

Various standards, as well as administrative rules and regulations, influence the design of ambulances and the medical equipment carried on each unit. Similar guidelines determine staffing levels and deployment of EMS agencies.

Because the oversight for EMS usually falls to provincial or territorial governments, many of the requirements for ambulance services are written in provincial or territorial statutes or regulations. However, national and international standards and trends do have an influence on the development of these laws. Typically, provincial and territorial legislation is broad, while corresponding regulations provide more specific guidelines or rules. For example, a public health law may authorize the ministry of health to issue regulations through its EMS bureau. These regulations, known as the "provincial EMS regulations," might then handle such matters as the essential equipment to be carried on every ambulance.

In most cases, government standards tend to be generic enough so that they are "palatable," affordable, and politically feasible to all EMS agencies. Provincial and territorial standards usually set minimum standards, rather than the "gold standard," for operation. In other words, they establish the lowest level at which units will be allowed to operate. When local and/or regional EMS systems get involved in regulation, their lists tend to be much more detailed and often approach a gold standard, which is the goal when ample resources are provided.

2. Discuss the importance of completing an ambulance equipment/supply checklist. pp. 122-123

Routine, detailed shift checks of the ambulance can minimize the issues associated with risk management. Many services, for example, hold a "stretcher day" once a week. By performing and documenting preventative maintenance on stretchers, it is less likely that a faulty stretcher will cause a patient to be dropped or EMS personnel to injure their backs. Medications carried on the paramedic unit expire. Therefore, expiration dates should be checked each shift, and the older unexpired drugs marked appropriately so that they will be used first. In services that utilize scheduled medications such as narcotics, the paramedics should sign for these medications at the beginning and at the end of each shift. In addition, the vehicle itself should be regularly checked so that it always in safe working order.

3. Discuss factors used to determine ambulance stationing and staffing within a community. pp. 124-125

Deployment

The strategy used by an EMS agency to maneuver its ambulances and crews in order to reduce response times is referred to as deployment. Deployment is based upon a number of factors—location of the facilities to house ambulances, location of hospitals, anticipated volume of calls, and the specific geographic and traffic congestion in your area.

The ideal deployment decisions must take into account two sets of data—past community responses and projected demographic changes. The highest volume of calls, or peak load, should be described both in terms of the day of the week and the time of day.

In communities that do not have multiple strategically located stations, services often deploy ambulances to wait for calls at specific high-volume locations. Such stationing locations are known as primary areas of responsibility (PAR).

Some technologically sophisticated systems use computers to assist the dispatch center in relocating ambulances. Vehicle tracking systems tell the computer exactly where each ambulance is located at a given time.

Operational staffing

In general, ambulance staffing should take into account the peak load of the system. Some services vary shift times to ensure ample coverage for the busiest days of the week and the busiest times of day. Services should also take into account the need for reserve capacity—the ability to muster additional crews when all ambulances are on call or when a system's resources are taxed by a multiple casualty incident. Some services fulfill this need by asking off-duty personnel to carry pagers or to volunteer for backup.

Whatever plan is adopted, each system must consider how they will deal with assigning paramedics. Clearly, an ambulance with two paramedics onboard is limited in the amount of care these two highly trained personnel can provide if they are the only available responders to cardiac arrests (meaning no backup for simultaneous additional emergencies). As a result, some communities prefer to combine a PCP with an ACP paramedic. Other communities, such as Calgary, specify that an ALS unit must have two ACP paramedics so that they can back each other up in making scene decisions.

Finally, each service needs to determine standards for ambulance operators and for driving the vehicle itself. As a rule, these standards are usually spelled out at the local service level.

4. Describe the advantages and disadvantages of air medical transport, and identify conditions/situations in which air medical transport should be considered. pp. 130-133

Advantages of air medical transport
• Rapid transport in situations where the time required for ground transport poses a threat to the patient's survival or recovery
• Access to rural or remote areas
• Access to specialty units—e.g., neonatal intensive care units, replantation units, transplant centers, burn centers, and so on
• Access to personnel with specialized skills—e.g., surgical airway, thoracotomy, rapid sequence intubation, critical care, and more
• Access to special supplies—e.g., aortic balloon pumps

Disadvantages of air medical transport
• Weather and environmental restrictions to flying
• Altitude limitations
• Air speed limitations
• Cabin sizes that sometimes restrict the number of crew members, the amount of onboard equipment,

stretcher configuration, and the procedures that can be preformed
• Lack of normal temperature control, especially in helicopters with their thin-walled fuselages
• Limited lighting (to prevent glare from entering the pilot's compartment)
• High cost of equipment, maintenance, and downtime, which puts air medical transport (especially helicopters) beyond the reach of some communities

Indications for air medical transport
• **Clinical criteria**
—Trauma score < 12
—Glasgow Coma Scale < 10
—Penetrating trauma to abdomen, pelvis, chest, neck, or head
—Spinal cord or spinal column injury or an injury producing paralysis or lateralizing signs
—Partial or total amputation of an extremity (excluding digits)
—Two or more long bone fractures or pelvis fracture
—Crush injury to abdomen, chest, or head
—Major burns or burns to face, hands, feet, or perineum; burns with respiratory involvement; electrical or chemical burns
—Patients in a serious traumatic event who are < 12 or > 55 years of age
—Patients with near-drowning injuries
—Adult patients with:
° Systolic BP < 90 mmHg
° Respiratory rate < 10 or > 35 per minute
° Heart rate < 60 or > 120 beats per minute
° Unresponsive to verbal stimuli
• **Mechanism of injury**
—Vehicle rollover with unbelted passengers
—Vehicle striking pedestrian > 30 kmh
—Falls > 3 m
—Motorcycle victim ejected at > 30 kmh
—Multiple victims
• **Difficult access situations**
—Wilderness rescue
—Ambulance egress or access impeded by road conditions, weather, or traffic
• **Time/distance factors**
—Transport to trauma center > 15 minutes by ground ambulance
—Transport time to local hospital by ground ambulance greater than transport time to trauma center by helicopter
—Patient extrication time > 20 minutes
—Utilization of local ground ambulance results in absence of ground ambulance coverage for local community

CONTENT SELF-EVALUATION

_____   **1.** EMS operations and standards in Canada are set by:
     A.   EMS operators.   **D.**   federal statute.
     B.   regional bodies.   **E.**   federal legislation.
     C.   provincial or territorial governments.

_____   **2.** A conventional truck cab-chassis with a modular ambulance body is a _____ ambulance design.
     A.   Type I   **D.**   medium duty
     B.   Type II   **E.**   heavy duty
     C.   Type III

_____   **3.** A specialty van with a forward control integral cab-body is a _____ ambulance design.

A.	Type I	**D.**	medium duty
B.	Type II	**E.**	heavy duty
C.	Type III		

_____ **4.** Lists of specific medications and protocols for use in an EMS system are generally set by:
- **A.** system medical director committees.
- **B.** the EMS administration.
- **C.** provincial licensing and certification bodies.
- **D.** the Canadian Medical Association.
- **E.** the Paramedic Association of Canada.

_____ **5.** Equipment lists calling for disinfecting agents, sharps containers, and other protective items onboard ambulances are generally established by:
- **A.** system medical director committees.
- **B.** EMS operators.
- **C.** provincial or territorial Workers' Compensation Boards.
- **D.** the Canadian Medical Association.
- **E.** the Paramedic Association of Canada.

_____ **6.** Who is responsible for reporting ambulance and equipment problems or failures?
- **A.** station administration officer
- **B.** ambulance crew
- **C.** ambulance supervisor
- **D.** fleet management personnel
- **E.** all of the above

_____ **7.** The expiration dates on medications carried on the paramedic unit should be checked:
- **A.** once a day.
- **B.** once a week.
- **C.** at the start of every shift.
- **D.** at the start of every month.
- **E.** every other day.

_____ **8.** An EMS agency uses deployment based on all of the following factors EXCEPT:
- **A.** anticipated call volume.
- **B.** local geographic and traffic conditions.
- **C.** location of hospitals.
- **D.** projected ethnic makeup of the population.
- **E.** location of facilities to house ambulances.

_____ **9.** A deployment strategy that uses a computerized personnel and ambulance deployment system is known as:
- **A.** a peak load system.
- **B.** a primary area of responsibility.
- **C.** system status management.
- **D.** primary deploy management.
- **E.** none of the above

_____ **10.** A system that allows multiple vehicles to arrive at an EMS call at different times is called a _____ system.
- **A.** multiple response
- **B.** tiered response
- **C.** primary response
- **D.** reserve capacity
- **E.** peak load

_____ **11.** According to one study, the majority of ambulance collisions occur:
- **A.** in patients' driveways.
- **B.** at intersections.
- **C.** backing into ambulance bays.
- **D.** at night.
- **E.** during inclement weather.

_____ **12.** A legal term found in the motor vehicle laws of most provinces or territories that sets up a higher standard for the operators of emergency vehicles is called:
- **A.** _res ispa loquitur._
- **B.** exempt rights.
- **C.** emergency power.
- **D.** due regard.
- **E.** special status.

13. Provincial and territorial laws typically exempt ambulance drivers who are operating in an emergency from all of the following traffic situations EXCEPT:

    A.   posted speed limits.

    B.   crossing railroad tracks with the gates down.

    C.   posted directions of travel.

    D.   parking regulations.

    E.   requirements to wait for red lights.

14. Which of the following is NOT true about the use of lights and sirens?

    A.   Motorists are less inclined to yield to an ambulance when the siren is continually sounded.

    B.   Many motorists feel that the right-of-way privileges given to ambulances are abused when sirens are sounded.

    C.   Inexperienced motorists tend to decrease their driving speed by 10 to 15 miles per hour when a siren is sounded.

    D.   The continuous sound of a siren can possibly worsen the condition of patients by increasing their anxiety.

    E.   Ambulance drivers may develop anxiety from using sirens on long runs.

15. Why do most EMS agencies no longer suggest the use of a police escort for ambulances?

    A.   Ambulances and police cars have different braking distances.

    B.   Motorists are often confused by escorts going through intersections.

    C.   Motorists often will not see the second vehicle and pull out in front of it.

    D.   Ambulance drivers may have trouble keeping up with police cars.

    E.   all of the above

16. When your ambulance is the first to arrive at the scene of a motor vehicle collision, you should park:

    A.   behind the wreckage.   **D.**   next to the wreckage on the side.

    B.   in front of the wreckage.   **E.**   across the road from the wreckage.

    C.   in a staging area.

17. The use of helicopters for medical rescue grew out of their proven benefit during:

    A.   the Vietnam War.   **D.**   World War II.

    B.   Operation Desert Storm.   **E.**   both A and C

    C.   the Korean War.

18. All of the following are advantages of air transport EXCEPT:

    A.   cost efficiency.

    B.   access to remote areas.

    C.   access to specialty units.

    D.   rapid transport when distance is a consideration.

    E.   access to specialty supplies.

19. A piece of equipment that can be affected by pressure changes during a flight is a(n):

    A.   IV bag.   **D.**   mobile radio.

    B.   capnograph.   **E.**   both A and C

    C.   PASG.

20. As a rule, a helicopter requires a landing zone of approximately:

    A.   100 by 100 feet.   **D.**   75 by 75 feet.

    B.   100 by 100 yards.   **E.**   15 large steps on each side.

    C.   75 by 75 yards.

True/False

21. Almost all communities in the Canada require two ACP paramedics aboard an ALS unit.

    A.   True

    B.   False

_____ **22.** Nowhere in the motor vehicle laws are drivers other than emergency vehicle operators held accountable for the safety of all other motorists.
    A.   True
    B.   False

_____ **23.** Always go around cars stopped at an intersection on their right (passenger's) side.
    A.   True
    B.   False

_____ **24.** The type of air transport that you will most likely encounter as a paramedic is fixed-wing aircraft.
    A.   True
    B.   False

_____ **25.** A number of local programs require physiological abnormalities in addition to MOI findings to activate air medical transport.
    A.   True
    B.   False

Matching

Write the letter of the term in the space provided next to the appropriate description.

A.	peak load		**F.**	gold standard
B.	primary area of responsibility		**G.**	spotter
C.	tiered response system		**H.**	reportable collisions
D.	deployment		**I.**	minimum standard
E.	demographic		**J.**	reserve capacity

_____ **26.** strategy used by an EMS agency to maneuver its ambulances and crews in an effort to reduce response times

_____ **27.** ultimate standard of excellence

_____ **28.** lowest or least allowable standards

_____ **29.** the highest volume of calls at a given time

_____ **30.** pertaining to population makeup or changes

_____ **31.** stationing of ambulances at specific high-volume locations

_____ **32.** allows multiple vehicles to arrive at an EMS call at different times, often providing different levels of care or transport

_____ **33.** the ability of an EMS agency to respond to calls beyond those handled by the on-duty crews

_____ **34.** collisions that involve over $1,000 in damage or a personal injury

_____ **35.** the person behind the left rear side of the ambulance who assists the operator in backing up the vehicle

Chapter 3

Operations

Part 2: Medical Incident Command

Review of Chapter Objectives

After reading this part of the chapter, you should be able to:

1. Explain the need for the incident management system (IMS)/incident command system (ICS) in managing emergency medical services incidents. **p. 134**

Traditional paramedic training focuses on the relationship between one or two patient-care providers and a single patient. In this setting, a paramedic has the ability to concentrate on the assessment and treatment of the patient. Occasionally, however, paramedics are called upon to treat more than one patient at a time. The multi-patient incident may result from a motor vehicle collision (MVC), an apartment fire, a gang fight, or any number of other scenarios.

Based on the confusion surrounding a number of major fires in the 1970s, the fire service took the lead in organizing responses to large-scale emergencies. The result was several versions of the Incident Command System (ICS)—a management program designed for controlling, directing, and coordinating emergency response resources. In recent years, the various ICS systems have been merged into the comprehensive, standardized Incident Management System (IMS). It is a system used for the management of multiple casualty incidents, involving assumption of responsibility for command and designation and coordination of such elements as triage, treatment, transport, and staging.

2. Define the terms multiple casualty incident (MCI), disaster management, open or uncontained incident, and closed or contained incident. **pp. 133, 137, 150**

• **Multiple casualty incident (MCI)**—incident that generates large numbers of patients and that often makes traditional EMS response ineffective because of special circumstances surrounding the event; also known as a mass casualty incident.
• **Disaster management**—management of incidents that generate large numbers of patients, often overwhelming resources and damaging parts of the infrastructure.
• **Open (uncontained) incident**—an incident that has the potential to generate additional patients; also known as an unstable incident.
• **Closed (contained) incident**—an incident that is not likely to generate any further patients; also known as a stable incident.

3. Describe essential elements of the scene size-up when arriving at a potential MCI. **pp. 136-137**

The first few minutes at an MCI can set the course of the next sixty minutes. The scene size-up is very important and should include three main priorities: life safety, incident stabilization, and property conservation.

Life safety

Life safety is always your top priority. If you arrive first on the scene of a high-impact incident, you must observe and protect all rescuers, including yourself, from hazards. Then, and only then, will you attend to patients who are in immediate life-threatening situations. Keep in mind, however, that the needs of the many usually outweigh the needs of the few. If you commit to caring for the first patient that you encounter, you may neglect the other critical patients lying nearby.

Incident stabilization

To achieve incident stabilization, quickly identify whether the situation is an open incident or a closed incident. Because an open incident can generate more patients at any time, it's better to call too many resources than call too few.

In the case of a closed incident, the injuries have usually already occurred by the time you arrive on-scene. Yet even a so-called closed incident carries the potential for additional hazards—an undetected gas leak, a distraught family member who rushes into traffic, or further injury to patients wandering about the scene. As a result, it only makes sense for an Incident Commander (IC) to expend effort stabilizing the incident. Preventing further injuries—either of patients or rescue personnel—helps to ensure a smoother and more successful management of an MCI.

Property conservation

At no time during an operation should rescue personnel damage property unless it is absolutely necessary for achieving the first two priorities—life safety and incident stabilization. Property conservation includes protection of the environment where operations are staged.

4. Describe the role of the paramedics and EMS system in planning for MCIs and disasters. pp. 135-136, 151, 152

The first step you can take in planning for MCIs and disasters is to familiarize yourself with the various laws, regulations, and standards that apply to procedures at an MCI. As a paramedic, you should research whether any of these stipulations apply to your province or territory. Pay particular attention to the presence of a scene-authority law—a legal statute specifying who has ultimate authority at an MCI.

With this information in mind, you can more effectively take part in developing a plan before an MCI or disaster actually occurs. Conduct a hazard analysis and then rate these hazards according to their likelihood. Anticipate any problems that could occur and work toward removing them. Anything that can be planned in advance should be planned in advance.

Once you have assessed potential hazards and any complicating problems, your agency should develop a plan that outlines the SOPs and protocols for the incidents that you have identified. Develop contingency plans for worst-case scenarios. Then, after you have completed your preplan, test it. Make sure that all personnel who could show up at any MCI or disaster are familiar with the preplan and, if possible, take part in practice drills. Start out small. Use local drills within your department to help familiarize personnel with the system. Then, aim for large-scale drills that involve outside agencies.

5. Describe the functional components (command, finance, logistics, operations, and planning) of the incident management system. pp.

To familiarize yourself with the components of the incident management system, use the mnemonic **C-FLOP,** which stands for the first letter in each of the following functions or roles:
• **Command**—individual or group responsible for coordinating all activities and who makes final decisions on the emergency scene; often referred to as the Incident Commander (IC) or Officer in Charge (OIC).
• **Finance/administration**—section responsible for maintaining records for personnel, time, and costs of resources/procurement; reports directly to the IC; rarely operates on small-scale incidents.

• **Logistics**—section that supports incident operations, coordinating procurement and distribution of all medical resources.
• **Operations**—section that fulfills directions from command and does the action work at an incident.
• **Planning**—section that provides past, present, and future information about an incident; operates on the principle of "anything that can go wrong, will go wrong," thus ensuring the necessary strategic support.

6. Differentiate between singular and unified command and identify when each is most applicable. p. 135-136

There are at least two different types of command: singular and unified command. To distinguish between these two types of command, keep these definitions in mind:
• **Singular command**—process where a single individual is responsible for coordinating an incident.
• **Unified command**—process in which managers from different jurisdictions—law enforcement agencies, fire, EMS—coordinate their activities and share responsibility for command.

At small incidents with limited jurisdictions, singular command usually works best. Such incidents have a smaller scope and usually do not involve outside agencies. In many incidents, however, a singular command will not be feasible because of overlapping responsibilities or jurisdictions. Instead, a unified command will be established. Examples of such incidents include terrorist attacks, explosions, sniper or hostage situations, and large-scale disasters. In each of these examples, the managers from several jurisdictions, law enforcement, fire, and EMS will coordinate their activities.

7. Describe the role of command, the need for command transfer, and procedures for transferring it.   pp. 135, 136, 138

The most important functional area in the Incident Management System is command. The Incident Commander is the individual who runs the incident. Most agencies have a single person who is the highest-ranking official. However, establishing command at a multi-agency, multi-jurisdictional incident can be complicated. Regional or local agencies often decide the issue in such situations. Otherwise, the decision should be reached by a pre-existing disaster plan. (See objective 4 on the importance of this plan.)

The determination of when to establish command and when to declare an MCI will vary from department to department. As a rule, the first arriving unit usually establishes command. Depending upon the scope of the incident and local protocols, you and your partner will most likely fill the roles of Incident Commander and Triage Officer—at least until other units arrive. If, or when, higher-ranking officers do arrive, command will be transferred. However, a higher-ranking officer does not become IC simply by his or her arrival. Command is only transferred face-to-face, with the current Incident Commander conducting a short but complete briefing on the incident status.

8. Differentiate between incident command structures used at small, medium, and large-scale incidents.   pp. 135-136

As already noted in objective 6, singular command works best at small incidents with limited jurisdiction. However, at incidents involving overlapping responsibilities or jurisdictions, a unified command will be established. In establishing a unified command, the co-managers will try to achieve balance in decision making. Together, they identify and access the appropriate agencies or specialized organizations that might be needed at the scene. When the Incident Management System is expanded or when the scene is large, co-managers may set up a command post—a place where command officers from various agencies can meet with each other and select a management staff.

In general, Incident Command is supported by four sections or functional areas: finance/administration, logistics, operations, and planning. Each section has a place within the Incident Management System and is headed by a Section Chief. However, all four areas may not be established at every incident. At small- or medium-sized incidents, for example, operations may be the only section implemented. At large-scale or long-term incidents, the Incident Management System may activate the areas of finance/administration, logistics, and planning. Depending upon the type of incident and structure of command, these sections may not be filled with EMS personnel. However, they help coordinate some EMS activities.

9. Explain the local/regional threshold for establishing command and implementation of the incident management system including MCI declaration. pp. 135-136

The threshold for establishing command and implementation of the IMS may differ from department to department, depending on the resources available at any given time. An example would be as follows:
Level 1: 3–10 patients
Level 2: 11–25 patients
Level 3: over 25 patients

10. List and describe the functions of the following groups and leaders in ICS as it pertains to EMS incidents: pp. 137-138, 140-1414, 142-150

The functions differ depending on which vest is being worn at an MCI. The following are examples of the sectors for which you, the paramedic, may be responsible for at the next MCI:

a. **Safety**
The Safety Officer may hold the most important role at an MCI. This person—or, in some cases, team of people—monitors all on-scene actions and ensures that they do not create any potentially harmful conditions.

b. **Logistics**
The logistics section supports incident operations. One of its most critical functions is fulfilling the Medical Supply Unit. In general, logistics coordinates the procurement and distribution of equipment and supplies at an MCI or disaster.

c. **Rehabilitation/rehab**
Medical personnel operating in the rehabilitation section assume responsibility for monitoring the well-being of rescuers. They take vital signs and watch for signs of fatigue or incident stress. A predetermined threshold should be established so that rescuers with abnormal vitals are removed from operation. This is especially important during extremely hot or cold conditions.

d. **Staging**
The Staging Officer supervises the staging area—the location where ambulances, personnel, and equipment are kept in reserve—and guards against premature commitment of resources. The Staging Officer makes every effort to prevent "freelancing" by EMS personnel.

e. **Treatment**
When the number of patients exceeds the number of ambulances available for support, you will need to collect patients in a treatment sector comprised of a red treatment unit, a yellow treatment unit, and a green treatment unit. Each of these units is supervised by a Treatment Unit Leader, who reports to the Treatment Group Supervisor—the person who controls all actions in the Treatment Group Sector.

The unit leader's job requires extreme flexibility to ensure that patients receive adequate care. Patient conditions can change and responders, equipment, or supplies may not be available in the sub-area. As a result, communications must be carefully coordinated. The Treatment Group Supervisor must be apprised of activities in each sub-area. He or she must also help coordinate operations with other functional areas, particularly command, triage, and transport.

f. **Triage**
Because triage will direct subsequent operations, it is one of the first functions performed at an MCI. As a result, all personnel should be trained in triage techniques and all response units should carry triage equipment. At small incidents, you or your partner may assume the role of triage. Larger incidents may require a Triage Group Supervisor, who may either act independently or supervise the Triage Group/Sector.

g. **Transportation**

The Transportation Supervisor coordinates operations with the Staging Officer and the Treatment Supervisor. His or her job is to get patients into the ambulances and routed to hospitals. If you are assigned to this role, you will need to be flexible in determining the order in which patients are packaged and loaded. You may, for example, elect to place two critical patients in one ambulance for transport to a trauma center. If you decide that the ambulance provider cannot adequately care for two critical patients, you may instead decide to transport one critical and one non-critical patient.

The routing of patients to hospitals is as important as getting them into the ambulance. Communication with local hospitals is essential to avoid overloading the resources of any one unit.

h. Extrication/rescue

In general, the Extrication/Rescue group removes patients from entanglements at the incident and arranges for them to be carried to treatment areas. The operation has many facets and may require specialized personnel and equipment.

i. Disposition of deceased/morgue

The Morgue Officer supervises the morgue—the area where the deceased victims of an incident are collected. This person may report to the Triage Officer or to the Treatment Officer. In many cases, these supervisors will in fact assist in selection and securing of an area for the morgue.

j. Communications

At large-scale incidents, the Incident Management System provides for an EMS Communications Officer, also known as the EMS COM or the MED COM. This person works closely with the Transportation Supervisor to notify hospitals of incoming patients. A dedicated radio channel works best for this purpose. The EMS COM will not deliver complete patient reports, which would increase communications traffic. Instead, he or she will transmit the basic information collected by the Transportation Supervisor, such as the number of Priority 1 patients en route to the hospital, the expected arrival time, and so on.

11. Describe the methods and rationale for identifying specific functions and leaders for the functions in ICS.   pp. 135-136, 138

The rationale for dividing tasks at an MCI has already been discussed in previous objectives. However, it is equally important that everybody knows who is charge of the various functions.

For an Incident Commander to manage an MCI, all personnel must be able to recognize the IC. At smaller, single-agency events, everyone may know the IC simply by his or her voice over the radio. However, at medium- or large-scale incidents, such recognition is often impossible. As a result, the Incident Management System calls for the IC and other officers to wear special reflective vests. The vests can be colour-coded to functional areas and may have the officer's title on the front and back. Such vests should be worn whenever IMS is utilized, even at smaller incidents. By making a basic set of vests, especially command and triage, available on every response unit, personnel will get in the habit of wearing and/or recognizing the vests prior to a major incident.

12. Describe the role of both command posts and emergency operations centers (EOC) in MCI and disaster management.   pp. 136, 138-139, 140-141

A command post (CP) provides a place where command officers from various agencies can meet with each other and select a management staff. Because a command post may operate for weeks, the site should be selected carefully. Access to telephones, restrooms, and shelters should be taken into account. Also, the command post should be close enough to the scene so that officers can monitor operations, but far enough away so that they are outside the direct operational area. Persons operating on the scene, members of the media, and bystanders should not have routine access to the CP.

In the case of long-term incidents or incidents over a wide geographical area, an emergency operations center (EOC) may be established. This is especially important in disasters such as hurricanes, floods, or large toxic spills. Arrangements should be made in case the primary communication system fails or if people need to be relocated. Set up guidelines for evacuation, the use of portable radios, and advising people on the best and safest action to take. When possible, every effort should be made to keep people in their natural social groupings. That is, provide home-based relocation instead of removing people to hospitals and clinics when they have not been injured.

13. Describe the role of the on-scene physician at multiple casualty incidents.   p. 147

At some high-impact or long-term incidents, physicians may be utilized outside the hospital to support EMS. Physicians may use their advanced medical knowledge and skills in several ways at an MCI. For example, they may be better able to make difficult triage decisions, perform advanced triage and treatment in the treatment area, or perform emergency surgery to extricate a patient as a last resort. Physicians also provide direct supervision and medical direction over paramedics in the treatment area, removing the need to operate under standing orders or radio contact. You should establish a contingency plan outlining when and how physicians respond to and operate at an MCI.

14. Define triage and describe the principles of triage. pp. 142, 145-146

Triage is the act of sorting patients based upon the severity of their injuries. The object of emergency medical services at an MCI is to do the most good for the most people. For this reason, you need to determine which patients need immediate care to live, which patients will live despite delays in care, and which patients will die despite receiving medical attention.

15. Describe the START (simple triage and rapid transport) method of initial triage.   pp. 143-145

The most widely used triage system is START, an acronym standing for Simple Triage and Rapid Transport. START's easy-to-use procedures allow for rapid sorting of patients into the categories in objective 16. START does not require a specific diagnosis on the part of the responder. Instead it focuses on these signs and symptoms: ability to walk, respiratory effort, pulses/perfusions, and neurological status.

16. Given colour-coded tags and numerical priorities, assign the following terms to each: pp. 143, 145-146

a.   Immediate
Patients in need of immediate treatment receive a red tag, indicating Priority-1 (P-1).

b.   Delayed
Patients whose treatment can be delayed (i.e., they do not have an immediately life-threatening injury or condition) receive a yellow tag, indicating Priority-2 (P-2).

c.   Hold
Patients who do not exhibit the signs and symptoms of START can have treatment withheld, even if they are injured, until a later time. They receive a green tag, indicating Priority-3 (P-3).

d.   Deceased
Patients who have died receive a black tag, indicating Priority-0 (P-0).

17. Define primary and secondary triage, and describe when primary and secondary triage techniques should be implemented.   pp. 143

Definitions
• **Primary triage**—triage that takes place early in the incident, usually upon first arrival.
• **Secondary triage**—triage that takes place after patients are moved to a treatment area to determine any change in status.

Implementation
Triage occurs in phases. Primary triage takes place early in the incident, when you first contact the patients. The action provides a basic categorization of sustained injuries. It must be done quickly and efficiently so that command can determine on-site treatment needs and resources. Universally recognized triage categories include those described in objective 16.

Secondary triage takes place throughout the incident as patients are collected, moved to treatment areas, and receive appropriate medical care. A patient's condition may change over time, requiring you to upgrade or downgrade his or her triage category.

18. Describe the need for and techniques used in tracking patients during multiple casualty incidents.   pp. 143-145

Triage helps the Transportation Supervisor to assign priorities for transport and to determine the types of treatment facilities to which patients should be sent. As you might suspect, the Transportation Supervisor needs to implement some type of tracking system or designation log. Ideally, the tracking sheet or log should include the following data:
• Triage tag number
• Triage priority
• Patient's age, gender, and major injuries
• Transporting unit
• Hospital destination
• Departure time
• Patient's name, if possible
    The tracking sheet not only helps to organize activities at an MCI, it also proves invaluable in reconstructing the incident at a later time. In addition, this record will help document on-scene patient care.

19. Describe techniques used to allocate patients to hospitals and track them.   p. 148

Early in the incident, the communications centre should contact local hospitals and determine how many patients in each triage category they can handle and what specialties (e.g. trauma centre, burn unit, neurological teams) are available. The Transportation supervisor then determines the appropriate destination hospital. The transport supervisor must also track and log the disposition of each patient. Ideally, this should include the patient's triage tag number, triage priority, age, gender, major injuries, transporting unit, hospital destination, and departure time. If possible, the patient's name should be included..

20. Describe modification of telecommunications procedures during multiple casualty incidents.   pp. 137-138, 149, 156

Modified telecommunications
Communication forms the cornerstone of the Incident Management System. Once command is established, the Incident Commander has a responsibility to relay this information to dispatch. After an MCI has been declared, further communication should be moved to a secondary, or tactical, channel. The Incident Commander must be able to supply the information necessary to coordinate resources. That is the whole purpose of the Incident Management System. Use of a secondary channel will also prevent an Incident Commander from interfacing with the communications by other jurisdictions or from overwhelming the primary EMS channel.
    When acting as an Incident Commander, remember that communication will involve units from different jurisdictions and perhaps different districts. One of the foundations of incident management is the use of a common terminology. When communicating, you should eliminate all radio codes and use only plain English. A radio code may have different meanings in different places. As an Incident Commander, you must eliminate any unnecessary confusion in an already complicated situation. In fact, it may be preferable to avoid radio codes even in routine operations. Then there will be no need to even think about switching to plain English when you assume command of an MCI.

Alternative means of communication
Also keep in mind the possibility of communications failure. Things can—and do—go wrong. Your primary radio system might not always work at an MCI. Disasters can knock out radio towers and power. Frequencies can be overwhelmed. Telephone lines can be down. Radio batteries can fail. As a result, alternative means of communication should be included in every MCI preplan and should be practiced regularly. You might use cellular phones, mobile data terminals, alphanumeric pages, fax

machines, or other technology to overcome the failure of your primary radio system. When all else fails, runners can be used to hand deliver messages around the incident scene. Although there are obvious limitations, it may be your last resort. So know how to use it.

21. List and describe the essential equipment to provide logistical support to MCI operations to include: airway, respiratory and hemorrhage control; burn management; patient packaging/immobilization. p. 146

You will need certain medical equipment to operate a treatment area properly. Essential equipment includes airway maintenance supplies, oxygen and oxygen delivery devices, bleeding control supplies, and burn management supplies. In addition, you will need patient immobilization and transportation devices such as stretchers, long spine boards, or other equipment to move patients. (For a more detailed list, see "The Right Equipment" in Chapter 11.)

22. List the physical and psychological signs of critical incident stress, and describe the role of critical incident stress management sessions in MCIs. pp. 140, 148-149, 152

Every EMS professional faces the possibility of critical incident stress (CIS)—the powerful emotional response to a catastrophic event. The response can begin during the event or immediately after. There can also be a delayed response, such as a flashback during a later call. Reactions can be physical, emotional, behavioral, or a combination of all three. (For information on the stress response, see Chapter 13)

You or your agency should make provisions for the use of specially trained Critical Incident Stress Management (CISM) teams. Such resources will provide access to mental health workers or other specially trained personnel who are familiar with emergency operations. CISM team members should circulate around the scene of a high-impact incident to spot anyone exhibiting a stress reaction. Other CISM members should be available for a debriefing after an event.

At smaller incidents, a CISM team will probably not be activated. For this reason, you and other members of your crew should be aware of the signs and symptoms of a stress reaction. Be ready to help each other, using the CISM techniques noted in Chapter 1.

23. Describe the role of table top exercises and small and large MCI drills. pp. 151-152

Table top exercises
As noted in objective 4, for any preplan to be effective, it must be tested and practiced. Tabletop drills are a good place to begin. Once you have worked out the wrinkles, distribute the plan to everyone in your department, the surrounding departments, local police, fire departments, hospitals—in short, to anyone who could be involved in the IMS in your area.

Small and large MCI drills
The next step is to make sure that all the personnel who could show up at an MCI have received training in the use of the IMS. Run or take part in drills so that you gain practice in MCI operations and large-scale use of the IMS. As mentioned in objective 4, start out small. Use local drills within your department and then plan large-scale, multi-agency drills. Never say "It will never happen here." Experience has proven time and again that mass casualty incidents and disasters can occur almost

CONTENT SELF-EVALUATION

_____ 1. An emergency event that involves six patients could be called a:
- **A.** disaster.
- **B.** critical stress incident.
- **C.** multiple casualty incident.
- **D.** mutual aid situation.
- **E.** all of the above

_____ 2. The ultimate authority for decision-making in Incident Command Systems is:

A.   the senior ambulance officer on scene.
B.   the senior fire officer on scene.
C.   the senior police or law enforcement official on scene.
D.   the incident commander.
E.   the senior officer on scene.

3. The most important functional area in the Incident Management System is:

A. logistics.	D. triage.
B. planning.	E. operations.
C. command.	

4. On average the span of control at an MCI is around:

A. 5.	D. 20.
B. 10.	E. 25.
C. 15.	

5. The process in which a single individual is responsible for coordinating an incident is known as:
A.   singular command.
B.   unified command.
C.   command and control.
D.   incident command.
E.   multi-agency command.

6. The process in which managers from different jurisdictions coordinate their activities and share responsibility for command is known as:
A.   singular command.
B.   unified command.
C.   command and control.
D.   incident command.
E.   multi-agency command.

7. A place where command officers from various agencies can meet with each other and select a management staff is called a(n):

A. command post.	D. incident management system.
B. coordination post.	E. direct operational area.
C. incident post.	

8. An incident that has the potential to generate additional patients is known as a(n):

A. open incident.	D. ICS.
B. MCI.	E. contained incident.
C. closed incident.	

9. The cornerstone of the Incident Command System (ICS) is:

A. leadership.	D. practice and drilling.
B. utilizing singular command.	E. communication.
C. having enough resources.	

10. The primary role of the Incident Commander is:
A.   recognizing unified command.
B.   identifying a staging area.
C.   using common terminology.
D.   the strategic deployment of all resources.
E.   directing the efficient movement of patients to the ER.

11. To ensure that units from different jurisdictions and agencies can communicate effectively, all radio communications should be:
A.   given in plain English, avoiding use of radio codes.
B.   use a common set of predetermined radio codes.
C.   relayed through a central dispatching authority.

D. coordinated by the incident commander.

E. conducted on the primary local channel, with routine communications moved to a secondary channel.

12. Before command can be transferred to another leader, it is necessary to report:

    A. face-to-face.

    B. via radio.

    C. in writing at the command post.

    D. via an indirect contact.

    E. none of the above—a higher-ranking officer automatically takes command upon arrival.

13. The Management, or Command, Staff handles all of the following EXCEPT:

    A. public information.   **D.** outside liaisons.

    B. safety.   **E.** critical stress debriefing.

    C. triage.

14. Under the Incident Management System, coordination with outside agencies such as disaster support networks, should be handled by the:

    A. liaison officer.   **D.** public information officer.

    B. safety officer.   **E.** communications officer.

    C. incident commander.

15. The person or group responsible for fulfilling the Medical Supply Unit is the:

    A. Facilities Unit.   **D.** Logistics Sector.

    B. Liaison Officer.   **E.** Planning Officer.

    C. Finance/Administration Sector.

16. Which of the following is the most task-specific section at an MCI?

    A. branch   **D.** unit

    B. group   **E.** sector

    C. division

17. Triage that takes place after patients are moved to a treatment area to determine any changes in their status is referred to as:

    A. secondary triage.   **D.** delayed triage.

    B. ongoing triage.   **E.** primary triage.

    C. sector triage.

18. Under the START system, a Triage Officer would focus on all of the following signs and symptoms EXCEPT:

    A. ability to walk.   **D.** ability to talk.

    B. respiratory effort   **E.** neurological status.

    C. pulses/perfusions.

19. Patients are able to walk should be tagged:

    A. red.   **D.** white.

    B. yellow.   **E.** black.

    C. green.

20. Patients with absent radial pulses should be tagged:

    A. red.   **D.** white.

    B. yellow.   **E.** black.

    C. green.

21. Patients with a radial pulse who can follow simple commands should be tagged:

    A. red.   **D.** white.

    B. yellow.   **E.** black.

    C. green.

22. Colour-coded tags that are placed on patients that have been sorted serve to:

A. track the patient.
B. prevent re-triage of the patient.
C. alert care providers to patient priorities.
D. record treatment information.
E. all of the above

23. One efficient way to speed up the triage process is to:
A. add extra personnel to triage.
B. do not use triage tags.
C. skip the primary triage.
D. do not triage the walking wounded.
E. ask the IC to assist in triage.

24. An ambulance crew who is dedicated to stand by in case a rescuer becomes ill or injured is called a _____ Team.
A. Rescue Response
B. Rehabilitation
C. Extrication
D. Rapid Intervention
E. TIP

25. As a general rule, disaster management occurs in which four stages?
A. mitigation, planning, response, recovery
B. request, response, react, recover
C. mitigation, react, recovery, recall
D. activation, planning, mitigation, recall
E. planning, response, react, reassess

25. CISM team members should circulate around the scene of a high-impact incident to spot anybody exhibiting a stress reaction.
A. True
B. False

True/False

26. Singular command, in many incidents, is not feasible because of overlapping responsibilities or jurisdictions.
A. True
B. False a 135

27. The command post at a large incident should remain within the direct operational area so that commanders can maintain control of operations.
A. True
B. False b 136

28. At an MCI, the needs of the many usually outweigh the needs of the few.
A. True
B. False a 137

29. The secondary staging area should be established in the opposite direction from the incident as the primary staging area.
A. True
B. Falsea a 137

30. To ensure flexibility, an Incident Commander should radio a brief progress report every 10 minutes until the event has been stabilized.
A. True
B. Falsea a 138

31. Under the Incident Management System, the Safety Officer has the authority to stop any action that is deemed as life-threatening.
A. True
B. False a 140

32. The term "sector" is interchangeable for a functional or geographical area.
   A. True
   B. False b 141

33. Capillary refill is an accure indicator of perfusion in adults.
   A. True
   B. False b 144

34. Ideally triage sould take less than 30 seconds per patient.
   A. True
   B. False a 146

35. CISM team members should circulate around the scene of a high-impact incident to spot anybody exhibiting a stress reaction.
   A. True
   B. False a 152

Matching

Write the letter of term in the space provided next to the appropriate description.

A.	Public Information Officer	F.	on site physicians
B.	closed incident	G.	demobilized
C.	Planning	H.	span of control
D.	C-FLOP	I.	Liaison Officer
E.	command post	J.	Staff Functions

36. mnemonic for the main functional areas within the IMS

37. officers who perform supervisory roles in the IMS rather than a task

38. coordinates all incident operations that involve outside agencies

39. the number of people a single individual can monitor

40. collects data about the incident and releases it to the media

41. an incident that is not likely to generate additional patients

42. release of resources no longer needed at an incident

43. provides past, present, and future information about the incident

44. provide direct supervision and medical direction in the treatment area

45. place where command officers from various agencies can meet

Chapter 3

Operations

Part 3: Rescue Awareness and Operations

Review of Chapter Objectives

After reading this part of the chapter, you should be able to:

1. **Define the term rescue, and explain the medical and mechanical aspects of rescue operations.**
   p. 153

According to the dictionary, rescue is "the act of delivering from danger or imprisonment." In the case of EMS, rescue means extricating and/or disentangling the victims who will become your patients.

Rescue involves a combination of medical and mechanical skills with the correct amount of each applied at the appropriate time. The medical aspects of rescue involve assessment and treatment of the patient. Mechanical aspects involve the tools and skills to disentangle the victim.

2. **Describe the phases of a rescue operation, and the role of the paramedic at each phase.**
   pp. 157-161

There are basically seven phases in a rescue operation. They include:

Arrival and size-up. Key to the success of any rescue operation is the prompt recognition of a rescue situation and the quick identification of the specific type of rescue required. You can then quickly notify dispatch of the magnitude of the event and summon the necessary resources. Now is the time to implement the IMS, any mutual-aid agreements, and the procedures for contacting off-duty personnel or backup ACP units. In calling for support, follow this precaution: "Don't undersell overkill."

Hazard control. On-scene hazards must be identified with speed and clarity. You must often deal with these hazards before even attempting to reach the patient. To do otherwise would place you and other personnel at risk. Control as many of the hazards as possible, but don't attempt to manage any conditions beyond your training or skills. Individual acts of courage may be called for, but safety comes first. If in doubt, err on the side of safety.

Patient access. After controlling hazards, you will then attempt to gain access to the patient or patients. Begin by formulating a plan. Determine the best method to gain access and deploy the necessary personnel. Make sure that you take steps to stabilize the physical location of the patient.

As you know, access triggers the technical beginning of the rescue. While gaining access, you must use appropriate safety equipment and procedures. This is the point when you and/or the Command and Safety Officer must honestly evaluate the training and skills needed to access the patient. During this phase, key medical, technical, and command personnel must confer with the Safety Officer on the strategy they will use to accomplish the rescue.

Medical treatment. After devising a rescue plan, medical personnel can begin to make patient contact. No personnel should enter an area to provide patient care unless they are physically fit, protected from hazards, and have the technical skills to reach, manage, and remove patients safely. In general, a paramedic has three responsibilities during this phase of operation. They are:

• Initiation of patient assessment and care as soon as possible
• Maintenance of patient care procedures during disentanglement
• Accompaniment of the patient during removal and transport

Disentanglement. Disentanglement involves the actual release from the cause of entrapment. This phase may be the most technical and time-consuming portion of the rescue. If assigned to patient care during this phase of the rescue, you have three responsibilities. They are:

• Personal and professional confidence in the technical expertise and gear needed to function effectively in the active rescue zone
• Readiness to provide prolonged patient care
• Ability to call for and/or use special rescue resources

If you or another member of the rescue team cannot fulfill these requirements, reassess available rescue personnel and call for backup.

Patient packaging. After disentanglement, a patient must be appropriately packaged to ensure that all medical needs are addressed. Some forms of packaging can be more complex than others, depending upon the specialized rescue techniques required to extricate the patient—e.g., being lifted out of a hole in a Stokes by a ladder truck. In situations where the patient may be vertical or suspended in a Stokes basket, it is paramount that the rescuer know how to properly package the patient to prevent additional injury.

Removal/transport. Removal of the patient may be one of the most difficult tasks to accomplish or it may be as easy as placing the person on a stretcher and wheeling it to a nearby ambulance. Activities involved in the removal of a patient will require the coordinated effort of all personnel. Transportation to a medical facility should be planned well in advance, especially if you anticipate any delays. Decisions regarding patient transport—whether it be by ground vehicle, by aircraft, or by physical carry-out—should be coordinated based on advice from medical direction. En route to the hospital, perform the ongoing assessment and treatment per the patient's condition.

3. List and describe the personal protective equipment needed to safely operate in the rescue environment to include: pp. 153-155

a.   Head, eye, and hand protection

Head. To protect the head, every unit should carry helmets, preferably ones with a four-point, non-elastic suspension system. A compact firefighting helmet that meets NFPA standards is adequate for most vehicle and structural applications. However, climbing helmets may work better for confined space and technical rescues, while padded rafting or kayaking helmets are more appropriate for water rescues.

Eye. Two essential pieces of eye gear include goggles, vented to prevent fogging, and industrial safety glasses. These should be ANSI approved. Do not rely on the face shields found in fire helmets. They usually provide inadequate eye protection.

Hand. Leather gloves usually protect against cuts and punctures. They allow free movement of the fingers and ample dexterity. As a rule, heavy gauntlet-style gloves are too awkward for most rescue work.

b.   Personal flotation devices

All PFDs should meet the Fisheries and Oceans Canada and Transport Canada standards for flotation and should be worn whenever operating on or around water. You should also attach a knife, strobe light, and whistle to the PFD so that they can be easily accessed.

c.   Thermal protection/layering systems

Appropriate clothing and gear should be worn for both flame/flash protection and insulation against extreme cold. Turnout gear, coveralls, or jumpsuits all offer some arm and leg protection. However, for limited flame protection, select gear made from Nomex, PBI, or flame-retardant cotton. For protection in cold or wet situations, such as remote wilderness areas, layer your clothing. Avoid cotton and choose synthetic materials that wick away moisture. Outer layers should be made from water- and wind-resistant fabrics such as Gore-Tex or nylon. Although insulated gear or jumpsuits are helpful in cold environments, they can also increase heat stress during heavy work or in high ambient temperatures.

d.   High visibility clothing

For high visibility, pick bright colours such as orange or lime and reflective trim or symbols. Some services, for example, have an SOP calling for highly visible gear and/or orange safety vests at all highway operations—both day and night.

4. Explain the risks and complications associated with rescues involving moving water, low head dams, flat water, trenches, motor vehicles, and confined spaces. pp. 161-167

Moving water. The force of moving water can be very deceptive. The hydraulics of moving water change with a number of variables, including water depth, velocity, obstructions to flow, changing tides, and more. Four swift-water rescue scenarios present a special challenge and danger to rescuers. They include:
• **Recirculating currents**—movement of currents over a uniform obstruction; also known as a "drowning machine"
• **Strainers**—a partial obstruction that filters, or strains, the water, such as downed trees or wire mesh; causes an unequal force on two sides
• **Low head dams/hydroelectric intakes**—structures that create the risk of recirculating currents (dams) and strainers (hydroelectric intakes)
• **Pins**—entrapped foot or extremity that exposes a person to the force and weight of moving water

Flat water. The greatest problem with flat water is that it looks so calm. Yet a large proportion of drowning or near-drowning incidents take place in flat or slow-moving water. Entry into the water exposes the rescuer to some of the same risks as the patient, such as hypothermia, exhaustion, and so on. Remember: REACH-THROW-ROW-GO, with "go" being absolutely the last resort.

Trenches. If a collapse has caused burial, a secondary collapse is likely. Therefore, your initial actions should be geared toward safety. While waiting for a rescue team to arrive, do not allow entry in the area surrounding the trench or cave-in. Safe access can take place only when proper shoring is in place.

Motor vehicles. Traffic flow is the largest single hazard associated with EMS highway operations. Studies have shown that drivers who are tired, drunk, or drugged actually drive right into the emergency lights. Spectators can worsen the situation by getting out of their cars to watch or even "help." Other hazards besides traffic flow include:
• fire and fuel
• alternative fuel systems
• sharp objects
• electric power (downed lines or underground feeds)
• energy-absorbing bumpers
• supplemental restraint systems
• hazardous cargoes
• rolling vehicles
• unstable vehicles

Confined spaces. Confined spaces present a wide range of risks. Some of the most common ones include:
• oxygen-deficient atmospheres
• toxic or explosive chemicals
• engulfment
• machinery entrapment
• electricity
• structural complications

5. Explain the effects of immersion hypothermia on the ability to survive sudden immersion and self rescue. pp. 161-162

Immersion can rapidly lead to hypothermia. As a rule, people cannot maintain body heat in water that is less than 33°C. The colder the water, the faster the loss of heat. In fact, water causes heat loss 25 times faster than the air. Immersion in 2°C water for 15 to 20 minutes is likely to kill a person. Factors contributing to the demise of a hypothermic patient include:
• Incapacitation and an inability to self rescue
• Inability to follow simple directions

• Inability to grasp a line or flotation device
• Laryngospasm (caused by sudden immersion) and greater likelihood of drowning

6. Explain the benefits and disadvantages of water-entry or "go techniques" versus the reach-throw-row-go approach to water rescue.   p. 162

The water rescue model is REACH-THROW-ROW-GO. All paramedics should be trained in reach-and-throw techniques. You should become proficient with a water-throw bag for shore-based operations. Remember: Boat-based techniques require specialized rescue training. Water entry ("go") is only the last resort—and is an action best left to specialized water rescuers. In all instances, a PFD should be worn in case you or another rescuer are pulled into the water, accidentally slip, and so on.

7. Explain the self rescue position if unexpectedly immersed in moving water. pp. 162, 165

If people suddenly become submerged, they can assume the Heat Escape Lessening Position (HELP). This position involves floating with the head out of the water and the body in a fetal tuck. Researchers estimate that someone who has practiced with HELP can reduce heat loss by almost 60 percent, as compared to the heat expended when treading water.

8. Describe the use of apparatus placement, headlights and emergency vehicle lighting, cones and flare placement, and reflective and high visibility clothing to reduce scene risk at highway incidents.   pp. 170-171

Apparatus placement. When apparatus arrives, ensure that it causes the minimum reduction of traffic flow. As much as possible, apparatus should be positioned to protect the scene. The ambulance loading area should NOT be directly exposed to traffic.

Headlights and emergency vehicle lighting. DO NOT rely solely on ambulance lights to warn traffic away. These lights are often obstructed when medics open the doors for loading. When deciding upon emergency lighting, use only a minimum amount of warning lights to alert traffic of a hazard and to define the actual size of your vehicle. Too many lights can confuse or blind drivers, causing yet other accidents. Experts strongly advise that you turn off all headlights when parked at the scene and rely instead on amber scene lighting.

Cones and flare placement. Be sure traffic cones and flares are placed early in the incident. If the police are not already on scene, this is your responsibility. As a first responder, you must redirect traffic away from the collision and away from all emergency workers. In other words, you need to create a safety zone. Make sure that you do not place lighted flares too near any sources of fuel or brush; otherwise you risk an explosion or fire. Once you light the flares, allow them to burn out. DO NOT try to extinguish them. Attempting to pick up a flare can cause a very serious thermal burn.

Reflective and high visibility clothing. As noted in objective 3, all rescuers should be dressed in highly visible clothing. Since many EMS, police, and fire agencies wear dark-coloured uniforms, you should don a brightly coloured turnout coat or vest with reflective tape. You can directly apply the tape at the scene.

9. List and describe the design element hazards and associated protective actions associated with autos and trucks, including energy-absorbing bumpers, air bag/supplemental restraint systems, catalytic converters, and conventional and non-conventional fuel systems.   pp. 171-172

Energy-absorbing bumpers. The bumpers on many vehicles come with pistons and are designed to withstand a slow-speed collision. Sometimes these bumpers become "loaded" in the crushed position and do not immediately bounce back out. When exposed to fire or even just tapped by rescue workers, the pistons can suddenly unload their stored energy. If you discover a loaded bumper, stay away from it unless you are specially trained to deal with this hazard.

Air bag/supplemental restraint systems. Air bags also have the potential to release stored energy. If they have not been deployed during the collision, they may do so during the middle of an extrication. As a result, these devices must be deactivated prior to disentanglement. Auto manufacturers can provide information about power removal or power dissipation for their particular brand of SRS. Also, keep in mind that many new model vehicles come equipped with side impact bags.

Catalytic converters. Remember that all automobiles manufactured since the 1970s have catalytic converters. They run at a temperature of around 650°C—hot enough to heat fuel to the point of ignition. Be especially careful when a vehicle has gone off the road into dry grass or brush. The debris can be just as dangerous as spilled fuel, especially when brought into contact with a blazing hot catalytic converter.

Conventional fuel systems. Fuel spilled at the scene increases the changes of fire. Be very careful whenever you smell or see pools of liquid at a collision. Keep in mind that bystanders who are smoking can cause a bigger problem than the original accident if they flick lighted ashes into a fuel leak. DO NOT drive your emergency vehicle over a fuel spill—or worse yet, park on one!

Non-conventional fuel systems. Be cautious of vehicles powered by alternative fuel systems. High-pressure tanks, especially if filled with natural gas, are extremely volatile. Even vehicles powered by electricity can be dangerous. The storage cells possess the energy to spark, flash, and more.

10. Given a diagram of a passenger auto, identify the A, B, C, and D posts, firewall, and unibody versus frame construction.   pp. 172-173

Basic vehicle constructions

Vehicles can have either a unibody or a frame construction. Most automobiles today have a unibody design, while older vehicles and lightweight trucks have a frame construction. For unibody vehicles to maintain their integrity, all the following features must remain intact: roof posts, floor, firewall, truck support, and windshield.

Both types of construction have roofs and roof supports. The support posts are lettered from front to back. The first post, which supports the roof at the windshield is called the "A" post. The next post is the "B" post. The third post, found in sedans and station wagons, is the "C" post. Station wagons have an additional rear post, known as the "D" post.

Firewalls

The firewall separates the engine compartment from the occupant compartment. Frequently, the firewall can collapse on a patient's legs during a high-speed head-on collision. Sometimes, a patient's feet may go through the firewall.

11. Explain the differences between tempered and safety glass, identify its locations on a vehicle, and describe how to break it.   p. 173

Safety glass

Safety glass is made from three layers of fused materials: glass–plastic laminate–glass. It is found in windshields and designed to stay intact when shattered or broken. However, safety glass can still produce glass dust or fracture into long shards. These materials can easily get into a patient's eyes, nose, or mouth and/or create cuts. As a result, be sure to cover a patient whenever you remove this type of glass. Safety glass is usually cut out with a GlasMaster saw or a flat-head axe.

Tempered glass

Tempered glass has high tensile strength. However, it does not stay intact when shattered or broken. It fractures into many small beads of glass, all of which can cause injuries or cuts. Tempered glass is usually broken using a spring-loaded center punch.

12. Explain typical door anatomy and methods to access through stuck doors.   p. 173

The doors of most new vehicles contain a reinforcing bar to protect the occupant in side-impact collisions. They also have a case-hardened steel "Nader" pin. Named after consumer advocate Ralph Nader, these pins help keep the doors from blowing open and ejecting the occupants. If the Nader pin has been engaged, it will be difficult to pry open the door. You must first disentangle the latch or use hydraulic jaws.

Before attempting to assist a patient through a door, you should be trained in proper extrication techniques. In general, follow these steps:
• Try all four doors first—a door is the easiest means of access.
• Otherwise, gain access through the window farthest away from the patient(s).

• Alternatively, use simple hand tools to peel back the outer sheet of metal on the door, exposing the lock mechanism. Unlock the lock and pry the cams from the Nader pin. Then pry open the door.

13. Describe methods for emergency stabilization using rope, cribbing, jacks, spare tires, and come-alongs for vehicles found in various positions.   pp. 172, 174-175

Motor vehicles can land in all kinds of unstable positions. They can roll over onto their side or roof. They can stop on an incline or unstable terrain. They can be suspended over a cliff or a river. They can come to rest on a patch of ice or on an on-site spill or leak.

As a result, vehicles must be stabilized before accessing the patient. Sometimes vehicle stabilization can be as simple as making sure the vehicle is in "Park" and chocking the wheels so it will not roll. Other times, such as in the case of an overturned vehicle, you might need to use ropes, cribbing, jacks, or even a spare tire to help prevent it from rolling over. If a vehicle is hanging over an embankment, you might use a combination of cribbing and a come-along tied onto the guard rail (if one is present). However, only attempt these techniques if you have the skills to do so. Otherwise, you need to request the necessary stabilization crews and/or equipment.

14. Describe electrical and other hazards commonly found at highway incidents (above and below the ground).   pp. 171-172

Contact with downed power lines or underground electrical feeds can be lethal. If a vehicle is in contact with electrical lines, consider it to be "charged" and call the power company immediately. In most newer communities, electric lines run underground. However, a vehicle can still run into a transformer or an electric feed box. As a result, make sure you look under the car and all around it during your scene size-up. DO NOT touch a vehicle until you have ruled out all electrical hazards. (Other hazards commonly found at highway incidents are listed/discussed in objectives 4 and 9.)

15. Define low-angle rescue, high-angle rescue, belay, rappel, scrambling, and hasty rope slide.   pp. 175-176

• **Low-angle rescue**—rescues up to 40° over faces that are not excessively smooth; requires rope, harnesses, hardware, and the necessary safety systems
• **High-angle rescue**—rescues involving ropes, harnesses, and specialized equipment to ascend and descend a steep and/or smooth face; also known as "vertical" rescue
• **Belay**—procedure for safeguarding a climber's progress by controlling a rope attached to an anchor; person controlling the rope is sometimes also called the belay
• **Rappel**—to descend by sliding down a fixed double rope, using the correct anchor, harness, and gear
• **Scrambling**—climbing over rocks and/or downed trees on a steep trail without the aid of ropes
• **Hasty rope slide**—using a rope to assist in balance and footing on rough terrain; rescuers do not actually "clip into" the rope as they do in low-angle and high-angle rescues

16. Describe the procedure for Stokes litter packaging for low-angle evacuations.   pp. 176-177

A Stokes litter is the standard stretcher for rough terrain evacuation. It provides a rigid frame for patient protection and is easy to carry with an adequate number of personnel. When using a Stokes litter (also called a Stokes basket stretcher) for high-angle or low-angle evacuation, take the following steps:
• Apply a harness to the patient.
• Apply leg stirrups to the patient.
• Secure the patient to a litter to prevent movement.
• Tie the tail of one litter line to the patient's harness.
• Use a helmet or litter shield to protect the patient.
• Administer fluids (IV or orally).
• Allow accessibility for taking BP, performing suction, and assessing distal perfusion.
• Apply extra strapping or lacing as necessary (for rough terrain evacuation and/or extrication).

17. Explain anchoring, litter/rope attachment, and lowering and raising procedures as they apply to low-angle litter evacuation. pp. 176, 178

Before beginning patient removal, rescuers must ensure that all anchors are secure. They must check their own safety equipment and recheck patient packaging. They must also have the necessary lowering and hauling systems in place, again doing the recommended safety checks.

Materials, especially ropes, should never be used if there is any question of their safety. If you see a frayed rope or any stressed or damaged equipment, do not hesitate to point it out to the rescuers in a polite, but professional, manner. Also, because hauling sometimes requires many "helpers," you may be asked to assist. Make sure you understand all directions given by the rescuers. Evacuation is a team effort.

18. Explain techniques used in non-technical litter carries over rough terrain. p. 178

When removing a patient in a non-technical litter over flat, rough terrain, make sure you have enough litter carriers to "leapfrog" ahead of each other to save time and to rotate rescuers. An adequate number of litter bearers would be two or, better yet, three teams of six. Litter bearers on each carry should be approximately the same height.

Several devices exist to ease the difficulty of a litter carry. For example, litter bearers can run webbing straps over the litter rails, across their shoulders, and into their free hands. This will help distribute the weight across the bearers' backs. Another helpful device is the litter wheel. It attaches to the bottom of a Stokes basket frame and takes most of the weight of the litter. Bearers must keep the litter balanced and control its motion. As you might suspect, the litter wheel works best across flatter terrain.

19. Explain non-technical high-angle rescue procedures using aerial apparatus. p. 178

When using aerial apparatus, it is necessary to provide a litter belay during movement to a bucket. Litters, of course, must then be correctly attached to the bucket. Use of aerial ladders can be difficult because upper sections are usually not wide enough to slot the litter. The litter must always be properly belayed if being slid down the ladder. Finally, ladders or other aerial apparatus should NOT be used as a crane to move a litter. They are neither designed nor rated for this work. Serious stress can cause accidents resulting in patient death.

20. Explain assessment and care modifications (including pain medication, temperature control, and hydration) necessary for attending entrapped patients. pp. 179–180

Protocols for extended care, which is often the case with entrapped patients, can vary substantially from standard EMS procedures. If SOPs for such situations do not already exist, procedures adopted from wilderness medical research will prove useful. Position papers written by the Wilderness Medical Society or the National Association for Search and Rescue can serve as guidelines for protocols.

In most situations, you should prepare for long-term hydration management. You should also look for signs and symptoms of hypothermia, which is not uncommon for these patients. You may have to apply non-pharmacological pain management (distracting questions, proper splinting, use of sensory stimuli) when doing painful procedures. Alternatively, you may need to turn to pharmacological pain management—morphine or nitrous oxide—depending upon the patient's condition, the length of entrapment, and/or advice from medical direction.

21. List the equipment necessary for an "off road" medical pack. pp. 155, 180

An off road medical pack should contain at least the following items:
• **Airway**—oral and nasal airways, manual suction, intubation equipment
• **Breathing**—thoracic decompression equipment, small oxygen tank/regulator, masks/cannulas, pocket mask/BVM
• **Circulation**—bandages/dressings, triangular bandages, occlusive dressings, IV administration equipment, BP cuff, and stethoscope
• **Disability**—extrication collars

• **Expose**—scissors
• **Miscellaneous**—headlamp/flashlight, space blanket, added aluminum splint (SAM splint), PPE (leather gloves, latex gloves, eye shields), provisions for drinking water, clothing for inclement weather, snacks for a few hours, temporary shelter, butane lighter, and some redundancy in lighting in case of light source failure

22. Explain the different types of "Stokes" or basket stretchers and the advantages and disadvantages associated with each. pp. 176-177

Stokes baskets come in wire and tubular as well as plastic styles. The older "military style" wire mesh Stokes basket will not accept a backboard. Newer models, however, offer several advantages. They include:
• Generally greater strength
• Less expense per unit
• Better air/water flow through the basket
• Better flotation, an important concern in water rescues

Plastic basket stretchers are usually weaker than their wire mesh counterparts. They are often rated for only 136 to 275 kg. However, they tend to offer better patient protection. In general, Stokes baskets with plastic bottoms and steel frames are best. These versatile units can also be slid in snow, when necessary.

23. Given a list of rescue scenarios, provide the victim survivability profile and identify which are rescue versus body recovery situations. pp. 152-180

During your classroom, clinical, and field training, you will be presented with a number of rescue scenarios in which you will be called upon to provide a victim survivability profile and to distinguish between rescue and body recovery situations. Use information presented in this text, the information on rescue operations presented by your instructors, and the guidance given by your clinical and field preceptors to develop a high level of rescue awareness and the skills needed to implement the various phases of a rescue operation. Continue to refine these skills once your training ends and you begin your career as a paramedic.

24. Given a series of pictures, identify those considered "confined spaces" and potentially oxygen deficient. pp. 168-170

Confined-space rescues present any number of potentially fatal threats, but one of the most serious is an oxygen-deficient environment. At first glance, most confined spaces might appear relatively safe. As a result, you might mistakenly think rescue procedures will be easier and/or less time-consuming and dangerous than they really are. Here's where rescue awareness comes in. Nearly 60 percent of all fatalities associated with confined spaces are people attempting to rescue a victim.

While "confined space" can have a variety of interpretations, BC Occupational Health and Safety Regulation 9.1 interprets the term to mean any space with limited access/egress that is not designed for human occupancy or habitation. In other words, confined spaces are not safe for people to enter for any sustained period of time. Examples of confined spaces include transport or storage tanks, grain bins and silos, wells and cisterns, manholes and pumping stations, drainage culverts, pits, hoppers, underground vaults, and the shafts of mines or caves. Before going into a confined space, special entry teams monitor the atmosphere to determine oxygen concentration, levels of hydrogen sulfide, explosive limits, flammable atmosphere, or toxic contaminants. They are also aware that increases in oxygen content for any reason—e.g., a gust of wind—can give atmospheric monitoring meters a false reading. The bottom line is this: Confined spaces often mean hazardous atmospheres.

CONTENT SELF-EVALUATION

_____ 1. As applied to rescue operations, awareness training involves a(n):
   A.   command of the technical skills to execute a rescue.
   B.   ability to recognize hazards.
   C.   realization of the need for additional resources.
   D.   detailed knowledge of rescue specialties.
   E.   both B and C

_____ 2. Which of the following items of personal protective equipment must EMS personnel unlikely be able to use in a rescue situation?.
   A.   Respiratory protection
   B.   SCBA
   C.   hearing and eye protection
   D.   helmets and gloves
   E.   EMS personnel must be able to use all of these items

_____ 3. The person who makes a "go/no go" decision in a rescue operation is the:
   A.   medical dispatcher.   D.   Safety Officer.
   B.   Incident Commander.   E.   first responders.
   C.   specialized rescue crew.

_____ 4. In what phase of a rescue operation does patient access take place?
   A.   first   D.   fourth
   B.   second   E.   fifth
   C.   third

_____ 5. The technical phase of a rescue begins with:
   A.   scene size-up.   D.   hazard control.
   B.   medical treatment.   E.   packaging.
   C.   access.

_____ 6. During an extended rescue, take all the following steps to calm patient fears EXCEPT:
   A.   explain all delays.
   B.   tell the patient you will not abandon him or her.
   C.   minimize the dangers of the situation.
   D.   explain unfamiliar technical aspects of the operation.
   E.   be sure the patient knows your name.

_____ 7. It is difficult for people to maintain their core body heat in water that is less than:
   A.   31 degrees Celsius.
   B.   33 degrees Celsius.
   C.   35 degrees Celsius.
   D.   37 degrees Celsius.
   E.   40 degrees Celsius.

_____ 8. Actions to delay the onset of hypothermia in water rescues include all of the following EXCEPT:
   A.   use of PFDs.   D.   treading water.
   B.   use of HELP.   E.   both C and D
   C.   huddling together.

_____ 9. The first action you should take in a water rescue is to:
   A.   reach for the patient with a pole.
   B.   swim to the patient.
   C.   row to the patient
   D.   throw a flotation device to the patient.

E. talk the patient into a self-rescue.

10. At a low head dam, one of the biggest dangers to rescue is a(n):
   A. strainer.   **D.** eddy.
   B. foot pin.   **E.** large rocks.
   C. recirculating current.

11. Factors that affect the survival of a patient in a near-drowning accident include:
   A. age.   **D.** posture.
   B. lung volume.   **E.** all of the above
   C. water temperature.

12. Which of the following factors is associated with 89% of boating fatalities in Canada?
   A. lack of PFDs.
   B. alcohol.
   C. cold water temperature.
   D. age (under 18).
   E. age (over 65).

13. The primary reason confined spaces present a potentially fatal threat is because:
   A. a patient cannot get out and panics.   **D.** faulty retrieval devices.
   B. a lack of WCB/OSH regulations.   **E.** none of the above
   C. the space is oxygen deficient.

14. Although all of the following present risks, the largest single hazard associated with EMS highway operations is:
   A. sharp objects.   **D.** hazardous cargoes.
   B. traffic flow.   **E.** alternative fuel systems.
   C. rollover situations.

15. The post that supports the roof at the windshield is the:
   A. "A" post.   **D.** "D" post.
   B. "B" post.   **E.** "E" post.
   C. "C" post.

16. The easiest means of accessing a motor vehicle patient is through the:
   A. windshield.   **D.** hatch.
   B. door.   **E.** rear window.
   C. window closest to the patient.

17. If you are unable to access a patient trapped in an automobile through the doors, you should enter through:
   A. the window closest to the patient.
   B. the window furthers from the patient.
   C. the front windshield.
   D. the rear windshiled.
   E. the largest available window.

18. Most plastic basket stretchers are rated for about:.
   A. 40 kg.
   B. 50 kg.
   C. 85 kg.
   D. 100 kg.
   E. 135 kg.

19. When involved in a rescue or extrication over hazardous terrain, you should:
   A. limit the use of BLS skills.
   B. limit the use of non-essential ALS skills.
   C. do not use ALS skills.
   D. do not use ALS or BLS skills.
   E. manage your patient using your full range of ALS and BLS skills.

20. Which of the following probably would NOT be found in a downsized backcountry pack?

    A. SAM splints   **D.** intubation equipment

    B. small oxygen tank/regulator   **E.** extrication collars

    C. ECG monitor

True/False

21. Most PPE used in rescue situations has been designed for the field of EMS.

    A. True

    B. False

22. Water causes heat loss 25 times faster than the air.

    A. True

    B. False

23. Entering the water for a rescue is always your last resort.

    A. True

    B. False

24. You should attempt resuscitation on any hypothermic and/or pulseless, nonbreathing patient who has been submerged in cold water.

    A. True

    B. False

25. When taking a patient on a backboard out of the water, always extricate the patient head first.

    A. True

    B. False

26. Federal law requires shoring or a trench box for any excavation deeper than 3 meters..

    A. True

    B. False

27. Removal of the patient from the vehicle almost always precedes patient care.

    A. True

    B. False

28. Each member of a high-angle rescue team must have complete competency in the ability to rig a hauling system.

    A. True

    B. False

29. Most Stokes stretchers are not equipped with adequate restraints.

    A. True

    B. False

30. Because they restrict mobility, cumbersome PPE such as heavy work gloves should not be used on extended rescues..

    A. True

    B. False

Matching

Write the letter of the term in the space provided next to the appropriate description.

    A. recirculating currents   **F.** HELP

    B. mammalian diving reflex   **G.** safety glass

    C. extrication   **H.** active rescue zone

    D. strainer   **I.** short haul

    E. eddies   **J.** tempered glass

_____ **31.** area where special rescue teams operate

_____ **32.** use of force to free a patient from entrapment

_____ **33.** an in-water, head-up tuck or fetal position designed to reduce heat loss

_____ **34.** movement of currents over a uniform obstruction

_____ **35.** type of glass with a high tensile strength that fractures into small beads when shattered

_____ **36.** helicopter extrication technique where a person is attached to a rope that is, in turn, attached to a helicopter

_____ **37.** partial obstruction that filters moving water

_____ **38.** water that flows around especially large objects and, for a time, flows upstream on the downside of the object

_____ **39.** a type of glass made from three layers of fused materials that is designed to stay intact when shattered

_____ **40.** the body's natural response to submersion in cold water, the end process of which increases blood flow to the heart and brain

Chapter 3

Operations

Part 4: Hazardous Materials Incidents

Review of Chapter Objectives

After reading this part of the chapter, you should be able to:

1. Explain the role of the paramedic/EMS responder at the hazardous material incident in terms of the following: pp. 181-182

a. Incident size-up

One of the most critical aspects of any hazmat response is the simple awareness that a dangerous substance may be present. Virtually every emergency site—residential, business, or highway—possesses the potential for hazardous materials. Always keep the possibility of dangerous substances in mind whenever you approach the scene of an emergency. In addition, learn the various placard systems and the resources for identifying them (see objective 1b).

Priorities at a hazmat incident are the same as for any other major incident: life, safety, and property conservation. However, you should be prepared for the special circumstances surrounding most hazmat emergencies. In performing early hazmat interventions, you face the challenge of avoiding exposure to the hazardous material yourself. As a result, never compromise scene safety during the early phase of a hazmat operation. In addition, expect a number of agencies to be involved in a hazmat incident. As a result, you should be skilled in the use of the Incident Management System (IMS) discussed in Part 2 of this chapter. As you learned in that part, you will need to quickly determine whether the hazmat emergency is an open or a closed incident. In reaching your decision, remember that some chemicals have delayed effects. Triage must be ongoing, as patient conditions can change rapidly. Finally, you must take into account certain conditions when choreographing the scene. The most preferable site for deploying resources will be uphill and upwind. This will help prevent contamination from ground-based liquids, high vapor density gases, run-off water, and vapor clouds. A backup plan for areas of operation must be determined early in the event. For example, what would you do if the wind direction suddenly shifted and a cloud of chlorine gas headed toward your staging area?

b. Assessment of toxicologic risk

To aid in the visual recognition of hazardous materials, two simple systems have been developed. CANUTEC, the US Department of Transportation (DOT), and the Secretariat of Communications and Transportation of Mexico have implemented placards to identify dangerous substances in transit, while the National Fire Protection Association (NFPA) has devised a system for fixed facilities.

When placards are used on vehicles, you can spot them easily by their diamond shape. Some placards also carry a UN number—a four digit number specific to the actual chemical. For quick reference, keep in mind these general classifications.

Hazard Classes and Placard Colours

Hazard Class	Hazard Type	Colour Code
1	explosives	orange
2	gases	red or green
3	liquids	red
4	solids	red and white
5	oxidizers and organic peroxides	yellow
6	poisonous and etiologic agents	white
7	radioactive materials	yellow and white
8	corrosives	black and white
9	miscellaneous	black and white

In addition to numbers and colours, placards also use symbols to indicate hazard types. For example, a flame symbol indicates a flammable substance, and a skull-and-crossbones symbol indicates a poisonous substance.

The NFPA 704 System identifies hazardous materials at fixed facilities. Like the DOT placards, the system uses diamond-shaped figures, which are divided into four sections and colours. The top section is red and indicates the flammability of the substance. The left section is blue and indicates the health hazards. The right segment is yellow and indicates the reactivity. The bottom segment is white and indicates special information such as water reactivity, oxidizer, or radioactivity.

Flammability, health hazard, and reactivity are measured on a scale of 0 to 4. A designation of 0 indicates no hazard, while a designation of 4 indicates extreme hazard.

See objective 2 for resources used to identify toxic substances and objective 3 for levels of toxicity.

c.   Appropriate decontamination methods

There are four methods of contamination—dilution, absorption, neutralization, and isolation. The method used depends upon the type of hazardous substance and the route of exposure. In many instances, rescuers will use two or more of these methods during the decontamination process.

d.   Treatment of semi-decontaminated patients

Remember that no patient who undergoes field decontamination is truly decontaminated. Field decontaminated patients, sometimes called semi-decontaminated patients, may still need to undergo a more invasive decontamination procedure at a medical facility.

When treating critically ill hazmat patients, it is important to perform a rapid risk-to-benefit assessment. Ask yourself these questions: How much risk of exposure will I incur by intubating a patient during decontamination? Does the patient really need an intravenous line established right now? Few ACP procedures will truly make a difference if performed rapidly, but one mistake can make any rescuer into a patient. Take a few moments and think before you act.

At incidents where patients are non-critical, rescuers can take a more contemplative approach, especially if they can identify the substance. Decontamination and treatment can proceed simultaneously, depending upon the substance. You might also have time to give special attention to other matters, such as containing run-off water, reclothing patients, isolating or containing patients, and so on.

e.   Transportation of semi-decontaminated patients

When transporting field-contaminated patients, always recall that they still have some contamination in or on them. For example, a patient may have ingested a chemical, which can be expelled if the patient coughs or vomits. As a result, use as much disposable equipment as possible. Keep in mind that any airborne hazard will not only incapacitate the crew in the back of the ambulance, but will affect the driver as well. Although it is not practical to line the ambulance in plastic, you can isolate the patient using a stretcher decontamination pool. The pool can help contain any potentially contaminated body fluids. Plastic can also be used to cover the pool—yet another protective barrier.

2. Identify resources for substance identification, decontamination, and treatment information. pp. 188-189

There are many sources for information that can be used to identify hazmat substances, methods of contamination, and treatment information. Some of the most common include:
• *Emergency Response Guidebook* (ERG)
• Shipping papers
• Material safety data sheets
• Monitors/chemical tests
• Databases (CAMEO)
• Hazmat telephone hotlines (CHEMTREC, CHEMTEL, Inc.)
• Poison control centers
• Toxicologists
• Reference books

3. Identify primary and secondary decontamination risk.   p. 192

Whenever people or equipment come in contact with a potentially toxic substance, they are considered to be contaminated. The contamination may be either primary or secondary.

Primary contamination occurs when someone or something is directly exposed to a hazardous substance. At this point, the contamination is limited—i.e., the exposure has not yet harmed others. *Secondary contamination* takes place when a contaminated person or object comes in contact with an uncontaminated person or object—i.e., the contamination is transferred. Touching a contaminated patient, for example, can result in a contaminated care provider. Although gas exposure rarely results in secondary contamination, liquids and particulate matter are much more likely to be transferred.

4. Describe topical, respiratory, gastrointestinal, and parenteral routes of exposure.   p. 193

There are four ways in which a patient can be exposed to a hazardous substance. The most common method is respiratory inhalation. Gases, liquids, and particulate solids can all be inhaled through the nose or mouth. Once substances enter the bronchial tree, they can be quickly absorbed, especially in oxygen-deficient atmospheres. The substance then enters the central circulation system and is distributed throughout the body. As a result, inhaled substances often trigger a rapid onset of symptoms.

Toxic substances may also be introduced into the body through the skin, either by topical absorption or parenteral injection. Any toxic substance placed topically on intact skin and transferred into the person's circulation is considered a medical threat. In the case of injections, poisons directly enter the body via a laceration, a burn, or a puncture.

In hazmat situations, the least common route of exposure is through gastrointestinal ingestion. In occupations involving hazardous materials, people can be exposed to poisons by eating, drinking, or smoking around deadly substances. Foodstuffs can be exposed to a chemical and then eaten. People can forget to wash their hands and introduce the substance into their mouths.

5. Explain acute and delayed toxicity, local versus systemic effects, dose response, and synergistic effects.   pp. 193

Basically, a poison's actions may be acute or delayed. Acute effects include those signs and symptoms that manifest themselves immediately or shortly after exposure. Delayed effects may not become apparent for hours, days, weeks, months, or even years.

Effects from a chemical may be local or systemic. Local effects involve areas around the immediate site and should be evaluated based upon the burn model. You can usually expect some skin irritation (topical) or perhaps acute bronchospasm (respiratory).

Systemic effects occur throughout the body. They can affect the cardiovascular, neurological, hepatic, and/or renal systems.

Once a substance is introduced into the body, it is distributed to target organs. The organs most commonly associated with toxic substances are the liver and kidneys. The liver metabolizes most substances by chemically altering them through a process known as biotransformation. The kidneys can usually excrete the substances through the urine. However, both the liver and kidneys can be adversely affected by chemicals as are other organ systems. In such situations, the body may not be able to eliminate substances, creating a life-threatening situation.

When treating patients exposed to toxic substances, keep in mind that two substances or drugs may work together to produce an effect that neither of them can produce on its own. This effect, known as synergism, is part of the standard pharmacological approach to medicine. Before administering any medication, be sure to consult with medical direction or the poison control center on possible synergistic effects or treatments.

6. Explain how the substance and route of contamination alters triage and decontamination methods. pp. 196

See objective 1c.

7. Explain the employment and limitations of field decontamination procedures. pp. 198-199

The decontamination method and type of PPE depend upon the substance involved. If in doubt, assume the worst-case scenario. When dealing with unknowns, do not attempt to neutralize. Brush dry particles off the patient before the application of water to prevent possible chemical reactions. Next, wash with great quantities of water—the universal decon agent—using tincture of green soap, if possible. Isopropyl alcohol is an effective agent for some isocyanates, while vegetable oil can be used to decon water-reactive substances.

As noted in objective 1d, field decontamination is never true contamination. Depending on the type of exposure, wounds may need debridement, hair or nails may need to be trimmed or removed, and so on. However, it is always better to deliver a grossly decontaminated living patient to the hospital than a perfectly decontaminated corpse. Just make sure that field-contaminated patients are transported to facilities capable of performing more thorough decon procedures.

8. Explain the use and limitations of personal protective equipment (PPE) in hazardous material situations. pp. 199-200

EMS personnel should not become involved in any hazmat situation without the proper PPE. All ambulances carry some level of PPE—even if not ideal. Hard hats, for example, protect rescuers against impacts to the head.

If the situation is emergent or the chemical unknown, use as much barrier protection as possible. Full turnout gear or a Tyvek suit is better than no gear at all. HEPA filter masks and double or triple gloves offer good protection against some hazards. Keep in mind that latex gloves are not chemically resistant. Instead, use nitrile gloves, which have a high resistance to most chemicals. Also remember that leather boots will absorb chemicals permanently, so be sure to don rubber boots. In general, there are basically four levels of hazmat protective equipment, ranging from Level A (the highest level) to Level D (the minimum level).
• **Level A**—provides the highest level of respiratory and splash protection. This hazmat suit offers a high degree of chemical breakthrough time and fully encapsulates the rescuer, even covering the SCBA. The sealed, impermeable suits are typically used by hazmat teams entering the hot zones with an unknown substance and a significant potential for both respiratory and dermal hazards.
• **Level B**—offers full respiratory protection when there is a lower probability of dermal hazard. The Level B suit is non-encapsulating but chemically resistant. Seams for zippers, gloves, boots, and mask interface are usually sealed with duct tape. The SCBA is worn outside the suit, allowing increased maneuverability and greater ease in changing SCBA bottles. The decon team typically wears Level B protective equipment.
• **Level C**—includes a non-permeable suit, boots, and gear for protecting eyes and hands. Instead of SCBA, Level C protective equipment uses an air-purifying respirator (APR). The APR relies on filters to protect against a known contaminant in a normal environment. As a result, the canisters in the APR must be specifically selected and are not usually implemented in a hazmat emergency response. Level C clothing is usually worn during transport of patients with the potential for secondary contamination.
• **Level D**—consists of structural firefighter, or turnout, gear. Level D gear is usually not suitable for hazmat incidents.

9. **List and explain the common signs, symptoms, and treatment of the following substances: pp. 193-196**

   a.   **Corrosives (acids/alkalis)**

Corrosives—acids and alkalis (bases)—can be inhaled, ingested, absorbed, or injected. Primary effects include severe skin burns and respiratory burns and/or edema. Some corrosives may also have systemic effects.

   When decontaminating a patient exposed to solid corrosives, brush off dry particles. In the case of liquid corrosives, flush the exposed area with large quantities of water. Tincture of green soap may help in decontamination. Irrigate eye injuries with water, possibly using a topic ophthalmic anesthetic such as tetracaine to reduce eye discomfort. In patients with pulmonary edema, consider the administration of furosemide (Lasix) or albuterol. If the patient has ingested a corrosive, DO NOT induce vomiting. If the patient can swallow and is not drooling, you may direct the person to drink 5cc/kg water up to 200 cc. As with other injuries, maintain and support the ABCs.

   b.   **Pulmonary irritants (ammonia/chlorine)**

Many different substances can be pulmonary irritants, including the fumes from chlorine and ammonia. Primary respiratory exposure cannot be decontaminated. However, you should remove the patient's clothing to prevent any trapped gas from being contained near the body. You should also flush any exposed skin with large quantities of water. Irrigate eye injuries with water, possibly using tetracaine to reduce eye discomfort. Treat pulmonary edema with furosemide, if indicated. Again, treatment includes maintaining and supporting the ABCs.

   c.   **Pesticides (carbamates/organophosphates)**

Toxic pesticides or insecticides primarily include carbamates and organophosphates. These substances can act to block acetylcholinesterase (AChE)—an enzyme that stops the action of acetylcholine, a neurotransmitter. The result is overstimulation of the muscarinic receptors and the SLUDGE syndrome: salivation, lacrimation, urination, diarrhea, gastrointestinal distress, and emesis. Stimulation of the nicotinic receptor may also trigger involuntary contraction of the muscles and pinpoint pupils.

   These chemicals will continue to be absorbed as long as they remain on the skin. As a result, decontamination with large amounts of water and tincture of green soap is essential. Remove all clothing and jewelry to prevent the chemical from being trapped against the skin. Maintain and support airway, breathing, and circulation. Secretions in the airway may need to be suctioned. The primary treatment for significant exposure to pesticides is atropinization. The dose should be increased until the SLUDGE symptoms start to resolve. For carbamates, Pralidoxime is NOT recommended. If an adult patient presents with seizures, administer 5 to 10 mg of diazepam. DO NOT induce vomiting if the patient has ingested the chemical. However, if the patient can swallow and has an intact gag reflex, you can administer 5 cc/kg up to 200 cc of water.

   d.   **Chemical asphyxiants (cyanides/carbon monoxide)**

The most common chemical asphyxiants include carbon monoxide (CO) and cyanides such as bitter almond oil, hydrocyanic acid, potassium cyanide, wild cherry syrup, prussic acid, and nitroprusside. Keep in mind that both CO and cyanides are byproducts of combustion, so patients who present with smoke inhalation may need to be assessed for these substances as well.

   These two chemicals have different actions once inhaled. Carbon monoxide has a high affinity for hemoglobin. As a result, it displaces oxygen in the red blood cells. Cyanides, on the other hand, inhibit the action of cytochrome oxidase. This enzyme complex enables oxygen to create the adenosine triphosphate (ATP) required for all muscle energy. Primary effects of CO exposure include changes in mental status and other signs of hypoxia such as chest pain, loss of consciousness, and seizures. Primary effects of cyanides include rapid onset of unconsciousness, seizures, and cardiopulmonary arrest.

   Decontamination of patients exposed to CO and cyanide asphyxiants is usually unnecessary. However, they must be removed from the toxic environment without exposing rescuers to inhalation. Take off the patient's clothing to prevent entrapment of any toxic gases while maintaining airway, breathing, and circulatory support. Definitive treatment for CO inhalation is oxygenation. In some cases, it may be provided through hyperbaric therapy.

Definitive treatment for cyanide exposure can be provided by several interventions carried in a cyanide kit. Basically follow these steps:
• Administer an ampule of amyl nitrite for 15 seconds.
• Repeat at one-minute intervals until the sodium nitrite is ready.
• Administer an infusion of sodium nitrite, 300 mg IV push over 5 minutes.
• Follow with an infusion of sodium thiosulfate, 12.5 g IV push over 5 minutes.
• Repeat at half the original doses, if necessary.

e. Hydrocarbon solvents (xylene, methylene chloride)

Many different chemicals can act as solvents, including xylene and methylene chloride. Usually found in liquid form, they give off easily inhaled vapors. Primary effects include dysrhythmias, pulmonary edema, and respiratory failure. Delayed effects include damage to the central nervous system and the renal system. If the patient ingests the chemical and vomits, aspiration may lead to pulmonary edema.

Treatment varies with the route of exposure. In cases of topical contact, decontaminate the exposed area with large quantities of warm water and tincture of green soap. If the patient has ingested the solvent, DO NOT induce vomiting. If the adult patient presents with seizures, administer 5–10 mg diazepam. In the case of inhalation, maintain and support the ABCs.

10. Describe the characteristics of hazardous materials and explain their importance to the risk assessment process. pp. 181, 182-190, 196-198

Keep in mind the definition of hazardous materials. A hazardous material can be regarded as "any substance that may pose an unreasonable risk to health and safety of operating or emergency personnel, the public, and/or the environment if not properly controlled during handling, storage, manufacture, processing, packaging, use, disposal, and transportation."

Some of the characteristics that will be important to consider when doing a risk assessment of chemicals include a material's boiling point, flammable/explosive limits, flash point, ignition temperature, specific gravity, vapor density, vapor pressure, and water solubility. These characteristics, as well as other on-scene factors and substance-specific qualities, will help you decide the best and safest mode of operation. In general, you will engage in either "fast-break" or long-term decision making. Fast-break decision making occurs at incidents that call for immediate action to prevent rescuer decontamination and/or to handle obvious life threats. Long-term decision making takes place at extended events in which hazmat teams retrieve patients, identify the substance(s), and determine methods of decontamination and treatment.

11. Describe the hazards and protection strategies for alpha, beta, and gamma radiation. p. 191

The levels of radiation and strategies for protection from their particles include:
• **Alpha radiation**—neutrons and protons released by the nucleus of a radioactive substance. These are very weak particles and will only travel a few inches in the air. Alpha particles are stopped by paper, clothing, or intact skin. They are hazardous if inhaled or ingested.
• **Beta radiation**—electrons released with great energy by a radioactive substance. Beta particles have more energy than alpha particles and will travel 2 to 3 m in the air. Beta particles will penetrate a few millimeters of skin.
• **Gamma radiation**—high-energy photons, such as X-rays. Gamma rays have the ability to penetrate most substances and to damage any cells within the body. Heavy shielding is needed for protection against gamma rays. Because gamma rays are electromagnetic (instead of particles), no decontamination is required.

12. Define the toxicologic terms and their use in the risk assessment process.   p. 192

Here are the most important toxicological terms used in the field during the risk assessment process:
• **Threshold limit value/time weighted average (TLV/TWA)**—maximum concentration of a substance in the air that a person can be exposed to for eight hours each day, forty hours per week, without suffering any adverse health effects. The lower the TLV/TWA, the more toxic the substance. The **Permissible Exposure Limit (PEL)** is a similar measure of toxicity.

• **Threshold limit value/short-term exposure limit (TLV/STEL)**—maximum concentration of a substance that a person can be exposed to for 15 minutes (time weighted), not to be exceeded or repeated more than four times daily with 60-minute rests between each of the four exposures.
• **Threshold limit value/ceiling level (TLV-CL)**—maximum concentration of a substance that should never be exceeded, even for a moment.
• **Lethal concentration/lethal doses (LCt/LD)**—concentration (in air) or dose (if ingested, injected, or absorbed) that results in the death of 50% of the test subjects. Also referred to as the LCt50 or LD50.
• **Parts per million/parts per billion (ppm/ppb)**—representation of the concentration of a substance in the air or a solution, with parts of the substance expressed per million or billion parts of the air or solution.
• **Immediately dangerous to life and health (IDLH)**—level of concentration of a substance that causes an immediate threat to life. It may also cause delayed or irreversible effects or interfere with a person's ability to remove himself or herself from the contaminated area.

13. Given a specific hazardous material, research the appropriate information about its physical and chemical properties and hazards, suggest the appropriate medical response, and determine the risk of secondary contaminations.   pp. 188-189

Once you have identified the hazardous material, it is necessary to research the appropriate information about the physical and chemical properties and hazards and then determine the appropriate medical response and any risk of secondary decontamination. It is strongly suggested that a number of resources be consulted in developing the plan of action. The resources include, but are not limited to, those listed in objective 2.

14. Identify the factors that determine where and when to treat a hazardous material incident patient.   pp. 189-190, 196-198

As noted in objective 10, EMS personnel generally engage in one of two modes of operation at hazmat incidents that generate patients: "fast-break" or long-term decision making.

Fast-break decision making
At hazmat incidents where patients are conscious, contaminated victims will often self-rescue. They will walk themselves from the primary incident site to the EMS unit. In such cases, you must make fast-break decisions to prevent rescuer contamination. Keep in mind that it may take time for a hazmat team to arrive and set up operations. In the interim, the conscious, contaminated patients may try to leave the scene entirely. As a result, all EMS units must be prepared for gross decontamination. Basic personal protection equipment should be on board and all personnel should be familiar with the two-step decontamination procedures (see objective 16).

Implement this mode of decision making at all incidents with critical patients and unknown life-threatening materials. Fire apparatus often respond very quickly and carry large quantities of water that can be used for decontamination. Remove patient clothing, treat life-threatening problems, and wash with water. While it is preferable to use warm water to prevent hypothermia, this option is not always available. Please remember that the first rule of EMS is NOT TO BECOME A PATIENT! At no time should you and other crew members expose yourselves to contaminants—even to rescue a critically injured patient. Instead, contain and isolate the patient as best as possible until the proper support arrives.

Long-term decision making
At more extended events, you will engage in long-term decision making. Traditionally, EMS personnel have not been trained or equipped to enter a contaminated area to retrieve patients. Instead, a hazmat team is summoned promptly, and the EMS crew awaits the team's arrival. The team will not make their entry until you or members of your crew perform the necessary medical monitoring and establish a decontamination corridor (see below). It often takes 60 minutes or more for actual team deployment.

Typically, three zones will be established at a hazmat incident:

• **Hot (red) zone:** This zone, also known as the exclusionary zone, is the site of contamination. Prevent anyone from entering this area unless they have the appropriate high-level PPE. Hold any patients that escape from this zone in the next zone, where contamination and/or treatment will be performed.

• **Warm (yellow) zone:** This zone, also called the contamination reduction zone, lies immediately adjacent to the hot zone. It forms a "buffer zone" in which a decontamination corridor is established for patients and EMS personnel leaving the hot zone. The corridor has both a "hot" and a "cold" end.

• **Cold (green) zone:** The cold zone, or "safe zone," is the area where the incident operation takes place. It includes the command post, medical monitoring and rehabilitation, treatment areas, and apparatus staging. The cold zone must be free of any contamination. No people or equipment from the hot zone should enter until undergoing the necessary decontamination. You and your crew should remain inside this zone unless you have the necessary training, equipment, and support to enter other areas.

15. Determine the appropriate level of PPE for various hazardous material incidents including: pp. 199-200

a.   Types, application, use, and limitations
See objective 8.

b.   Use of a chemical compatibility chart
When chemicals can be identified, consult a permeability chart to determine the breakthrough time on a hazmat site. No single material is suitable to all hazmat situations. Some materials are resistant to certain chemicals and non-resistant to others.

16. Explain decontamination procedures including: p. 198

a.   Critical patient rapid two-step decontamination process
Use the two-step decontamination process for gross decontamination of patients who cannot wait for a more comprehensive decontamination process, usually patients at a fast-break incident. Remove all clothing, including shoes, socks, and jewelry. (Remember to have some method of accounting for personal effects BEFORE hazmat incidents occur.) Wash and rinse the patients with soap and water, making sure that they do not stay in the run-off. Repeat the process, paying particular attention to the body areas noted in objective 18.

b.   Non-critical patient eight-step decontamination process
The eight-step process takes place in a complete decontamination corridor and is much more thorough. To leave the hot zone, the hazmat rescuers follow these steps:
• **Step 1:** Rescuers enter the decontamination area at the hot end of corridor and mechanically remove contamination from the victims.
• **Step 2:** Rescuers drop equipment in a tool-drop area and remove outer gloves.
• **Step 3:** Decontamination personnel shower and scrub all victims and rescuers, using gross decontamination. As surface decontamination is removed, the run-off is conducted into a contained area. Victims may be moved ahead to Step 6 or Step 7.
• **Step 4:** Rescuers remove and isolate their SCBA. If re-entry is necessary, the team dons new SCBA from a non-contaminated side.
• **Step 5:** Rescuers remove all protective clothing. Articles are isolated, labeled for disposal, and placed on the contaminated side.
• **Step 6:** Rescuers remove all personal clothing. Victims who have not had their clothing removed have it taken off here. All items are isolated in plastic bags and labeled for later disposal or storage.
• **Step 7:** Rescuers and patients receive a full-body washing, using soft scrub brushes or sponges, water, and mild soap or detergent. Cleaning tools are bagged for later disposal.
• **Step 8:** Patients receive rapid assessment and stabilization before being transported to hospitals for further care. EMS crews medically monitor rescuers, complete exposure records, and transport rescuers to hospitals as needed.

These procedures are not set in stone. Small variations may exist from system to system. You should become familiar with the specific procedures in the jurisdiction where you work.

17. Identify the four most common solutions used for decontamination.   p. 198

The most common solutions used for decontamination are water, tincture of green soap, isopropyl alcohol, and vegetable oil.

18. Identify the body areas that are difficult to decontaminate.   p. 198

Body areas that are difficult to decontaminate include:
• Scalp and hair
• Ears
• Nostrils
• Axilla
• Fingernails
• Navel
• Genitals
• Groin
• Buttocks
• Behind the knees
• Between the toes
• Toenails

19. Explain the medical monitoring procedures for hazardous material team members. pp. 200

Entry readiness
Prior to entry, you or other EMS crew members will assess rescuers and document the following information on an incident flow sheet: blood pressure, pulse, respiratory rate, temperature, body weight, ECG, and mental/neurological status. If you observe anything abnormal, do not allow the hazmat team member to attempt a rescue.

After-exit "rehab"
After the hazmat team exits the hot zone and completes decontamination, they should report back to EMS for post-entry monitoring. Measure and document the same parameters on the flow sheet. Rehydrate the team with more water or diluted sports drink. You can use weight changes to estimate fluid losses. Check with medical direction or protocols to determine fluid replacement by means of PO or IV. Entry teams should not be allowed to re-enter the hot zone until they are alert, non-tachycardic, normotensive, and within a reasonable percentage of their normal body weight.

**20. Explain the factors that influence the heat stress of hazardous material team personnel.
        p. 200**

To evaluate heat stress, you will need to take into account many factors. Primary considerations include temperature and humidity. Prehydration, duration and degree of activity, and the team member's overall physical fitness will also have a bearing on your evaluation. Keep in mind that Level A suits protect a rescuer, but prevent cooling. A rescuer essentially works inside an encapsulated sauna. The same suit that seals out hazards also prevents heat loss by evaporation, conduction, convection, and radiation. Therefore, place heat stress at the top of your list of tasks for post-exit medical monitoring.

21. Explain the documentation necessary for hazmat medical monitoring and rehabilitation operations. pp. 200

The documentation for hazmat medical monitoring and rehabilitation operations should include the following: blood pressure, pulse, respiratory rate, temperature, body weight, ECG, and mental status. (See objective 19.)

22. Given a simulated hazardous substance, use reference material to determine the appropriate actions.   pp. 188-189

Begin by collecting any information provided on the placards—numbers, symbols, colours, and so on. Then use several of the references identified in objective 2 to augment this information. Become familiar with the latest edition of the *Emergency Response Guidebook,* which should be aboard the EMS unit at all times.

23. Integrate the principles and practices of hazardous materials response in an effective manner to prevent and limit contamination, morbidity, and mortality. pp. 181-201

As a paramedic, you will play an important role at any hazmat incident. You may establish command, make the first incident decisions, and help protect all on-scene personnel, including the hazmat team. As a result, you should practice skills that you can expect to use in most hazmat incidents.

Here are some things that you should routinely do. Put on and take off Level B hazmat protective equipment. Set up a rapid two-step decontamination process and an eight-step decontamination process, preferably with the help of the local hazmat team. With a crew member, identify a simulated chemical, determine the correct PPE, and establish the proper decontamination methods. Practice pre-entry and post-exit medical monitoring and documentation. Prepare a patient and ambulance for transport. As these skills may be rarely used except in the busiest EMS systems, you should work closely with your local hazmat team to practice these skills on a regular basis.

24. Size up a hazardous material (hazmat) incident and determine: pp. 182-190, 192-200

a. Potential hazards to the rescuers, public, and environment

Sizing up a hazmat incident is a very difficult task. You often receive inaccurate or incomplete information. Plus events tend to develop very quickly during each phase of the incident. Also, you can expect other agencies to be involved in the event.

As indicated in objective 1a, you must remember that almost every emergency response has the potential for hazardous materials. For example, most households keep ammonia and liquid bleach in the kitchen or laundry room. When combined, these substances can produce a toxic gas. Homes with kerosene heaters or blocked flues can be filled with carbon monoxide. Don't take any chances. Always keep the possibility of dangerous substances in mind whenever you approach the scene of an emergency.

Transportation incidents. Be especially wary of any transportation accident—automobile, truck, or railroad. Maintain a high degree of hazmat awareness whenever you are summoned to MVCs involving commercial vehicles, pest control vehicles, tanker trucks, tractor-trailers, or cars powered by alternative fuels. Do not rule out the presence of hazardous materials just because you do not see a warning placard. Hospitals and laboratories, for example, routinely and legally transport medical radioactive isotopes in unmarked passenger cars.

Railroad accidents merit special attention for two reasons. First, railroad cars can carry large quantities of hazardous materials. Second, there may be several tank cars hitched together on a freight train. Obviously there is a greater chance for a major incident if one or more of these tanks rupture during an accident.

Incidents at fixed facilities. Hazmat incidents can take place in a variety of fixed facilities where hazardous substances are stored. Chemical plants and all manufacturing operations have tanks, storage vessels, and pipelines used to transport products and/or wastes. Additional fixed sites with possible hazardous materials include warehouses, hardware or agricultural stores, water treatment centers, and loading docks. If you work in a rural area, keep in mind the number of places where you can find hazardous materials on a farm or ranch—silos, barns, greenhouses, and more.

Terrorist incidents. As a last note, remember that a new type of hazmat incident has emerged in recent years in the form of terrorism. The terrorists may use any variety of chemical, biological, or nuclear devices to strike at government or high-profile targets.

b. Potential risk of primary contamination to patients

In sizing up a hazmat incident (real or simulated), remember that whenever people or equipment come in contact with potentially toxic substances they should be considered contaminated. Direct contact, as indicated in objective 3, means primary contamination.

c. Potential risk of secondary contamination to rescuers

See objectives 3 and 14. Keep in mind the high risk of secondary contaminations to rescuers in "fast-break" situations.

25. Given a contaminated patient, determine the level of decontamination necessary and: pp. 193-200

a.   Level of rescuer PPE

See objective 8 for the information that you will be applying.

b.   Decontamination methods

See objectives 1c, 7, 9, 16, 17, and 18 for the information that you will be applying.

c.   Treatment

See objectives 1d, 5, 9, and 14 for the information that you will be applying.

d.   Transportation and patient isolation techniques

See objective 1e for the information that you will be applying.

26. Determine the hazards present to the patient and paramedic given an incident involving a hazardous material.   pp. 181-200

During your classroom, clinical, and field training, you will given a chance to participate in, or observe, all of the phases of a hazmat incident. Use the information presented in this text chapter, the information on hazardous materials presented by your instructors, and guidance given by your clinical and field preceptors to develop good safety skills at a hazmat incident. Continue to refine these skills once your training ends and you begin your career as a paramedic.

CONTENT SELF-EVALUATION

1. Upon arriving at the scene of a potential hazmat incident, the first step you should take is to:
   - A.   size up the scene.
   - B.   don PPE.
   - C.   activate the IMS.
   - D.   request additional resources.
   - E.   establish command.

2. Which first responders need to be trained to the hazmat Awareness Level?
   - A.   all EMS personnel
   - B.   police officers
   - C.   firefighters
   - D.   A and C
   - E.   A, B, and C

3. The most preferable site for deploying resources at a hazmat scene is:
   - A.   uphill and downwind.
   - B.   uphill and upwind.
   - C.   across the street from the incident.
   - D.   one mile away.
   - E.   30 meters away.

4. The basic IMS at a hazmat incident will require all of the following EXCEPT a:
   - A.   staging area.
   - B.   decontamination corridor.
   - C.   transport zone.
   - D.   command post.
   - E.   treatment area.

5. One of the most critical aspects of any hazmat response is:
   - A.   working with unified command.
   - B.   establishing the time the incident began.
   - C.   transporting all patients who have been exposed.
   - D.   the awareness that a dangerous substance is present.
   - E.   treating critically injured patients.

6. A diamond-shaped graphic placed on vehicles to indicate hazard classification is a(n):

A.	placard.	D.	CANUTEC label.
B.	MSDS.	E.	Emergency Response Guide code.
C.	UN number sign.		

7. One of the most difficult aspects of dealing with a hazmat incident is:
   A. reading hazmat references.
   B. identifying the particular substance.
   C. working with uncooperative patients.
   D. establishing EMS command.
   E. communicating with the media.

8. Data sheets containing detailed information about all potentially hazardous substances found at a work site are called:

A.	placards.	D.	CANUTEC label.
B.	MSDS.	E.	Emergency Response Guide code.
C.	UN number signs.		

9. Shipping papers that contain accurate information about a transported substance are known as:

A.	transport vouchers.	D.	cargo filing.
B.	MSDS.	E.	special protection information.
C.	bills of lading.		

10. Workplace Hazardous Materials Information System programs are established through:
    A. federal legislation.
    B. provincial occupational health and safety agencies.
    C. provincial and territorial legislation.
    D. Health and Transport Canada.
    E. international trade agreements.

11. Which safety zone is also called the contamination reduction or buffer zone?

A.	hot zone	D.	treatment zone
B.	warm zone	E.	extrication zone
C.	cold zone		

12. Which of the following is least likely to result in secondary contamination?

A.	acids and alkalis	D.	liquid corrosives
B.	carbon monoxide	E.	carbamates
C.	organophosphates		

13. In hazmat situations, the least common route(s) of exposure is (are) through:

A.	respiratory inhalation.	D.	gastrointestinal ingestion.
B.	parenteral injection.	E.	direct contact.
C.	topical absorption.		

14. In a hazmat situation, the most common route(s) of exposure is (are) through:

A.	respiratory inhalation.	D.	gastrointestinal ingestion.
B.	parenteral injection.	E.	direct contact.
C.	topical absorption.		

15. If a patient was exposed to a hazardous gas and developed acute bronchospasm, this could be called a _____ effect.

A.	local.	D.	synergistic.
B.	systemic.	E.	secondary.
C.	biotransformation.		

16. Cyanide is an example a:
    A. chemical asphyxiate.
    B. corrosive.
    C. pulmonary irritant.

    D.   solvent.

    E.   organophosphate.

17. Definitive treatment for CO inhalation is:

A. oxygenation.	**D.** infusion of sodium thiosulfate.
B. hyperbaric therapy.	**E.** none of the above
C. use of a cyanide kit.	

18. All of the following are methods of decontamination EXCEPT:

A. stabilization.	**D.** isolation.
B. dilution.	**E.** neutralization.
C. absorption.	

19. Which priority should guide your decision making while performing decontamination?

A. life safety	**D.** triage
B. incident stabilization	**E.** neutralization
C. property conservation	

20. All the following are common decontamination solvents EXCEPT:

A. water.	**D.** baking soda.
B. tincture of green soap.	**E.** vegetable oil.
C. isopropyl alcohol.	

21. Two methods for decontamination in the field are the:

    A.   two-step and twelve-step processes.

    B.   complete and incomplete methods.

    C.   gross decontamination and neutralizing methods.

    D.   two-step and eight-step processes.

    E.   fast-break and long-term methods.

22. The lowest level of hazmat protective equipment is:

A. Level A.	**D.** Level D.
B. Level B.	**E.** Level E.
C. Level C.	

23. The highest level of hazmat protective equipment uses a(n):

A. HEPA filter mask.	**D.** SCUBA.
B. air-purifying respirator.	**E.** PBI flash protector.
C. SCBA.	

24. Which of the following should be consulted to determine the breakthrough time of a specific chemical on a hazmat suit?

A. CAMEO website	**D.** OSHA publication CFR 1910.120
B. *Emergency Response Guidebook*	**E.** NFPA table
C. permeability chart	

25. What precaution should hazmat team members make to prevent dehydration?

    A.   prehydrate with 250 – 500 ml of water or sports drink

    B.   prehydrate with 500 – 750 ml of water or sports drink

    C.   prehydrate with 1 to 2 litres of water or sports drink

    D.   take salt supplements

    E.   take breaks for rehydration every 20 minutes

True/False

26. The *Emergency Response Guide* is produced by CANUTEC, the US DOT, and the Secretariat of Communications and Transportation of Mexico.

    A.   True

    B.   False

27. Hazmat monitoring devices should be routinely used by EMS personnel for quick identification of a substance.
    A.   True
    B.   False

28. Your most critical action at a hazmat response is to recognize that a dangerous substance is present.
    A.   True
    B.   False

29. A placard that displays a "W" with a line through it indicates that the substance will react with water.
    A.   True
    B.   False

30. Hazmat monitoring devices should be routinely used by EMS personnel for quick identification of a substance.
    A.   True
    B.   False

31. CHEMTREC maintains a database describing the health hazards and principles for managing exposure to specific chemicals.
    A.   True
    B.   False

32. The upper range of vapour concentration in the air at which an ignition will initiate combustion is known as the flash point.
    A.   True
    B.   False

33. The threshold limit value is the concentration or dose that results in the death of 50 percent of those who are exposed to it.
    A.   True
    B.   False

34. The most common route of exposure of cyanides is through inhalation, although cyanides can also be ingested, absorbed, or injected.
    A.   True
    B.   False

35. One of the primary roles of EMS personnel at a hazmat incident is medical monitoring of entry personnel.
    A.   True
    B.   False

Matching

Write the letter of the term in the space provided next to the appropriate description.

Term

A.	boiling point	**F.**	ignition temperature
B.	warm zone	**G.**	cold zone
C.	CHEMTREC	**H.**	warning placard
D.	hazardous material	**I.**	MSDS
E.	flash point	**J.**	hot zone

Description

36. any substance that causes adverse health effects upon human exposure

_____ **37.** diamond-shaped graphic placed on vehicles to indicate hazmat classification

_____ **38.** easily accessible sheets of detailed information about chemicals found at fixed facilities

_____ **39.** Chemical Transportation Emergency Center that maintains a 24-hour toll-free hazmat information hotline

_____ **40.** the location where the hazardous material and the highest levels of contamination exist

_____ **41.** the location where the decontamination corridor should be set up

_____ **42.** the area at a hazardous material incident where the command post and sectors are set up

_____ **43.** the lowest temperature at which a liquid will give off enough vapors to ignite

_____ **44.** the temperature at which a liquid becomes a gas

_____ **45.** the lowest temperature at which a liquid will give off enough vapors to support combustion

Chapter 3

Operations

Part 5: Crime Scene Awareness

Review of Chapter Objectives

After reading this part of the chapter, you should be able to:

1. Explain how EMS providers are often mistaken for the police. **pp. 202, 207**

Depending upon your uniform colours and the use of badges, people might mistake you for the police—especially if you exit from a vehicle with a flashing lights and siren. They might expect you to intervene in a violent situation, or they might direct aggression toward you as an authority figure.

When entering gang territory, you are especially at risk if your uniform resembles that of the police. Gangs with a history of arrest may in fact make every effort to prevent you from transporting one of their members to a hospital or any other place beyond their reach. Do not force the situation if your safety is at stake.

2. Explain specific techniques for risk reduction when approaching the following types of routine EMS scenes: **pp. 202-204, 204-208**

a. Highway encounters

To make a safe approach to a vehicle at a roadside emergency, follow these steps:

• Park the ambulance in a position that provides safety from traffic.

• Notify dispatch of the situation, location, the vehicle make and model, and the province and number of the license plate.

• Use a one-person approach. The driver should remain in the ambulance, which is elevated and provides greater visibility.

• The driver should remain prepared to radio for immediate help and to back or drive away rapidly once the other medic returns.

• At nighttime, use the ambulance lights to illuminate the vehicle. However, do not walk between the ambulance and the other vehicle. You will be backlit, forming an easy target.

• Since police approach vehicles from the driver's side, you should approach from the passenger's side, which is an unexpected route.

• Use the A, B, and C door posts for cover.

• Observe the rear seat. Do not move forward of the C post unless you are sure there are no threats in the rear seat or foot wells.

• Retreat to the ambulance (or another strategic position of cover) at the first sign of danger.

• Make sure you have mapped out your intended retreat and escape with the ambulance driver.

b. Violent street incidents

You can encounter many different types of violence while working on the streets. Incidents can range from random acts of violence against individual citizens to organized efforts at domestic or international terrorism. In responding to scene of any violent crime, keep these precautions in mind:

• Dangerous weapons may have been used in the crime.
• Perpetrators may still be on-scene or could return on-scene.
• Patients may sometimes exhibit violence toward EMS personnel, particularly if they risk criminal penalties as a result of the original incident.

When on the streets, you must remain constantly aware of crowd dynamics. Crowds can quickly become larger and volatile, especially in the case of a hate crime. Violence can be directed against anyone or anything in the path of an angry crowd. Your status as an EMS provider does not give you immunity against an out-of-control mob. Whenever a crowd is present, look for these warning signs of impending danger:

• Shouts or increasingly loud voices
• Pushing or shoving
• Hostilities toward anyone on-scene, including the perpetrator of a crime, the victim, police, and so on
• Rapid increase in crowd size
• Inability of law enforcement officials to control bystanders

To protect yourself, constantly monitor the crowd and retreat if necessary. If possible, take the patient with you so that you do not have to return later. Rapid transport may require limited or tactical assessment at the scene, with more in-depth assessment done inside the safety of the ambulance. Be sure to document reasons for the quick assessment and transport.

c. Residences and "dark houses"

Domestic violence needs to be a consideration whenever you approach a residence and detect yelling, screaming, or any other signs of fighting. Sometimes you might spot clues such as broken glass or blood on the sidewalk. If you approach a "dark house," especially one where the front door is ajar, be very cautious—it could a set-up. In such cases, ask the dispatcher to call the residence and request that occupants turn on lights and meet you at the front door, if possible. When entering a residence, look around for any potential weapons that may be used against you. If you are unsure of the safety of the scene, call for police backup. If there is a fight going on as you approach the residence, retreat and request police to secure the scene.

3. Describe the warning signs of potentially violent situations.   pp. 202-204, 204=208

You should remain alert throughout a call, especially in areas with a history of violence. You may enter the scene and spot weapons or drugs. Additional combative people may arrive on the scene. The patient or bystanders may become agitated or threatening. Even if treatment has begun, you must place your own safety first. You may have just two tactical options: quickly package the patient and leave the scene with the patient or retreat without the patient.

4. Explain emergency evasive techniques for potentially violent situations, including: pp. 201-213

a. Threats of physical violence
See objectives 2, 5, and 6.

b. Firearms encounters
See objectives 5b and 6c.

c. Edged weapon encounters
Your best tactical response to an edged weapon is observation. If you suspect violence with any kind of weapon, stay out of danger in the first place—i.e., retreat. Ideally you will retreat to the ambulance so that you can summon help. If the attacker pursues you, follow the evasive strategies listed in objective 6c.

5. Explain EMS considerations for the following types of violent or potentially violent situations: pp. 204-208

a. Gangs and gang violence

Street gangs can be found in big cities, suburban towns, and, lately, in rural communities. No EMS unit is totally immune from gang activity. In fact, some gangs have purposely branched out into smaller towns in an effort to escape surveillance and expand their illicit businesses. Commonly observed gang characteristics include:

• **Appearance:** Gang members frequently wear unique clothing specific to the group. Because the clothing is often a particular colour or hue, it is referred to as the gang's "colours." Wearing a colour, even a bandana, can signify gang membership. Within the gang itself, members sometimes wear different articles to signify rank.

• **Graffiti:** Gangs have definite territories or "turfs." Members often mark their turf with graffiti broadcasting the gang's logo, warning away intruders, bragging about crimes, insulting rival gangs, or taunting police.

• **Tattoos:** Many gang members wear tattoos or other body markings to identify their gang affiliation. Some gangs even require these tattoos. The tattoos will be in the gang's colours and often contain the gang's motto or logo.

• **Hand signals/language:** Gangs commonly create their own methods of communication. They give gang-related meanings to everyday words or create codes. Hand signals provide quick identification among gang members, warn of approaching law enforcement, or show disrespect to other gangs. Gang members often perform signals so quickly that an uninformed outsider may not spot them, much less understand them.

Always remember that gang members are usually armed and expect your respect. Do not cut their "colours" or clothing without permission, or you will be displaying a public show of disrespect. Finally, keep in mind the attitudes toward authority mentioned in objective 1.

### b.	Hostages/sniper situations

The provision of care in hostage/sniper situations often necessitates risks far beyond those found on most EMS calls. Medical personnel assigned to such incidents require special training and authorization. Like hazmat teams, they must don special equipment, function with compact gear, and, in most cases, work as medical adjuncts to the police or military.

If you find yourself in one of these situations, be sure to stage your ambulance outside the "kill zone," or the range of a typical rifle. If you are unsure of the distance, ask the police. Do not approach the scene, as you may end up being taken as a hostage also. A good precaution for any dangerous situation is the use of prearranged verbal and nonverbal clues. Be sure to alert dispatch to the meaning of spoken clues. Choose signals that indicate a variety of circumstances while sounding harmless to an attacker. This can be a life-saving technique in situations where you find yourself, the crew, and/or the patient held hostage. Your so-called "routine" radio reports can spell out the nature of the trouble and summon help from a Special Weapons and Tactics (SWAT) team.

### c.	Clandestine drug labs

Drug raids on clandestine ("clan") labs have a way of turning into hazmat operations. All too often, the labs contain toxic fumes and volatile chemicals. The people on-scene complicate matters by fighting or shooting at the rescuers who come to extricate them from the toxic environment. As they retreat, drug dealers may also trigger booby traps or wait for police or EMS personnel to trigger them. If you ever come upon a clan lab, take these actions:

• Leave the area immediately.
• Do not touch anything.
• Never stop any chemical reactions already in progress.
• Do not smoke or bring any source of flame near the lab.
• Notify the police.
• Initiate ICS and hazmat procedures.
• Consider evacuation of the area.

Remember that laboratories can be found anywhere—on farms, in trailers, in city apartments, and more. They may be mobile, roaming from place to place in a camper or a truck. Or they may be disassembled and stored in almost any variety of locations. The job of raiding clan labs belongs to specialized personnel—not EMS.

### d.	Domestic violence

Domestic violence involves people who live together in an intimate relationship. The violence may be physical, emotional, sexual, verbal, or economic. It may be directed against a spouse or partner, or it may involve children and/or older relatives who live at the residence.

When called to the scene of domestic violence, the abuser may turn on you or other members of the crew. You have two main concerns: your own personal safety and protection of the patient from further harm. For more on the indications of domestic violence and the appropriate actions of EMS crews, see Chapter 44, "Abuse and Assault."

e.   Emotionally disturbed people

The prudent strategy is to retreat whenever you spot indicators of violence or physical confrontations with an emotionally disturbed person. Conduct the retreat in a calm but decisive manner. Be aware that the danger is now at your back and integrate cover into your retreat. For information on emotionally disturbed patients, see Chapter 38, Division 4.

6. Explain the following techniques: pp. 208-213

a.   Field "contact and cover" procedures during assessment and care

The concept of "contact and cover" comes from a police procedure developed in San Diego, California. When adapted to EMS practice, the procedure assigns the roles shown in the following table.

Contact Provider	Cover Provider
• Initiates and provides direct patient care.	• Observes the scene for danger while the "contact" cares for the patient.
• Performs patient assessment.	• Generally avoids patient care duties that would prevent observation of the scene.
• Handles most interpersonal scene contact.	• In small crews, may perform limited functions such as handling equipment.

As with any tactic adopted from another discipline, contact and cover has obvious correlations and drawbacks. The tactic is ideal for street encounters with intoxicated persons or subjects acting in a suspicious manner. An obvious drawback is that two medics working on a cardiac arrest will not be able to designate one person to act solely as a "cover" medic.

Perhaps the best application of this police procedure to EMS is its emphasis on the importance of observation and teamwork. A crew that works well together will assign roles—formally or informally—to guarantee safety and patient care. In its most basic form, contact and cover means that you will watch your partner's back while he or she watches yours.

b.   Evasive tactics

Some specific techniques to avoid violence include:
- Throwing equipment to trip, slow, or distract an aggressor
- Wedging a stretcher in a doorway to block an attacker
- Using an unconventional path while retreating
- Anticipating the moves of the aggressor and taking counter moves
- Overturning objects in the path of the attacker
- Using preplanned tactics with your partner to confuse or "throw off" an aggressor

Key to the success of these safety tactics is your own physical well-being. Regular exercise and good health ensure that you will have the strength to outrun or, if necessary, defend yourself against an attacker. Some units provide basic training in self-defense or have protocols on its use. Make sure you take advantage of this training and/or know the protocols related to the application of force.

c.   Concealment techniques

When faced with danger, two of your most immediate and practical strategies are cover and concealment. Concealment hides your body, as when you crouch behind bushes, wallboards, or vehicle doors. However, most common objects do not stop bullets. During armed encounters, seek cover by hiding your body behind solid and impenetrable objects such as brick walls, rocks, large trees, telephone poles, and the engine block of vehicles.

For cover and concealment to work, they must be used properly. In applying these safety tactics, keep in mind the following general rules.

• As you approach any scene, remain aware of the surroundings and any potential sources of protection in case you must retreat or are "pinned down."

• Choose your cover carefully. You may have only one chance to pick your protection. Select the item that hides your body adequately while shielding you against bullets.

• Once you have made your choice of cover, conceal as much of your body as possible. Be conscious of any reflective clothing that you may be wearing. Armed assailants can use it as a target, especially at night.

• Constantly look to improve your protection and location.

7. Describe police evidence considerations and techniques to assist in evidence preservation. pp. 213-215

When on the scene of a call where a crime has been committed, the paramedic should never jeopardize patient care for the sake of evidence. However, do not perform patient care with disregard of the criminal investigation that will follow. Remember that EMS and the police are on the same side—so work together. If you are the first person on the scene of a crime, be aware that anything you touch, walk on, pick up, cut, wipe off, or move could be evidence. Developing an awareness of evidence will even affect the way you treat patients. You will need to observe the patient carefully and to disturb as little direct evidence as possible. Also, when examining a patient, remember that you may be at risk. The patient may have a concealed weapon, such as a knife or gun.

Types of evidence
Gathering evidence is a specialized and time-consuming job. While it is unrealistic to train EMS personnel in the details of police work, it is not unrealistic to ask them to develop an awareness of the general types of evidence that they may expect to encounter at a crime scene. Some of the main categories of evidence include prints, blood and body fluids, and particulate evidence.

On-scene observations
Everything that you and other members of the EMS crew see and hear can serve as evidence. Your observations on the scene will become part of the police record—and ultimately part of the court record. Be sure to look for and record the following information:

• Conditions at the scene—absence or presence of lights, locked or unlocked doors, open or closed curtains, and so on
• Position of the patient/victim
• Injuries suffered by the patient/victim
• Statements of persons on the scene
• Statements by the patient/victim
• Dying declarations
• Suspicious persons at, or fleeing from, the scene
• Presence and/or location of any weapons

Documenting evidence
Record only the facts at the scene of a crime and record them accurately. Otherwise, they might be thrown out of court as evidence. Use quotation marks to indicate the words of bystanders and any remarks made by the patient. Avoid opinions not relevant to patient care. If the patient has died, do not offer any judgments that might contradict later findings by the medical examiner.

Finally, follow local policies and regulations regarding confidentiality surrounding any crime case. Any offhand remarks that you make might later become testimony in a courtroom, along with other documents that you prepare at the scene.

8. Given several crime scene scenarios, identify potential hazards and determine if the scene is safe to enter, then provide care preserving the crime scene as appropriate. pp. 201-215

During your classroom, clinical, and field training, you will have a chance to practice your approach to violent or potentially violent crime scenes. Use the information presented in this text chapter, the information on crime scene awareness presented by your instructors, and the guidance given by your clinical and field preceptors to develop the skills to protect yourself and your partner, as well as to preserve on-scene evidence. Continue to refine these skills once your training ends and you begin your career as a paramedic.

CONTENT SELF-EVALUATION

_____ **1.** In 2002 in British Columbia, 84% of all violent crimes were committed by men aged:
　　　A. 10 to 17.　　　　　　**D.** 51 to 65.
　　　B. 18 to 34.　　　　　　**E.** over age 65.
　　　C. 35 to 50.

_____ **2.** A computer-aided dispatch (CAD) program can assist in preventing an attack on EMS personnel by:
　　　A. predicting when crimes are most likely to occur.
　　　B. noting addresses with a history of violence.
　　　C. maintaining a list of known criminals.
　　　D. linking an EMS unit to a special forces team.
　　　E. all of the above

_____ **3.** If dispatch advises you that there is a potential for violence at the scene, you should.
　　　A. cancel the call until police request EMS assistance.
　　　B. wait out of sight until police have secured the scene.
　　　C. wait and approach the scene with the police units.
　　　D. park in front of the scene with your lights on to alert the next arriving units.
　　　E. park beyond the scene and approach from an unconventional direction.

_____ **4.** One of the main purposes of the scene survey at a crime scene is to search for:
　　　A. possible evidence.　　　　**D.** law enforcement officials.
　　　B. alleged assailants.　　　　**E.** a way to rescue the victim.
　　　C. hazards.

_____ **5.** If you are with the patient and bystanders become agitated or threatening, your best tactical option is to.
　　　A. quickly package the patient or retreat without the patient.
　　　B. call for additional resources while you quickly complete your treatment.
　　　C. have your partner deal with the disruptive person while you continue treatment.
　　　D. use the minimum amount of force required to subdue the agitated person.
　　　E. all of these are acceptable options

_____ **6.** When approaching a residence that may be hazardous, you should:
　　　A. be careful not to backlight yourself.
　　　B. hold your flashlight to the side.
　　　C. take an unconventional approach to the door.
　　　D. keep your partner in sight.
　　　E. all of the above

_____ **7.** Before knocking on the door, you should do all of the following EXCEPT:
　　　A. stand on the hinge side of the door.
　　　B. listen for loud noises.
　　　C. listen for items breaking.
　　　D. listen for the lack of any sounds at all.
　　　E. look in the windows for the presence of weapons.

_____ **8.** If you must approach a stopped vehicle at night, you should:
　　　A. approach from one side of the vehicle and have your partner approach from the other side.
　　　B. use your ambulance lights to illuminate the vehicle.

C. stay between the vehicle and your ambulance lights.
D. approach the patient from the driver's door.
E. B and C are correct

9. To make a safe approach to a suspicious roadside emergency, you should take all of the following safety steps EXCEPT:
A. use a one-person approach.
B. use the ambulance lights to illuminate the vehicle.
C. approach the vehicle from the driver's side.
D. use the A, B, and C posts for cover.
E. observe the rear seat.

10. Most homicides in Canada are committed using:
A. handguns.
B. knives.
C. fists and feet.
D. blunt objects.
E. impromptu weapons.

11. Crimes committed against a person solely on the basis of the individual's actual or perceived race, colour, national origin, ethnicity, gender, disability, or sexual orientation are know as:
A. bias crimes.   **D.** selective crimes.
B. hate crimes.   **E.** none of the above
C. non-discriminatory crimes.

12. When responding to the scene of any violent crime, you should remember that:
A. dangerous weapons may have been used in the crime.
B. perpetrators may still be on-scene.
C. patients may sometimes exhibit violence toward EMS personnel.
D. perpetrators may return to the scene.
E. all of the above

13. Warning signs of impending danger from a crowd include all of the following EXCEPT:
A. a rapid increase in the crowd size.
B. hostility toward anyone on the scene.
C. pushing or shoving.
D. inability of police to control bystanders.
E. a decreasing level of noise.

14. A gang's "colours" refers to their:
A. clothing.   **D.** graffiti.
B. flag.   **E.** logo.
C. language.

15. Which of the following are used by gang members to identify themselves.
A. appearance, including clothing
B. tattoos
C. hand signals
D. special language or phrases
E. all of the above

16. One of the most common substances manufactured in clandestine drug labs is:
A. cocaine.   **D.** methadone.
B. methamphetamine   .   **E.** morphine.
C. heroin.

17. If you ever come upon a clan lab, all of the following are appropriate actions EXCEPT to:
A. leave the area immediately.
B. stop any chemical reactions in progress.

C.   notify the police.
D.   initiate ICS and hazmat procedures.
E.   evacuate the area.

18. Clandestine labs generally have the following requirements:

A.   privacy.   **D.**   heating mantles or burners.
B.   utilities.   **E.**   all of the above
C.   glassware.

19. All of the following strategies can be employed as safety tactics in a potentially violent situation EXCEPT:

A.   retreat.   **D.**   distraction and evasion.
B.   cover and concealment.   **E.**   contact and cover.
C.   confrontation and interrogation.

20. Hiding your body behind solid and impenetrable objects such as brick walls is known as:

A.   cover..
B.   concealment.
C.   contact and cover.
D.   distraction.
E.   evasion.

True/False

21. The EMS unit should follow the police units to the scene.

A.   True
B.   False

22. Even if a scene has been declared secure by the police, violence may still occur.

A.   True
B.   False

23. If you must defend yourself, use the maximum amount of force possible.

A.   True
B.   False

24. The most common violent crimes are aggravated assaults.

A.   True
B.   False

25. Gang activities are confined to urban areas and are of minimal concern to EMS units outside cities.

A.   True
B.   False

26. Concealment is hiding your body behind solid and impenetrable objects such as brick walls.

A.   True
B.   False

27. When using a cover and contact strategy, the contact provider is responsible for observing for danger and maintaining radio contact with dispatch..

A.   True
B.   False

28. Medical personnel assigned to a tactical emergency medical service may be expected to extricate patients from the hot zone.

A.   True
B.   False

29. The goal of EMS at a crime scene is to provide high-quality patient care while preserving evidence.
    A.   True
    B.   False

30. When documenting a call involving violence, you should describe the shape and anatomical location of a laceration rather than characterizing it as a knife wound.
    A.   True
    B.   False

Matching

Write the letter of the term in the space provided next to the appropriate description.

A.	TEMS	F.	EMT-Ts
B.	particulate evidence	G.	blood splatter evidence
C.	concealment	H.	cover
D.	SWAT	I.	CONTOMS
E.	body armor	J.	graffiti

_____ 31. painting on walls to mark a gang's territory, membership, or threats

_____ 32. trained police unit equipped to handle hostage takers and other difficult law enforcement situations

_____ 33. hiding the body behind objects that shield a person from view but offer little or no protection against bullets or other ballistics

_____ 34. vest made of tightly woven, strong fibers that offers protection against handgun bullets, most knives, and blunt trauma

_____ 35. counter-narcotics tactical operations program that manages training and certification of EMT-Ts and SWAT-medics

_____ 36. hairs or fibers that cannot be readily seen with the human eye

_____ 37. a specially trained unit that provides on-site medical support to law enforcement

_____ 38. hiding the body behind solid and impenetrable objects that protect a person from bullets

_____ 39. pattern that blood forms when it is dropped at the scene of a crime

_____ 40. EMS personnel trained to serve with a law enforcement agency

Essentials of Paramedic Care

Division 2

Patient Assessment

Chapter 4

Therapeutic Communications

Review of Chapter Objectives

With each chapter of the Workbook, we identify the objectives and the important elements of the text content. You should review these items and refer to the pages listed if any points are not clear.

After reading this chapter, you should be able to:

1. Define communication.   p. 219

Communication is the exchange of information through the use of common symbols—written, spoken, or of other kinds. The basic elements of communication include a sender, an encoded message, a receiver, and feedback. The sender encodes a written, spoken, signed, or other message to the receiver. The receiver decodes the message to derive his interpretation of the content. He then provides feedback to the sender. If, because of the feedback, the sender believes the communication was accurately received, the communication was successful.

2. Identify internal and external factors that affect a patient/bystander interview.   pp. 219-221, 226-227

There are several reasons why communications can be ineffective or fail. They include prejudice, lack of empathy or understanding, lack of (or a perceived invasion of) privacy, or internal or external distractions. If the sender, receiver, or both are subject to these influences, the communication is likely to be ineffective. On the other hand, trust and rapport between sender and receiver can facilitate communication. Common errors in interviewing include providing false assurances, giving advice, going on a "power trip," using avoidance language, standing too close or too far from patients, using professional jargon, talking too much, interrupting the patient, and using too many "why" questions.

3. Identify the strategies for developing rapport with the patient.   pp. 219-220, 226

Developing rapport with a patient is dependent upon truly feeling empathy for the patient and observing several principles of good interpersonal communication. Use your patient's name frequently with the proper form of address (Mr., Ms., or Mrs.). Use a professional but compassionate tone of voice and explain what you are doing and why, and be honest about what is happening. Keep a kind, calming, and caring facial expression, use the appropriate style of communication, and listen carefully to what your patient says.

Using the following techniques can provide feedback to your interviewee and thus help develop rapport:
- **Silence** gives your patient time to gather his thoughts and complete his answer.
- **Reflection,** your echoing of the patient's response, assures you understand the interviewee's answer.
- **Facilitation** encourages the patient to make further responses.
- **Empathy** is using your body language and your speech to assure the patient you are interested and

concerned.
• **Clarification** involves asking the interviewee to explain answers you don't understand.
• **Confrontation** is a technique in which you ask direct questions about confusing or contradictory statements by the patient.
• **Interpretation** is a statement of your understanding of the events and circumstances of which the interviewee has offered an explanation.
• **Explanation** is a technique in which you share objective information you gather with the interviewee.
• **Summarization** is your brief review of all the pertinent information you have gathered from the interviewee.

4. Discuss open-ended and closed-ended questions.   pp. 224-225

Open-ended questions provide the patient with the opportunity to respond to your question with an unguided, spontaneous answer. An example is "What happened to cause you to call for an ambulance?" or "Describe what you had for lunch." Closed, or direct, questions guide the patient to an answer of yes or no or some other short response. The question does not allow for an explanation of the circumstance. Examples of closed or direct questions are "Do you have any chest pain?" and "Does it hurt to breathe?" Use open-ended questions when possible. Use closed-ended questions when necessary to obtain specific information.

5. Discuss common errors made when interviewing patients. p. 226-227

Common errors associated with interviewing include providing false assurance, giving inappropriate advice, using authority inappropriately, using avoidance language, improperly distancing yourself from the interviewee, using professional jargon, talking instead of listening, interrupting the interviewee, and using questioning language that implies guilt (using "why" questions).

6. Identify the nonverbal skills used in patient interviewing.   pp. 222-223

Distance. The distance at which you place yourself from the patient during the interview process is an important tool in making the patient comfortable and in defining your role as a caregiver. The closer you come to the patient, the more personal and intimate your conversation. However, unwanted entry into someone's personal space can be perceived as threatening.
Relative level. The relative difference between a caregiver's eye level and the patient's is important. When the care giver's eye level is above the patient's, it reflects a state of authority; an eye level equal with the patient's indicates equality; while an eye level below the patient's indicates a willingness to let the patient have some control over the interview. Each position has advantages and disadvantages when interviewing the emergency patient.
Stance. A closed stance (arms crossed, fists clenched, and the body square to the patient) suggests disinterest, discomfort, fear, or anger. An open stance (open hands, relaxed muscles, and a nodding head) suggests comfort, interest, and confidence.
Eye contact. Eye contact with a patient suggests interest and an entry into the patient's personal space. It is a powerful communication tool and a way to convey the caregiver's empathy with the patient.
Touching. Touching is also a way to communicate empathy and concern. Like eye contact, however, it can be threatening when not used in the right circumstances.

7. Identify interview methods used to assess mental status.   pp. 224-225

By carefully watching the patient's body language and attending to his verbal and nonverbal responses to questioning, you can assess his level of responsiveness and his ability to concentrate. Be especially watchful of speech and how the patient phrases sentences and articulates. Also note how well he answers questions and the appropriateness of questions he asks.

8. Discuss strategies for interviewing a patient who is not motivated to talk.   pp. 225, 227-228

Be sure the patient understands your questions and why you are asking them. If the patient is acting out and hostile, point out their behaviour in a professional manner. Use the feedback techniques explained in objective 3. Take the time to develop rapport and trust with the patient and to communicate your empathy toward his situation. Assure there is no language barrier and that you and the patient are isolated so that information given is confidential. Provide supportive feedback to encourage freer communication. If information is unavailable from the patient, ask family or bystanders to help provide it.

9. Describe the use of, and differentiate between facilitation, reflection, clarification, empathetic responses, confrontation, and interpretation. p. 226

There are several feedback techniques to use during an interview, including:

Facilitation—encouraging the speaker to provide more information
Clarification—asking the speaker to help you understand confusing parts of his or her response
Empathetic responses—showing you understand the patient
Confrontation—focusing the speaker on a particular part of his or her response
Interpretation—relating your interpretation of the speaker's information

10. Differentiate strategies used for interviewing hostile and cooperative patients. pp. 225, 231

The uncooperative patient is one who simply does not want to help with, participate in, or permit your assessment or care for him. A hostile patient displays anger and may be a risk to you. Work carefully to establish rapport with each type, but recognize that the hostile patient may endanger you and your crew. Always maintain distance from the hostile patient and have an escape route ready should a threat of violence become an attempt.

11. Summarize developmental considerations that influence patient interviewing. pp. 222, 225, 228-229

Your interviewing techniques must be flexible to accommodate the developmental considerations that influence patient assessment and care. Be patient, understanding, and empathetic and listen carefully to what the patient says. Adjust your interviewing technique, intensity, eye contact, eye level, touch, and stance to meet the needs of your patient. Be simple and straightforward with young children, and build a good rapport with their caregivers, as they are the ones the children look to for guidance. With age, children become more objective, realistic, trusting, and cooperative. With the elderly, show respect and appreciate the difficulties pre-existing diseases and reduced hearing and eyesight can have on their ability to understand what is happening to them.

12. Define the unique interviewing techniques for patients with special needs. pp. 227-233

Patients with special needs include children, the elderly, patients with sensory impairments, and those with language or cultural considerations. Generally an empathetic and calm approach to any of these patients will be helpful, combined with special strategies for each group.
Children Effective interviewing techniques depend on a child's age, as they grow quickly from infancy to childhood, to adolescence, and to adulthood. Begin by talking with and establishing a rapport with the child's care givers (parents and family) and gradually approach the patient. Keep your eye level close to the child's and speak choosing your words carefully so the patient can understand and is not threatened. Explain what you are doing and why, being honest and truthful. Build trust and use a toy to distract younger children from their symptoms and your intrusion into their personal space.
Elderly patients require respect, the proper form of address, slower explanations, and patience. Take along their living assists—eyeglasses, hearing aids, etc.—if you must transport them, and always respect their dignity.
Sensory impairment can make communication more difficult and requires careful explanations of what is going to happen to the patient and why. Guide the sightless patient with an arm and provide written or signed communication for the hearing impaired. If the patient can lip read, assure your face

is illuminated and facing directly toward him when you speak.

Language and cultural barriers are obstacles to effective communication that can only be overcome with patience and compassion. Do not judge a patient's values or try to impose yours on him. Use an interpreter (family member or sibling) and phrase questions and statements carefully, addressing both the patient and interpreter. Recognize that eye contact and personal distances may mean different things in different cultures. Respect cultural folk medicines and beliefs.

13. Discuss cross-cultural interviewing considerations. pp. 230-231

When interviewing across cultures, be patient, understanding, and empathetic. Understand the differences in how the culture perceives eye contact and personal distances and resist making judgments due to stereotyping. Respect folk medicine practices and beliefs.

14. Describe the basic principles of conflict resolution. pp. 231 –233

Conflict is the stress, tension, or negative feelings that occur when people perceive opposition between their needs, values, or interests. You may encounter conflict in your relationships with partners, other rescuers, other health care providers, patients, and bystanders. There are five basic styles of approaching conflict. These approaches can be employed in cooperative or adversarial manners.

Competing/controlling: characterized by a focus on your own interests
Avoiding: characterized by a focus away from conflict
Accommodating: focus is more on the other person and less on yourself
Compromising: focuses on satisfying both parties, but with a preference towards yourself
Collaborating: focuses on satisfying both parties to the greatest degree possible.

When dealing with conflict, avoid focusing on positions, as this frames the discussion in terms of "right" and "wrong." Rather, explore the interest, or underlying reasons and rationale that support each party's position. In general, collaborative approaches are best for meeting the needs of all parties. However, in many EMS situations this is not desirable or even possible.

15. Given several preprogrammed simulated patients, provide a patient interview using therapeutic communications. pp. 219 - 233

During every day of your career as a paramedic, you will attend patients and their families to determine what is wrong with the patient and then to provide care. These encounters will, from time to time, be with patients who do not trust you, do not understand you, are threatened by you, are frightened by you, or do not understand what is happening to them. They present a challenge to good communication that you must overcome to extract information from them and begin your care. The impression you leave with these patients is the impression they will carry of the emergency medical service system until they again call on the system for assistance. During your classroom, practical, and clinical experience, work to develop your interviewing skills, especially with troublesome patients, so you present a good image to the people who use our services.

CONTENT SELF-EVALUATION

Multiple Choice

_____ 1. In communication theory, creating a message is also known as:
A.	alliterating.	D.	feedback.
B.	encoding.	E.	drafting.
C.	receiving.		

_____ 2. In communication theory, responding to a received message is also known as:

	A.	alliterating.	D.	feedback.
	B.	encoding.	E.	drafting.
	C.	receiving.		

_____ 3. Which of the following represents an example of an external distraction to communication?

A.	lack of empathy	D.	thinking about family or the job
B.	prejudice	E.	all of the above
C.	loud music		

_____ 4. Which of the following is NOT one of the elements necessary for a paramedic to make a good first impression?

A.	clean, neat uniform	D.	consideration for the patient
B.	arrogant demeanor	E.	good personal hygiene
C.	interested and caring facial expression		

_____ 5. Which of the following techniques is NOT considered to be a way to build patient trust and rapport?

- A. using your patient's name
- B. explaining what you are doing and why
- C. addressing your patient as "honey" or "sweetie"
- D. modulating your voice
- E. using an appropriate style of communication

_____ 6. Which of the following techniques is a preferred method for building patient trust and rapport on approach to the patient?

- A. introduce yourself, your partner, and other rescuers
- B. standing above the patient's level to establish a zone of control
- C. kneeling beside the person but remaining at least 3 meters away
- D. speaking slowly, loudly, and avoiding modulations in your voice
- E. addressing elderly patients by their first names

_____ 7. The gestures, mannerisms, and postures by which a paramedic communicates with others is known as:

A.	demeanor.	D.	social interaction.
B.	stance.	E.	communication style.
C.	nonverbal communication.		

_____ 8. The interpersonal zone that extends 1.2 to 3.5 m from the patient is:

A.	the intimate zone.	D.	public distance.
B.	personal distance.	E.	none of the above
C.	social distance.		

_____ 9. The interpersonal zone that is best for assessing breath and body odours is known as:

A.	the intimate zone.	D.	public distance.
B.	personal distance.	E.	none of the above
C.	social distance.		

_____ 10. The interpersonal zone that is normally used for conducting a patient interview is known as:

A.	the intimate zone.	D.	public distance.
B.	personal distance.	E.	none of the above
C.	social distance.		

_____ 11. The interpersonal zone that is normally used for conducting most patient assessment is known as:

A.	the intimate zone.	D.	public distance.
B.	personal distance.	E.	none of the above
C.	social distance.		

12. The interpersonal zone that is normally used for interacting with impersonal interactions with others is known as:

A.   the intimate zone.
B.   personal distance.
C.   social distance.
D.   public distance.
E.   none of the above

13. Which of a caregiver's eye levels imparts authority and may intimidate the patient?

A.   one higher than the patient's eye level
B.   one lower than the patient's eye level
C.   one on the same level with the patient's
D.   both A and B
E.   Both B and C

14. A body position or posture that is relaxed and suggests confidence, ease, warmth and attentiveness is called a/an:

A.   reflective stance.
B.   empathic stance.
C.   personal stance.
D.   closed stance.
E.   open stance.

15. Which of the following statements about eye contact is correct?

A.   you must always maintain eye contact while interviewing your patient
B.   eye contact is a power communication tool and should be used as much as possible
C.   many European cultures find eye contact discomforting
D.   direct eye contact is intimidating and should be avoided as much as possible
E.   eye contact builds trust, but does not generally convey impressions or meaning

16. Questions that are framed to guide the direction of a patient's answer are known as:

A.   open-ended.
B.   closed.
C.   reflective.
D.   facilitating.
E.   leading.

17. Questions that ask for specific information and require only very short or yes/no answers are known as:

A.   open-ended.
B.   closed.
C.   reflective.
D.   facilitating.
E.   leading.

18. Questions that permit unguided, spontaneous answers are known as:

A.   open-ended.
B.   closed.
C.   reflective.
D.   facilitating.
E.   leading.

19. If your patient is uncomfortable being the centre of attention, and constantly shifts focus away from your questions, you should:

A.   back off a bit, reassure the patient, then return to the topic from a different angle
B.   be firm and let the patient know that their behaviour is defeating the purpose of the call for help
C.   provide additional reassurance and leave that line of questioning out of your interview
D.   move back from the patient, but persist with your line of questioning until you obtain the answers you need
E.   continue with your physical assessment and return to the patient interview later in the call

20. The listening and feedback technique in which the interviewer encourages the speaker to provide more information is:

A. summarization. **D.** clarification.
B. explanation. **E.** facilitation.
C. reflection.

21. Common errors made when interviewing patients include all of the following EXCEPT:
    A. using professional jargon.
    B. echoing back the patient's statements as part of the reflection technique.
    C. inappropriate distancing.
    D. inappropriate advice.
    E. providing false assurances.

22. A difficult patient interview may stem from which of the following?
    A. a disease process   D. cultural differences
    B. fear   E. all of the above
    C. language differences

23. When interviewing young children, you should:
    A. start by talking to the caregiver, then gradually approach the child.
    B. confine your interview to the caregiver unless the child offers to answer.
    C. avoid explanations or descriptions of your actions as these may frighten the child.
    D. complete all physical assessment before trying to question the child.
    E. explain your needs to the caregiver and let him/her ask the child the questions.

24. The viewing of one's own life as more desirable or acceptable or best is:
    A. ethnicity.   **D.** cultural imposition.
    B. cultural diversity.   **E.** cultural arrogance.
    C. ethnocentrism.

25. The approach to conflict that is most focused on the other person and least on the self is:
    A. cooperative.   **D.** accommodating.
    B. compromising.   **E.** collaborating.
    C. avoiding.

True/False

26. Empathy is the identification with and understanding of another's situation, feelings, and motives.
    A. True
    B. False

27. Sunglasses often help reduce the intimidation of eye contact and should be kept on when possible.
    A. True
    B. False

28. Nothing builds trust and rapport, of calms patients, faster than the power of compassionate touch.
    A. True
    B. False

29. Closed questions direct the patient and elicit very specific responses; since this is not desired during an interview, these questions should be avoided at all costs.
    A. True
    B. False

30. Interrupting a patient to guide him to the information you need is both a useful tool in the interview process and a good listening skill.

    A. True
    B. False

_____ **31.** When interviewing a patient who is acting out and hostile, you should leave the scene immediately and call for further assistance.
    A. True
    B. False

_____ **32.** When interviewing a patient who is not responding to your questions, you should first consider and rule out language barriers and hearing impairments.
    A. True
    B. False

_____ **33.** When treating a child you must also consider treating the caregivers since they may be upset and concerned.
    A. True
    B. False

_____ **34.** Asian, Aboriginal, Indochinese, and Arab people may find direct eye contact impolite or aggressive.
    A. True
    B. False

_____ **35.** Framing discussion in terms of what is "right" and "wrong" allows you to get at the root issues of a conflict.
    A. True
    B. False

Matching

Write the letter of the question type in the space provided next to the question to which it applies.

Role

    A. Open-ended
    B. Closed
    C. Leading

Function

_____ **36.** Can you tell my why you called for the ambulance today?

_____ **37.** Where does it hurt the most?

_____ **38.** Is the pain steady, or does it come and go?

_____ **39.** Has this ever happened to you before?

_____ **40.** How would you describe the pain?

Write the letter of the appropriate term in the space provided next to the definition to which it applies.

Term

    A. Competing
    B. Avoiding
    C. Accommodating
    D. Compromising
    E. Collaborating

Definition

_____ **41.** most cooperative style, focused on satisfying both parties to the greatest degree possible.

_____ **42.** can be either cooperative or adversarial and is characterized by a focus away from the conflict.

_____ **43.** most adversarial approach, characterized by a focus on your own interests.

_____ **44.** can be either cooperative or adversarial and is most focused on the other person and least on the self.

_____ **45.** can be cooperative or adversarial, and focuses on satisfying both parties, with a preference toward the self.

Chapter 5

History Taking

Review of Chapter Objectives

With each chapter of the Workbook, we identify the objectives and the important elements of the text content. You should review these items and refer to the pages listed if any points are not clear.

After reading this chapter, you should be able to:

1. **Describe the techniques of history taking.**   **pp. 235 - 238**

   For successful history taking, establish a rapport with the patient to gain his confidence and to set the stage for investigation of the chief complaint and medical history. Factors that will help in establishing rapport include:
   • Well-groomed initial appearance
   • Positive body language
   • Good eye contact with the patient
   • Professional demeanor
   • Demonstration of interest in the patient
        Your introduction should convey your interest in helping the patient and begin the two-way communication. It should convey your care and compassion for the patient and begin to build his trust in you. Once you have introduced yourself and established your intent to help the patient, begin your questioning. Determine the formal chief complaint and investigate the current and past medical history. Pose questions in a way the patient understands, using terminology and the English language at the patient's level of comprehension.
   Questioning frequently involves asking the patient personal, and possibly embarrassing, questions. At such times, ask these questions in a sensitive, nonthreatening way. "Ease into" the discussion of sensitive topics and use questions that are nonjudgmental. You may suggest to the patient that the issue of concern to him is common to many people in our society. Practice in questioning will help you develop the most effective approach. Be prepared to explain that the answers to questions are used for the patient's care and are not communicated beyond the necessary care providers.

2. **Describe the structure, purpose, and how to obtain a comprehensive patient history.**
   pp. 235 - 251

   The comprehensive health history establishes a relationship between you and the patient and draws out pertinent information about the patient's medical history. This information may explain the current problem or guide further care in either the prehospital or in-hospital settings. The comprehensive patient history is gained by investigative questioning of the patient about past and current medical problems, including the chief complaint, the present illness (OPQRST-ASPN), the past medical history, current health status, and a review of systems.

3. **List the components of a comprehensive history of an adult patient.**   **pp. 238 - 246**

   The comprehensive patient history includes the following:
   • Preliminary data (age, race, sex, etc.)

• The chief complaint
• The present illness or problem (including investigation of onset, provocation, quality, region/radiation, severity, time, as well as associated symptoms and pertinent negatives—OPQRST-ASPN)
• Past medical history (including the patient's general health, childhood and adult illnesses, psychiatric illness, serious accidents or injuries, and surgeries and hospitalizations)
• Current health status (including patient medications, allergies, use of tobacco, alcohol, and drugs, diet, recent screening tests and immunizations, exercise, leisure and sleep patterns, and environmental hazard/safety measures, family history, and psychosocial history)
• A review of systems (including, as appropriate, general physical information; skin; head, eyes, ears, nose, throat (HEENT); respiratory, cardiac; gastrointestinal; urinary; genital; peripheral vascular; musculoskeletal; neurologic; hematologic; endocrine; psychiatric)

The following objectives, while not listed in the chapter, will help in your understanding of the chapter content.

*   Describe the review of systems and explain how it assists in identifying the patient's primary medical problem.   pp. 244-246

The review of systems is an examination of each body system during the patient history. It is performed to rule out or further investigate medical problems and to assure that pertinent information is not overlooked during the assessment. Systems examined include:
• Skin
• Head, eyes, ears, nose, throat (HEENT)
• Respiratory
• Cardiac
• Gastrointestinal
• Urinary
• Genital
• Peripheral vascular
• Musculoskeletal
• Neurologic
• Hematologic
• Endocrine
• Psychiatric

*   Identify techniques for working with patients with special challenges.   pp. 246-250

Silent patient. Be patient yourself. Speak reassuringly. Gently shake the patient. Consider a neurologic problem.
Overly talkative patient. Focus the patient on the important areas. Summarize what he or she says. Be patient.
Numerous symptoms. Be more clear in questioning; suspect an emotional problem.
Anxious patient. Encourage free conversation and reassure the patient.
Patient needing reassurance. Ask about his anxieties. Offer emotional support.
Anger and hostility. Accept the patient's responses without becoming defensive or angry.
Intoxicated patient. Be friendly and nonjudgmental. Listen to what the patient says, not how he says it. Make your safety and scene safety priorities.
Crying patient. Be patient. Accept the crying as a natural venting of emotions and be supportive.
Depression. Recognize the condition as a serious medical problem. Ask the patient whether he has had suicidal thoughts.
Sexually attractive or seductive patient. Maintain a professional relationship. Try to have a partner present.

Confusing behaviors or histories. Suspect mental illness, dementia, or delirium. Pay careful attention to the patient's mental status. Be reassuring.

Patient of limited intelligence. Try to evaluate the patient's mental abilities. Show genuine interest and establish a positive relationship. Elicit what information you can.

Language barriers. Seek out an interpreter. Be aware that important information is likely to be lost in translation.

Patient with hearing problems. Speak to the patient's best ear. If he reads lips, position yourself directly in front of him in good lighting, and speak slowly in a low-pitched voice. Consider writing your questions.

Patient who is blind or has limited vision. Identify yourself immediately and explain why you are there. Explain what you are doing before you do it.

Family and friends. If gaining pertinent information directly from the patient is difficult, talk to family members or friends on the scene.

CONTENT SELF-EVALUATION

Each of the chapters in this Workbook includes a short content review. The questions are designed to test your ability to remember what you read. At the end of this Workbook, you can find the answers to the questions as well as the pages where the topic of the question was discussed in the text. If you answer the question incorrectly or are unsure of the answer, review the pages listed.

_____ 1. In the majority of medical cases, the basis of the paramedic's field diagnosis is the:
A.   chief complaint.   D.   patient history.
B.   index of suspicion.   E.   vital signs.
C.   mechanism of injury.

_____ 2. Which of the following factors should influence the sequence and selection of questions in your history-taking?
A.   age of the patient   D.   you should not alter the sequence
B.   patient's cultural background   E.   all of the above
C.   your patient's answers to previous questions

_____ 3. The term differential field diagnosis refers to the:
A.   underlying cause of the patient's presenting complaint.
B.   list of possible causes for your patient's symptoms.
C.   reason that the patient called EMS today.
D.   patient's primary problem.
E.   patient's presenting complaint.

_____ 4. If an emergency medical responder gives you a report with the patient's chief complaint and medical history, you should:
A.   accept the information and proceed with your secondary assessment.
B.   perform your own patient interview before considering the information in their report.
C.   disregard the information and perform your own patient interview.
D.   accept the report, and briefly reconfirm the key points with the patient.
E.   accept the report, but reconfirm all information during your patient interview.

_____ 5. Which of the following is NOT an active listening skill:
A.   recitation.   D.   reflection.
B.   facilitation.   E.   all of the above are active listening skills
C.   clarification.

_____ 6. If you feel uneasy following a line of questioning on a sensitive topic such as sexual activities, bodily functions, or family violence, you should:

A.	complete the other components of the history and return to these topics last.
B.	explore the sensitive areas first, then complete the other components of your history.
C.	complete your history-taking without exploring these topics.
D.	leave that line of questioning for the medical staff.
E.	remain calm, objective, and non-judgmental, but continue asking the questions.

7.	Determining your patient's age, sex, race, birthplace, and occupation are part of the:
A.	primary problem.	D.	mechanism of injury.
B.	chief complaint.	E.	preliminary data.
C.	nature of the illness.

8.	The reason (pain, discomfort, or dysfunction) that the patient or other person summons emergency medical services is termed the:
A.	primary problem.	D.	mechanism of injury.
B.	chief complaint.	E.	none of the above
C.	nature of the illness.

9.	The underlying cause of the patient's pain, discomfort, or dysfunction is called the:
A.	primary problem.	D.	mechanism of injury.
B.	chief complaint.	E.	none of the above
C.	nature of the illness.

10.	The OPQRST–ASPN mnemonic is used to explore which element of the patient's history?
A.	chief complaint	D.	current health status
B.	present illness	E.	systems inquiry
C.	past history

11.	Which of the following is an important part of the past medical history?
A.	radiation of the pain	D.	quality of the pain
B.	last oral intake	E.	all of the above
C.	surgeries or hospitalizations

12.	A prescribed medication may account for medical problems due to which of the following?
A.	over-medication	D.	untoward reaction
B.	under-medication	E.	all of the above
C.	allergic reaction

13.	Drug allergies that may affect emergency care include all of the following EXCEPT:
A.	the "caine" family.	D.	narcotics.
B.	tetanus toxoid.	E.	antibiotics such as penicillin.
C.	glucose.

14.	A patient who has smoked 21 packs of cigarettes a week for 10 years has a pack history of:
A.	7 pack/years.	D.	30 pack/years.
B.	10 pack/years.	E.	210 pack/years.
C.	21 pack/years.

15.	Administer the CAGE questionnaire to screen for:
A.	adult onset diabetes.	D.	depression.
B.	alcoholism.	E.	substance abuse.
C.	asthma or immune system conditions.

16.	In which of the following situations should you explore the medical history of your patient's immediate family?
A.	45 year-old patient with chest pain
B.	65 year-old patient with emphysema
C.	patient with suspected acute alcohol intoxication

D. 40 year old woman with an upper GI bleed
E. all of the above patients

17. The purpose of the review of systems is to:
    A. explore the body system(s) associated with the patient's chief complaint.
    B. ensure that all associated symptoms are found.
    C. generate a list of differential diagnoses.
    D. identify problems your patient has not already mentioned.
    E. determine the patient's past medical history.

18. Which of the following is NOT a system examined during the review of systems?
    A. skin   **D.** hematologic system
    B. lymphatic system   **E.** endocrine system
    C. musculoskeletal system

19. Which step below would you attempt with the patient who suddenly goes silent?
    A. Stay calm and observe for nonverbal clues.
    B. Arrange for air medical transport.
    C. Terminate the interview immediately.
    D. Attempt to walk the patient back and forth a few times.
    E. Rapidly provide oral glucose.

20. Which of the following strategies is suggested for the patient who is overly talkative?
    A. Document the patient's answers and lack of cooperation.
    B. Focus on vital signs and physical assessment clues rather than the history.
    C. Focus on important history topics and ask closed-ended questions.
    D. Allow the patient to tell his or her story in their own way.
    E. Cut the patient short whenever the answer strays off topic.

True/False

21. Always accept information from previous caregivers gratefully, but briefly reconfirm it with the patient.
    A. True
    B. False

22. Always use appropriate language during the interview to establish a closer, more trusting relationship.
    A. True
    B. False

23. It is best to form a prearranged list of specific questions to assure you cover all bases while interviewing your patient.
    A. True
    B. False

24. One way of dealing with taking a history on sensitive topics is to develop and practice using some opening questions that will put your patient at ease and encourage him or her to talk.
    A. True
    B. False

25. Common sense and clinical experience will help determine how much of the history to take on every call.
    A. True
    B. False

26. Referred pain is pain that is elicited through deep palpation.
    A. True
    B. False

27. Pertinent negatives are symptoms that are not associated with the chief complaint but may indicate the presence of other conditions.
- **A.** True
- **B.** False

28. Untoward reactions or anaphylaxis due to penicillin, the "caine" family (local anesthetics) tetanus toxoid, or narcotics are known as environmental allergies.
- **A.** True
- **B.** False

29. The system-by-system questions asked in the systems review are more specific than those asked in the basic history.
- **A.** True
- **B.** False

30. Crying is a form of venting emotional stress; be patient and provide a patient who is crying with supportive remarks.
- **A.** True
- **B.** False

Matching

Classify each question or statement under the OPQRST category that best applies by writing the letter of the category in the space provided.

- **O.** Onset
- **P.** Provocation/palliation
- **Q.** Quality
- **R.** Region/radiation
- **S.** Severity
- **T.** Time

31. How does this compare to the worst pain you have ever felt?

32. Does rest lessen your pain?

33. Point to where you feel pain.

34. Does this pain feel crushing in nature?

35. Does deep breathing increase the pain?

36. Did this pain begin suddenly or gradually?

37. Where does this pain travel to?

38. When did the first symptoms begin?

39. Describe how the pain feels.

40. Were you walking or running when this pain first began?

Write the letter of the appropriate term in the space provided next to the definition to which it applies.

Term

- **A.** para
- **B.** gravida

C. hymoptysis
D. hematemesis
E. dyspnea
F. orthopnea
G. polyuria
H. nocturia
I. dysmenorrhea

Definition

_____   **41.** excessive urination

_____   **42.** menstrual difficulties

_____   **43.** difficulty in breathing while lying supine

_____   **44.** coughing up blood

_____   **45.** how many times a woman has been pregnant

Chapter 6

Physical Assessment Techniques

Review of Chapter Objectives

With each chapter of the Workbook, we identify the objectives and the important elements of the text content. You should review these items and refer to the pages listed if any points are not clear.

After reading this section of the chapter, you should be able to:

1. **Define and describe the techniques of inspection, palpation, percussion, and auscultation. pp. 254-258**

   Inspection is the process of informed observation, viewing the patient for anatomical shape, colouration, and movement. It is the least invasive examination tool, yet may provide the most patient information.

   Palpation is the use of touch to gather information regarding size, shape, position, temperature, moisture, texture, movement, and response to pressure. The fingertips are most sensitive, while the palm best evaluates vibration and the back of the hand, temperature.

   Percussion is the production of a vibration in tissue to elicit sounds. These sounds—dull, resonant, hyperresonant, tympanic, and flat—identify the nature of the tissue underneath. The vibration is generated by striking the first knuckle of a finger placed against the area to be percussed with the fingertip of the other hand.

   Auscultation is listening for sounds within the body, most frequently with a stethoscope. The intensity, pitch, duration, quality, and timing of sounds in the patient's lungs, heart, blood vessels, and intestines are compared against normal sounds.

2. **Describe the evaluation of mental status. pp. 319-321**

   The evaluation of the mental status begins with your interview. The evaluation permits you to determine your patient's level of responsiveness, general appearance, behavior, and speech. You specifically look at his appearance and behavior, speech and language skills, mood, thought and perception, insight and judgment, and memory and attention.

3. **Evaluate the importance of a general survey. pp. 266-273**

   The general survey is the first part of the comprehensive exam. It is made up of your evaluation of the patient's appearance—including level of consciousness, expression, state of health, general characteristics (weight, height, etc.), posturing, dress, grooming, etc.—the vital signs, and additional assessments such as pulse oximetry, cardiac monitoring, and blood glucose determination. The survey helps you form a general impression of your patient's health.

4. **Describe the examination of the following body regions, differentiate between normal and abnormal findings, and define the significance of abnormal findings:**

Skin, hair, and nails   pp. 274-279

Observe the skin carefully for colour, especially in the nail beds, lips, conjunctiva, and mucous membranes of the mouth. Pink skin reflects good oxygenation, while pale skin reflects poor blood flow from hypovolemia, hypothermia, compensatory shock, or anemia. A bluish-coloured skin, cyanosis, suggests blood is low in oxygen. A yellow sclera or general discolouration, jaundice, is due to liver failure. Other skin observations may include petechiae, small round, flat purplish spots caused by capillary bleeding from a variety of etiologies, and ecchymosis, a larger, black-and-blue discolouration that is often the result of trauma or bleeding disorders. Moisture, temperature, texture, mobility, and turgor are also evaluated. Skin lesions are disruptions in normal tissue that may take on almost any shape, colour, or arrangement.

Inspect and palpate the hair to determine colour, quality, distribution, quantity, and texture and inspect and palpate the scalp for scaling, lesions, redness, lumps, or tenderness. Generalized hair loss may reflect chemotherapy; failure to develop normal hair patterns may be caused by a pituitary or hormonal problem; and unusual facial hair in women suggests a hormonal imbalance. Mild scalp flaking suggests dandruff; heavy scaling, psoriasis; and greasy scaling, seborrheic dermatitis. Lice eggs (nits) may be found firmly attached to the hair shafts. Normal hair texture is smooth and soft in Caucasians; in people of African descent, the texture is coarser. Dry, brittle, or fragile hair is abnormal.

Inspect the finger and toenails for colour. Note any discolourations, lesions, ridging, grooves, depressions, or pitting. Depressions suggest systemic disease. Compress the nail and bed to determine its adherence and look for nail hygiene. Any bogginess suggests cardiorespiratory disease.

Head, scalp, and skull   p. 280

Observe and palpate the skull and facial region for symmetry, smoothness, wounds, bleeding, size, and general contour. Examine the hair and scalp as described above. Check the eyes for bilateral periorbital and mastoid ecchymosis, "raccoon eyes" and "Battle's sign," respectively. They suggest basilar skull fracture and occur an hour or so after injury. Palpate the facial region for crepitation, false motion, or instability suggesting fracture. Evaluate the temporomandibular joint for pain, tenderness, swelling, and range of motion. Have the patient open and close his mouth and jut and retract his jaw. Any loss of normal function suggests injury.

Eyes, ears, nose, mouth, and pharynx   pp. 280-289

Examine for visual acuity as described below (objective 5), then evaluate for peripheral vision. While the patient faces you, have him look at your nose while you extend your arms, bend your elbows and wiggle the fingers. If he notices the fingers moving in all four directions (up, down, left, and right) for each eye, his peripheral vision is grossly normal. Inspect the eyes for symmetry, shape, inflammation, swelling, misalignment (disconjugate gaze), lesions, and contour. Examine the eyelids, open and closed, for swelling, discolouration, droop (ptosis), styes, and lash positioning. Observe the tearing or dryness of the eyes. Gently retract the lower eyelid while asking the patient to look through a range of motion. Examine the sclera for signs of irritation, cloudiness, yellow discolouration (jaundice), any nodules, swelling, discharge, or hemorrhage into the scleral tissue. With an oblique light source, inspect the cornea for opacities. Inspect the size, shape, symmetry, and reactivity of the pupils. Note the pupils' direct and consensual response to increased light intensity. A sluggish pupil suggests pressure on CN-III; bilateral sluggishness suggests global hypoxia or depressant drug action. Constricted pupils suggest opiate overdose, while dilated and fixed pupils reflect brain anoxia. Ask the patient to focus on your finger close at hand, then move the hand to his nose, then away. The eyes should converge, while the pupils should constrict slightly. Then have him follow your finger as you move it through an "H" pattern. The eyes should move smoothly together. Nystagmus is a jerky movement at the distal extremes of ocular movement. Gently touch the cornea with a strand of cotton. The patient should respond with a blink. Using an ophthalmoscope, look into the eye's anterior chamber for signs of blood (hyphema), cells, or pus (hypopyon), and check the cornea for lacerations, abrasions, cataracts, papilledema (from increased ICP), vascular occlusions, and retinal hemorrhage.

Examine the ears by looking for symmetry from in front of the patient, then examine each ear separately. Examine the external portion (auricle) for shape, size, landmarks, and position on the head. Examine the surrounding area for deformities, lesions, tenderness, and erythema. Pull the helix upward and outward, press on the tragus and on the mastoid process and note any discomfort or pain suggesting otitis or mastoiditis. Some pain may be associated with toothache, a cold, sore throat, or cervical spine injury. Inspect the ear canal for discharge (pus, mucus, blood, or cerebral spinal fluid [CSF]) and inflammation. Trauma can account for blood, mucus, and CSF in the ear canal. Check hearing acuity by covering one ear and whispering, then speaking into the other. Hearing loss may be accounted for by trauma, accumulation of debris (often cerumen), tympanic membrane rupture, drug use, and prolonged exposure to loud noise. Visualize the inner canal with the otoscope. With the largest speculum that will fit the canal, turn the patient's head away from you, pull the auricle slightly up and backward, and insert the otoscope. Inspect for wax (cerumen), discharge, redness, lesions, perforations, and foreign bodies. Then focus on the tympanic membrane. It should be a translucent pearly gray. Color changes suggest fluid behind the eardrum or infection. Also check for bulging, protractions, or perforations.

Visualize the patient's nose from the front and sides to determine any asymmetry, deviation, tenderness, flaring, or abnormal colour. Tilt your patient's head back slightly and examine the nostrils. Insert the otoscope and check for deviation of the septum and perforations. Examine the nasal mucosa for colour, and the colour, consistency, and quantity of drainage. Rhinitis (a runny nose) suggests seasonal allergies; a thick yellow discharge, infection; and blood, epistaxis from trauma or a septal defect. Test each side of the nose for patency by occluding the other side during a breath. There is normally some difference in patency between the sides. Palpate the frontal sinuses for swelling and tenderness.

Begin assessment of the mouth by observing the lips for colour and condition. They should be pink, smooth, symmetrical, and without lesions, swelling, lumps, cracks, or scaliness. Using a bright light and tongue blade, examine the oral mucosa for colour, lesions, white patches, or fissures. The mucosa should be pinkish-red, smooth, and moist. The gums should be pink with clearly defined margins around the teeth. The teeth should be well formed and straight. If the gums are swollen, bleed easily, and are separated from the teeth, suspect periodontal disease. Ask the patient to stick his tongue out and note its velvety surface. Hold the tongue with a 20 3 20 gauze pad and inspect all sides and the bottom. All surfaces should be pink and smooth. Then examine the pharynx and have the patient say "aaaahhh" while you hold the tongue down with a tongue blade. Watch the movement of the uvula and the colouration and condition of the palatine tonsils and posterior pharynx. Look for any pus, swelling, ulcers, or drainage. Also notice any odors including alcohol, feces (bowel obstruction), acetone (diabetic ketoacidosis), gastric contents, coffee-grounds-like material (gastric hemorrhage), pink-tinged sputum (pulmonary edema), or the smell of bitter almonds (cyanide poisoning).

Neck   pp. 289-291
Inspect your patient's neck for symmetry and visible masses. Note any deformity, deviations, tugging, scars, gland enlargement, or visible lymph nodes. Examine for any open wounds and cover them with an occlusive dressing. Examine the jugular veins for distention while the patient is seated upright and at a 45° incline. Palpate the trachea to assure it is inline. Palpate the thyroid while the patient swallows to assure it is small, smooth, and without nodules. Palpate each lymph node to determine size, shape, tenderness, consistency, and mobility. Tender, swollen, and mobile nodes suggest inflammation from infection, while hard and fixed ones suggest malignancy.

Thorax (anterior and posterior)   pp. 291-296
To assess the chest, you need a stethoscope with a bell and diaphragm. Expose the entire thorax with consideration for the patient's dignity and modesty, and inspect, palpate, percuss, and auscultate. Compare findings from one side of the chest to the other and from posterior to anterior. Look for general shape and symmetry as well as for the rate and pattern of breathing. Observe for retractions and the use of accessory muscles (suggestive of airway obstruction or restriction), and palpate for deformities, tenderness, crepitus (suggestive of rib fracture), and abnormal chest excursion (suggestive of flail chest or spinal injury). Feel for vibrations associated with air movement and speech. Percuss the chest for dullness (hemothorax, pleural effusion, or pneumonia), resonance, and hyperresonance (pneumothorax or tension pneumothorax). Finally, auscultate the lung lobes for normal breath sounds,

crackles (pulmonary edema), wheezes (asthma), rhonchi, stridor (airway obstruction), and pleural friction rubs.

Arterial pulse including rate, rhythm, and amplitude pp. 296-300
Locate a soft and pulsing carotid artery in the neck, just lateral to the cricoid cartilage to avoid pressure on the carotid sinus. Carefully press down until the pulse wave just lifts your finger off the artery. Determine the rate and carefully evaluate for regularity. Irregularity may be caused by dysrhythmia, while variation in strength may be due to such phenomena as pulsus paradoxus, increasing strength with exhalation and decreasing with inhalation. Also note any thrills (humming or vibration) and listen with the stethoscope for bruits (sounds of turbulent flow).

Jugular venous pressure and pulsations   pp. 296-300
Examine the anterior neck and locate the jugular veins. Position your patient with his head elevated 30° and turned away from you. Look for pulsation just above the suprasternal notch. Identify the highest point of pulsation and measure the distance from the sternal angle. The highest point of pulsation is usually between 1 and 2 cm from the sternal angle. (Distension when the patient is elevated at higher angles may reflect tension pneumothorax or pericardial tamponade, while flat veins at lower angles may suggest hypovolemia.)

Heart and blood vessels   pp. 296-300
The normal heart produces a "lub-dub" sound heard through the disk of the stethoscope with each cardiac contraction. The "lub" and "dub" may split when valves close out of sync, "la-lub-dub" reflects an S_1 split while "lub-da-dub" is an S_2 split. S_2 splitting is normal in children and young adults, though abnormal in older adults if expiratory or persistent splitting occurs. S_3 splitting produces a "lub-dub-dee" cadence like the word "Kentucky." It occurs commonly in children and young adults, but reflects blood filling a dilated ventricle and may suggest ventricular failure in the patient over 30. The S_4 heart sound is the "dee" sound of "dee-lub-dub" with a cadence similar to the word "Tennessee." It develops from vibrations as the atrium pushes blood into a ventricle that resists filling, suggestive of heart failure.

Abdomen   pp. 300-301
Question your patient regarding any pain, tenderness or unusual feeling, and recent bowel and bladder function. Carefully inspect the area for scars, dilated veins, stretch marks, rashes, lesions, and pigmentation changes. Discolouration around the umbilicus (Cullen's sign) or over the flanks (Grey-Turner's sign) suggest intra-abdominal hemorrhage. Assess the size and shape of the abdomen, determining whether it is scaphoid (concave), flat, round, or distended, and look for any bulges or hernias. Ascites result in bulges in the flanks and across the abdomen suggesting congestive heart or liver failure, while suprapubic bulges suggest a full bladder or pregnant uterus. Look also for any masses, palpations, or peristalsis. A slight vascular pulsing is normal, but excessive movement suggests an aneurysm. Auscultate and percuss as described earlier. Then depress each quadrant gently and release. Look for patient expression or muscle guarding suggestive of injury or peritonitis.

Male and female genitalia   pp. 301-303
Assure patient privacy, a warm environment, and patient modesty during the exam; also be sure the patient has emptied his or her bladder before beginning. Expose only those body areas that you must, and explain what you are going to do before you do it. Inspect the genitalia for development and maturity. Visually inspect the mons pubis, labia, and perineum of the female patient for swelling, lesions, or irritation suggestive of a sebaceous cyst or sexually transmitted disease. Check the hair bases for small red maculopapules suggestive of lice. Retract the labia and inspect the inner labia and urethral opening. Examine for a white curdy discharge (fungal infection) or yellow-green discharge (bacterial infection). For the male, inspect the penis and testicles, noting inflammation and lesions suggestive of sexually transmitted disease. Check for lice and examine the glans for degeneration, inflammation, or discharge. Yellow discharge is reflective of gonorrhea.

Anus and rectum   pp. 303-304
Position your patient on his or her left side with legs flexed and buttocks near the edge of the stretcher. Be sensitive to the patient's feelings and drape or cover any areas not being observed. With

a gloved hand, spread the buttocks apart and examine the area for lumps, ulcers, inflammations, rashes, or lesions. Palpate any areas carefully, noting inflammation or tenderness. If appropriate, obtain a fecal sample for testing.

Peripheral vascular system   pp. 314, 316-318, 301-305

Examine the upper, then the lower extremities and compare them, one to another, for the following: size, symmetry, swelling, venous congestion, skin and nail bed colour, temperature, skin texture, and turgor. Yellow brittle nails, swollen digit ends (clubbing), or poor nailbed colour suggest chronic arterial insufficiency. Assess the distal circulation, noting the strength, rate, and regularity of the pulse and comparing pulses bilaterally. If you have difficulty palpating a pulse or can't find one, palpate a more proximal site. Feel the spongy compliance of the vessels, note their colouration, and examine for inflammation along the vein, indicative of deep vein thrombosis. Gently feel for edema and pitting edema in each distal extremity.

Musculoskeletal system   pp. 304-305

Advancing age causes changes in the musculoskeletal system including shortening and increased curvature of the spine, a reduction in muscle mass and strength, and a reduction in the range of motion. Observe the patient's general posture, build, and muscular development as well as the movement of the extremities, gait, and position at rest. Then inspect all regions of the body for deformities, symmetry and symmetrical movement, joint structure, and swelling, nodules, or inflammation. Deformities are often related to misaligned articulating bones, dislocations, or subluxations. Impaired movement is usually related to arthritis; nodules related to rheumatic fever or rheumatoid arthritis; and redness related to gout, rheumatic fever, or arthritis. Compare dissimilar joints to determine what structures might be affected. Assess range of motion by moving the limb, ask the patient to move the limb, and then ask the patient to move the limb against resistance. Note any asymmetry and inequality between active and passive motion. Also examine for crepitation (a grating vibration or sound) that may suggest arthritis, an inflamed joint, or a fracture. Avoid manipulating a deformed or painful joint. Perform a physical exam on each joint, moving it through its normal range of motion and noting any deformities, limited or resistant movement, tenderness, and swelling.

Nervous system   pp. 318-324

To evaluate mental status and speech, examine your patient's appearance and behavior, speech and language, mood, thoughts and perceptions, and memory and attention. Observe the patient's appearance and behavior, level of consciousness, posture and motor behavior, appropriateness of dress, grooming and personal hygiene, and the patient's facial expression. Note any abnormal speech pattern and observe the patient's attitude toward you and others expressed both verbally and non-verbally. Note any excessive emotion or lack of emotion. Assess the patient's thoughts and perceptions. Are they realistic and socially acceptable? Question for any visions, voices, perceived odors, or feelings about things that are not there. Examine the patient's insights and judgments to determine if he knows what is happening. Assess the patient's memory and attention and determine his orientation to time, place, and person (sometimes considered as person and own person). Then test immediate, recent, and remote memory. Any deviation from a normal and expected response is to be noted and suggests illness or psychiatric problem.

Begin the examination of the motor system by observing the patient for symmetry, deformities, and involuntary movements. Tremors or fasiculations while the patient is at rest suggest

Parkinson's disease, while their occurrence during motion suggests postural tremor. Determine muscle bulk, which is classified as normal, atrophy, hypertrophy, or pseudotrophy (bulk without strength as in muscular dystrophy). Unilateral hand atrophy suggests median or ulnar nerve paralysis. Check tone by moving a relaxed limb through a range of motion. Describe any flaccidity or rigidity and then examine muscle strength starting with grip strength and continuing through all limbs. Again note any asymmetry (the patient's dominant side should be slightly stronger). Observe the patient's gait and have him walk a straight line (heel to toe). Any ataxia suggests cerebellar disease, loss of position sense, or intoxication. Also have the patient walk on his toes, then heels, hop on each foot, and then do a shallow knee bend. Perform a Romberg test (have him stand with his feet together and eyes closed for 20 to 30 seconds). Any excessive sway (a positive Romberg test) suggests ataxia from loss of position sense, while inability to maintain balance with eyes open represents cerebellar ataxia. Ask the patient to hold his arms straight out in front with his palms up and eyes closed. Pronation suggests mild hemiparesis, drifting sideways or upward suggests loss of positional sense. Ask your patient to perform various rapid alternating movements and observe for smoothness, speed, and rhythm. The dominant side should perform best, and any slow, irregular or clumsy movements suggest cerebellar or extrapyramidal disease. Have your patient touch his thumb rapidly with the tip of the index finger, place his hand on his thigh and rapidly alternate from palm up to down, and assess for point-to-point testing (touch his nose, then your index finger several times rapidly, or, for the legs, have him touch heel to knee, then run it down the shin). Any jerking, difficulty in performing the task, or tremors suggest cerebellar disease. For position testing, have the patient perform the leg test with his eyes closed.

Evaluate the sensory system by testing sensations of pain, light touch, temperature, position, vibration, and discrimination. Compare responses bilaterally and from distal to proximal, then associate any deficit discovered with the dermatome it represents. Test superficial and deep tendon reflexes and note a dulled (cord or lower neuron damage) or hyperactive response (upper neuron disease).

Cranial nerves   pp. 321-324

CN-I is checked by evaluating the ability to sense odors in each nostril.

CN-II is checked by testing for visual acuity and field of view.

CN-III is checked by examining pupillary direct and consensual response.

CN-III, IV, and VI are checked by testing for smooth and unrestricted extraocular motion.

CN-V is checked by testing the masseter muscle strength and sensation on the forehead, cheek, chin, and cornea.

CN-VII is checked by examining the patient's face during conversations, looking for any asymmetry, eyelid droop, or abnormal movements.

CN-VIII is checked by evaluating for hearing and balance (with his eyes closed).

CN-IX and X are checked by evaluating speech, swallowing, saying "aaahhh," and the gag reflex.

CN-XI is checked by testing trapezius and sternocleidomastoid muscles at rest and by evaluating head turning and shoulder raising.

CN-XII is checked by evaluating speech and having the patient extend his tongue outward.

Any deviation from a normally expected response is a reason to suspect a cranial nerve injury.

5.   Describe the assessment of visual acuity.   pp. 280, 282

Visual acuity is the ability to read detail. A wall chart with lines of progressively smaller letters is placed at 20 feet from the patient. He then reads to the smallest line in which he can recognize at least one half the letters. The result is recorded as the distance from the chart and the distance at which a person with normal sight could distinguish the letters, 20/20 for normal or 20/60 for someone who reads what is normally read at 60 feet.

6.   Explain the rationale for the use of an ophthalmoscope and otoscope.   pp. 264, 283-284

The ophthalmoscope is a light source and a series of lenses that permit you to examine the interior of the patient's eyes. It allows you to examine the retina, blood vessels, and optic nerve at the back of the posterior chamber of the eye.

The otoscope is a light source and a magnifying lens that permits examination of a patient's ears and nose. It allows you to examine the external auditory canal and the tympanic membrane for trauma, irritation, or infection.

7.   Describe the survey of respiration.   pp. 259-261, 292-296

The survey of the chest assesses the thorax and respiration by inspection, palpation, percussion, and auscultation. Compare findings side to side and anterior to back. Visualize and auscultate the five lung lobes during your exam. Examine the patient's respiration, looking for increased inspiratory or expiratory time or any sounds indicating upper or lower airway obstruction. Examine the chest for symmetry and symmetry of motion and any retraction or any anterior-posterior dimension abnormality. Also feel for any unusual vibrations associated with speech. Percuss the chest and note any hyperresonance or dullness. Listen through the stethoscope for lung sounds over each lobe and note any crackles or wheezes. Identify the respiratory rate and volume of each breath and determine the minute volume.

8. Describe percussion of the chest. pp. 293,294, 296

Percuss both the anterior and posterior chest surfaces, examining for resonant (normal), hyperresonant (air-filled pneumothorax or tension pneumothorax) or dull sounds. Percuss both sides symmetrically from the apex to the base at 5 centimeter intervals, avoiding the scapula. Determine the boundaries of any hyperresonance or dullness.

9. Differentiate the percussion notes and their characteristics.   pp. 256-257

Percussion provides three basic sounds; dull, resonant, and hyperresonant. Dull reflects a density and is a medium-pitched thud. It is usually caused by a dense organ (like the liver) or fluid, like blood, underneath. Resonant sounds are generally associated with a less dense tissue, like the lungs, and are lower-pitched and longer lasting sounds. Hyperresonant sounds reflect air, or air under pressure, and are the lowest-pitched sounds and the ones that diminish in volume most slowly.

10. Describe special examination techniques related to the assessment of the chest.   pp. 291-296

Chest excursion
Place your hands with the fingers spread at the 10th intercostal space and feel for chest excursion as the patient breathes deeply. Your hand should move equally about 3 to 5 cm with each breath.

Fremitus
Place a cupped hand against the chest wall at various locations and feel for vibrations while the patient says "ninety-nine" or "one-on-one." These vibrations should be equal throughout the chest. Note any enhanced, decreased, or absent fremitus.

Diaphragm excursion
Percuss the border of the rib cage for the dullness of the diaphragm during quiet breathing. Then mark the highest and lowest movement during respiration. Repeat the process on the other side of the chest. This excursion should be about 6 cm and equal on each side.

11. Describe the auscultation of the chest, heart, and abdomen.   pp. 293-299, 300-301

Chest
Have your patient breathe more deeply and slowly than normal with an open mouth. Using the stethoscope's disk, auscultate each side of the chest from the apex to the base every 5 cm, listening at each location for one full breath.

Heart
Using the diaphragm of the stethoscope, listen for heart sounds at the 2nd through 5th intercostal spaces at both sternal borders and at the point of maximum impulse (PMI). Repeat the process using the bell of the stethoscope to discern lower-pitched sounds.

Abdomen
Using the stethoscope's disk, auscultate each abdominal quadrant for at least 30 seconds to 1 minute.

12. Distinguish between normal and abnormal auscultation findings of the chest, heart, and abdomen and explain their significance.   pp. 293-299, 300-301

Chest
Normal breath sounds are the quiet sounds (almost low-pitched sighs) of air moving. Abnormal breath sounds are termed adventitious, and include the following. Any crackles (a light crackling, popping,

non-musical sound) suggest fluid in the smaller airways. Late inspiratory crackles suggest heart failure or interstitial lung disease, while early crackles suggest heart failure or chronic bronchitis. Wheezes (more musical notes) denote obstruction of the smaller airways. The closer they appear to inspiration, the more serious the obstruction is. Stridor is a high-pitched, loud inspiratory wheeze reflective of laryngeal or tracheal obstruction. Grating or squeaking sounds describe pleural friction rubs and occur as the pleural layers become inflamed, then rub together. You may also listen for sound transmission while the patient speaks. Bronchophony occurs when you hear the words "ninety-nine" abnormally clearly through the stethoscope, a suggestion that blood, fluid, or a tumor has replaced normal tissue. Assess for whispered pectoriloquy by asking the patient to whisper "ninety-nine"; unusually clear sounds indicate an abnormal condition. Egophony occurs when you can hear the sound of long "e" as "a" when vocal resonance is abnormally increased.

Heart

The normal heart produces a "lub-dub" sound heard through the disk of the stethoscope with each cardiac contraction. The "lub" and "dub" may split when valves close out of sync, "la-lub-dub" reflects an S_1 split while "lub-da-dub" is an S_2 split. S_2 splitting is normal in children and young adults, though abnormal in older adults if expiratory or persistent splitting occurs. S_3 splitting produces a "lub-dub-dee" cadence like the word "Kentucky." It occurs commonly in children and young adults, but reflects blood filling a dilated ventricle and may suggest ventricular failure in the patient over 30. The S_4 heart sound is the "dee" sound of "dee-lub-dub" with a cadence similar to the word "Tennessee." It develops from vibrations as the atrium pushes blood into a ventricle that resists filling, suggestive of heart failure.

Abdomen

Normal bowel sounds consist of a variety of high-pitched gurgles and clicks that occur every 5 to 15 seconds. More frequent activity suggests an increase in bowel motility and especially loud and prolonged gurgling sounds (borborygmi) indicate hyperperistalsis. Decreased or absent sounds suggest a paralytic ileus or peritonitis. You may also hear swishing sounds (bruit) over the major vessels suggesting vascular defect such as aneurysm or stenosis.

13. Describe special techniques of the cardiovascular examination. pp. 293-299, 300-301

Inspection for signs of cardiovascular insufficiency

Examine the extremities for signs of insufficiency including pallor, delayed capillary refill, temperature variation, and dependent edema. Then assess the carotid arteries for pulse strength, rate, and rhythm. Does the rate or strength vary with respirations? Do you feel thrills (feel a humming sensation)? If so, auscultate for bruits.

Jugular vein distention

Position the patient supine with the head elevated 30° and turned away from the side being assessed. Look for pulsations of the external jugular vein on either side of the trachea just before it passes behind the manubrium. Locate the highest point of pulsation and measure the distance from the sternal angle. Normal venous pressure distends the vein above the clavicle between 1 to 2 cm. Examine both jugulars for symmetrical pulsing and distention.

Point of maximum impulse (PMI)

Have the patient lie comfortably with his head elevated 30°. Inspect and palpate the chest for the apical impulse or the PMI. It is normally at the 5th intercostal space, mid-clavicular line. In muscular or obese patients, you may need to percuss the point (dull vs. resonant).

14. Describe the general guidelines of recording examination information.   pp. 338-339

Use a standard format to organize the information. Use appropriate medical terminology and language. Present your findings legibly, accurately, and truthfully, remembering that your record will become a legal document. Include all data discovered in your assessment.

The standard organization for medical documentation is the S (Subjective), O (Objective), A (Assessment), and P (Plan) format (SOAP format):

Subjective information is what your patient or others tell you, including the chief complaint and the past and present medical history.

Objective information is that which you observe or determine during the scene size-up, initial assessment, focused history and physical exam, detailed assessment, and ongoing assessments.

Assessment summarizes the findings to suggest a field diagnosis.

Plan is the further diagnosis, treatment, and patient education you intend to offer.

15. Discuss the examination considerations for an infant or child.   pp. 333-338

Children are not small adults, but patients with special physiological and psychological differences. In general, remain calm and confident, establish a rapport with the parents, and have them help with the exam. Provide positive feedback to both the child and parents.

The transition from newborn to adulthood is a continuum of development, both physically and emotionally. When assessing pediatric patients, keep the following differences from adults in mind:

The bones of the skull do not close until about 18 months and joints remain cartilaginous until 5 years.

The child's airway is narrow and will be more quickly and severely obstructed than the adult's. Instead of listening for verbal complaints, note the child's eyes, expression, and the degree of activity it takes to distract him from the problem as an indication of its seriousness.

Rib fractures are rare due to the cartilaginous nature of the ribs, though the tissue underneath is more prone to injury.

The liver and spleen are proportionally large and are more subject to injury.

Children are more likely to experience bone injury rather than ligament and tendon injury.

Normal vital signs for children will change through the stages of their development.

The following objectives, while not listed in the chapter, will help in your understanding of the chapter content.

*   Identify and describe the vital signs.   pp. 258-262

Pulse is the wave of pressure generated by the heart as it expels blood into the arterial system. It is measured by palpating a distal artery (or auscultated during blood pressure determination) and is evaluated for rate, rhythm, and quality (strength). The normal pulse is strong, regular, and has a rate of between 60 and 80 beats per minute.

Respiration is the movement of air through the airway and into and out of the lungs. It is evaluated by observing and/or feeling chest excursion and listening to air movement. The rate, effort, and quality (depth and pattern) of respirations are determined. Normal respiration moves a tidal volume of 500 mL at a rate of 12 to 20 times per minute with symmetrical chest wall movement.

Blood pressure is the force of blood against the arterial wall during the cardiac/pulse cycle. It is measured using a sphygmomanometer (blood pressure cuff) and stethoscope. The maximum or systolic blood pressure—the reading obtained when the ventricles contract, the lower or diastolic blood pressure—the reading obtained when the ventricles relax, and the difference between them, the pulse pressure, are evaluated. The systolic pressure is usually between 100 and 135, and the diastolic, between 60 and 80.

Temperature is the body core temperature and is the product of heat-creating metabolism and body heat loss. It is measured by a glass or electronic thermometer placed in the axilla, mouth, or rectum. Normal body temperature is 37°C (98.6°F).

*   Identify and explain the importance of additional assessment techniques.   pp. 269-273

Pulse oximetry is the noninvasive measurement of oxygen saturation in the tissue of a distal extremity. It provides a real-time evaluation of oxygen delivery to the distal circulation. Normal readings are between 96 and 100 percent. Readings below this reflect problems with either respiration or circulation and demand intervention.

Cardiac monitoring uses electronics to display the electrical activity of the heart. The monitor shows an electronic or paper tracing of the heart's activity, either a normal rhythm, a dysrhythmia, or no activity—asystole. This information is essential to identifying when to shock the heart back to a normal rhythm or to treat it through the use of medication.

Blood glucose determination is performed by using a glucometer, a small electronic device that evaluates the colour of a blood-stained reagent strip. The glucose level can rule out or identify hypoglycemia in a patient with a lowered level of consciousness or in the known diabetic.

CONTENT SELF-EVALUATION

1. Of the physical examination techniques used in prehospital care, which is the least invasive?
   A. inspection
   B. auscultation
   C. palpation
   D. percussion
   E. C and D

2. "Crackles" would be found using which of the following assessment techniques?
   A. palpation
   B. auscultation
   C. inspection
   D. percussion
   E. none of the above

3. "Guarding" would be discovered using which of the following assessment techniques?
   A. palpation
   B. auscultation
   C. inspection
   D. percussion
   E. none of the above

4. Which of the following techniques should be performed first during the physical examination?
   A. palpation
   B. auscultation
   C. inspection
   D. percussion
   E. none of the above

5. Which part of the hands and fingers is best suited to evaluate tissue consistency?
   A. tips of the fingers
   B. pads of the fingers
   C. palm of the hand
   D. back of the hands or fingers
   E. none of the above

6. Which part of the hands and fingers is best suited to evaluate vibration?
   A. tips of the fingers
   B. pads of the fingers
   C. palm of the hand
   D. back of the hands or fingers
   E. none of the above

7. The loud, hollow sound produced by percussing an air-filled region is:
   A. hyperresonance.
   B. dull.
   C. resonance.
   D. flat.
   E. none of the above

8. The booming sound produced by percussing an air-filled region is:
   A. hyperresonance.
   B. dull.
   C. resonance.
   D. flat.
   E. none of the above

9. The only region where you perform auscultation as other than the last step of assessment is the:

A. anterior thorax.
B. neck.
C. abdomen.
D. peripheral arteries.
E. posterior thorax.

10. A heart rate above 100 is known as a:

A. bradycardia.
B. tachycardia.
C. hypercardia.
D. tachypnea.
E. bradypnea.

11. One likely cause of bradycardia is:

A. fever.
B. pain.
C. parasympathetic stimulation.
D. fear.
E. blood loss.

12. Which of the following is NOT an aspect of pulse evaluation?

A. volume
B. rhythm
C. quality
D. rate
E. none of the above

13. Normal exhalation is:

A. an active process involving accessory muscles.
B. an active process involving the diaphragm and intercostal muscles.
C. active in its early stages and passive in later stages.
D. passive in its early stages and active in later stages.
E. a passive process.

14. For a patient with an airway obstruction, exhalation is likely to be:

A. an active process involving accessory muscles.
B. an active process involving only the diaphragm and intercostal muscles.
C. active in its early stages and passive in later stages.
D. passive in its early stages and active in later stages.
E. a passive process.

15. The amount of air a patient moves into and out of his lungs in one breath is the:

A. normal volume.
B. respiratory volume.
C. residual volume.
D. tidal volume.
E. minute volume.

16. The pressure of the blood within the blood vessels while the ventricles are relaxing is the:

A. Korotkoff blood pressure.
B. systolic blood pressure.
C. diastolic blood pressure.
D. asystolic blood pressure.
E. atrial blood pressure.

17. The diastolic blood pressure represents a measure of:

A. systemic vascular resistance.
B. the cardiac output.
C. the viscosity of the blood.
D. the strength of ventricular contraction.
E. relative blood volume.

18. Which of the following are likely to influence a patient's blood pressure?

A. anxiety
B. position (lying, sitting, standing)
C. recent smoking
D. eating
E. all of the above

19. Generally, hypertension in a healthy adult is any blood pressure higher than:

    A.   120/80.   **D.**   180/100.

    B.   140/90.   **E.**   200/100.

    C.   160/90.

20. What is the pulse pressure in a patient with the following vital signs: pulse 82 and strong; respirations 14 and full: and blood pressure 144/96?

    A.   14   **D.**   96

    B.   40   **E.**   120

    C.   48

21. In the tilt test, what vital sign change is a positive sign of hypovolemia?

    A.   blood pressure drops by 10 to 20 mmHg

    B.   blood pressure rises by 10 to 20 mmHg

    C.   pulse rate drops by 10 to 20 beats per minute

    D.   pulse rate rises by 10 to 20 beats per minute

    E.   either A or D

22. Hyperthermia can result from all of the following EXCEPT:

    A.   high environmental temperatures.   **D.**   drugs.

    B.   infections.   **E.**   increases in metabolic activity.

    C.   reduced metabolic activity.

23. What technique of stethoscope use best transmits low-pitched sound to the ear?

    A.   light pressure on the diaphragm   **D.**   light pressure on the bell

    B.   firm pressure on the diaphragm   **E.**   strong pressure on the bell

    C.   moderate pressure on the bell

24. The bell of a stethoscope is best for listening to the sounds of:

    A.   blood vessel bruits.   **D.**   the lung.

    B.   the blood pressure.   **E.**   none of the above

    C.   the heart.

25. Which of the following is NOT a characteristic of a good stethoscope?

    A.   thick, heavy tubing   **D.**   a bell with a rubber-ring edge

    B.   long tubing (70 to 100 cm)   **E.**   all of the above

    C.   snug-fitting earpieces

26. Generally, each narrow line on a sphygmomanometer represents what pressure difference?

    A.   1 mmHg   **D.**   5 mmHg

    B.   2 mmHg   **E.**   10 mmHg

    C.   4 mmHg

27. If a patient has a regular and strong pulse, you should determine the pulse rate by assessing the number of beats in:

    A.   two minutes and dividing by 2.

    B.   three minutes.

    C.   30 seconds and multiplying by 2.

    D.   15 seconds and multiplying by 4.

    E.   10 seconds and multiplying by 5.

28. Use of which of the following pulse points is recommended with a small child?

    A.   radial   **D.**   popliteal

    B.   brachial   **E.**   dorsalis pedis

    C.   carotid

29. Use of which of the following pulse points does not give you information about your patient's hemodynamic status?

A. radial
B. brachial
C. carotid
D. apical
E. dorsalis pedis

30. The proper position of the patient's arm when taking the blood pressure is:

A. arm slightly flexed.
B. palm up.
C. fingers relaxed.
D. clothing removed from the upper arm.
E. all of the above

31. The sphygmomanometer should be inflated to what level beyond the point at which the patient's radial pulse disappears?

A. 10 mmHg
B. 20 mmHg
C. 30 mmHg
D. 40 mmHg
E. between B and C

32. Which of the following types of thermometer should be left in place for 2 to 3 seconds?

A. tympanic
B. oral
C. axilla
D. rectal
E. none of the above

33. When using the oral glass thermometer, it should be left in the mouth for what period of time?

A. 30 to 45 seconds
B. 30 to 60 seconds
C. 1 to 2 minutes
D. 2 minutes
E. 3 to 4 minutes

34. The normal patient oxygen saturation without supplemental oxygen at sea level should be:

A. between 90 to 95 percent.
B. below 95 percent.
C. 100 percent.
D. 96 to 100 percent.
E. below 90 percent.

35. A patient suffering from carbon monoxide poisoning will likely have a pulse oximetry reading that is:

A. accurate.
B. falsely high.
C. falsely low.
D. erratic and inaccurate.
E. unreadable.

36. The ECG of a cardiac monitor can tell you all of the following EXCEPT:

A. the heart rate.
B. the sequence of cardiac events.
C. the timing of cardiac events.
D. the pumping ability of the heart.
E. both A and C

37. Evaluation of the skin involves evaluating its:

A. moisture.
B. temperature.
C. turgor.
D. colour.
E. all of the above

38. Pale skin is least likely to be caused by which of the following?

A. increased deoxyhemoglobin
B. a cold environment
C. shock compensation
D. anemia
E. hypovolemic shock

39. Which of the following skin discolourations represents a yellow hue?

A. cyanosis

B. jaundice

C. eccyhmosis

D. erythema

E. pallor

40. A heavy scaling of the skin under the hair is:

A. dandruff.

B. nits.

C. seborrheic dermatitis.

D. psoriasis.

E. none of the above

41. The bluish discolouration around the orbits of the eyes, suggestive of a basilar skull fracture, is called:

A. "raccoon eyes."

B. "Battle's sign."

C. periorbital ecchymosis.

D. retroauricular ecchymosis.

E. either A or C

42. The characteristic of the unaffected eye responding to stimuli in the affected eye is:

A. consensual response.

B. direct response.

C. simultaneous response.

D. ipsilateral response.

E. none of the above

43. About 20 percent of the population have a noticeable difference in the size of the pupils, a condition called:

A. hyphema.

B. anisocoria.

C. glaucoma.

D. hypopyon.

E. none of the above

44. Otorrhea is a discharge from the ear that may contain:

A. pus.

B. mucus.

C. blood.

D. cerebrospinal fluid.

E. all of the above

45. The term for a common nosebleed is:

A. epistaxis.

B. otorrhea.

C. rhinorrhea.

D. rhinitis.

E. none of the above

46. A likely location to notice retraction during forced inspiration is:

A. the suprasternal notch.

B. the intercostal spaces.

C. the supraclavicular space.

D. all of the above

E. none of the above

47. The type of motion associated with a free segment of the chest where the segment moves opposite to the rest of the chest during breathing is:

A. symbiotic.

B. paradoxical.

C. antagonistic.

D. retractive.

E. traumatic.

48. During the palpation of the chest, you should feel for which of the following?

A. tenderness

B. deformities

C. depressions

D. asymmetry

E. all of the above

49. During the check for chest excursion, the distance between your thumbs should increase by what amount during the patient's inspiration?

A. 2 cm

B. 3 to 5 cm

C. 5 to 6 cm

D. 10 to 12 cm

E. the hands should not move

50. Increased tactile fremitus suggests which of the following conditions?

A. pneumonia D. emphysema
B. pneumothorax E. all of the above
C. pleural effusion

51. Which condition is most likely to cause an area of the lung that is dull to percussion?
   A. pneumothorax D. pericardial tamponade
   B. tension pneumothorax E. friction rubs
   C. hemothorax

52. Light popping, nonmusical sounds heard in the chest during inspiration are known as:
   A. rhonchi. D. wheezes.
   B. stridor. E. none of the above
   C. crackles.

53. The "lub" of the heart sounds represents which event of the cardiac cycle?
   A. ejection of blood from the ventricles
   B. ventricular contraction
   C. ventricular filling
   D. closing of the aortic and pulmonic valves
   E. closing of the tricuspid and mitral valves

54. An eccyhmotic discolouration over the umbilicus is:
   A. Grey-Turner's sign. D. Cullen's sign.
   B. borborygami. E. none of the above
   C. Hering-Breuer sign.

55. Auscultation of high-pitched gurgles and clicks every 5 to 15 seconds in the abdomen indicates:
   A. borborygmi. D. normal bowel sounds.
   B. increased bowel motility. E. ascites.
   C. absent bowel sounds.

56. The sound or feeling caused by unlubricated bone ends rubbing together is:
   A. palpable fremitus. D. friction rub.
   B. crepitation. E. the pooh-pooh sign.
   C. bruit.

57. Carpal tunnel syndrome involves which nerve?
   A. brachial D. ulnar
   B. median E. olecranon
   C. radial

58. A lateral curvature of the spine is:
   A. lordosis. D. spina bifida.
   B. scoliosis. E. none of the above
   C. kyphosis.

59. Tenderness at a vertebral process and in the surrounding musculature of the lumbar spine is most likely due to:
   A. vertebral process fracture. D. herniated intervertebral disk.
   B. ligamentous injury. E. none of the above
   C. paravertebral muscular spasm.

60. Your patient has a pulse rate of 64. However, you note that every fourth beat is missing. This is described as a:
   A. regular pulse. D. regularly irregular pulse.
   B. irregular pulse. E. regularly dropped pulse.
   C. irregularly irregular pulse.

61. A normal pulse quality would be reported as:
- **A.**   0.
- **B.**   1+.
- **C.**   2+.
- **D.**   3+.
- **E.**   4+.

62. Which of the following is NOT a sign of proximal arterial occlusion?
- **A.**   thrills
- **B.**   pulse deficit
- **C.**   cold limb
- **D.**   poor colour in the fingertips
- **E.**   slow capillary refill

63. Pitting edema that depresses 1 to 2.5 cm is reported as:
- **A.**   0.
- **B.**   1+.
- **C.**   2+.
- **D.**   3+.
- **E.**   4+.

64. The pitting of edema will usually disappear within how many seconds after the release of pressure?
- **A.**   2
- **B.**   4
- **C.**   6
- **D.**   8
- **E.**   10

65. A complete neurological exam includes which of the following areas?
- **A.**   cranial nerves
- **B.**   motor system
- **C.**   reflexes
- **D.**   sensory system
- **E.**   all of the above

66. A patient who is drowsy but answers questions is considered to be:
- **A.**   lethargic.
- **B.**   obtunded.
- **C.**   stuporous.
- **D.**   comatose.
- **E.**   none of the above

67. Normal speech is:
- **A.**   inflected.
- **B.**   clear and strong.
- **C.**   fluent and articulate.
- **D.**   varies in volume.
- **E.**   all of the above

68. The term dysphonia refers to which of the following?
- **A.**   defective speech caused by motor deficits
- **B.**   voice changes due to vocal cord problems
- **C.**   defective language due to neurologic problem
- **D.**   voice changes due to aging
- **E.**   none of the above

69. The term aphasia refers to which of the following?
- **A.**   defective speech caused by motor deficits
- **B.**   voice changes due to vocal cord problems
- **C.**   defective language due to a neurologic problem
- **D.**   voice changes due to aging
- **E.**   none of the above

70. Which of the following is one of the three basic grades of memory:
- **A.**   intermediate.
- **B.**   verifiable.
- **C.**   redux.
- **D.**   remote.
- **E.**   retrograde.

71. A question about a patient's wife's birthday tests which of the following types of memory?
- **A.**   intermediate
- **B.**   verifiable
- **C.**   redux
- **D.**   remote
- **E.**   retrograde

72. During the test of extraoccular eye movement you should trace which figure in front of your patient's eyes?

    A.   an "X"   **D.**   a large "O"
    B.   an "H"   **E.**   any of the above
    C.   a "+"

73. Stimulation for a blink by touching the eye's surface with fine cotton fibers tests which of the following?

    A.   corneal reflex   **D.**   the trigeminal nerve
    B.   ptosis   **E.**   none of the above
    C.   EOM

74. When a person loses his sense of balance, which cranial nerve has most likely been injured?

    A.   equilibrial   **D.**   vagus
    B.   glossopharyngeal   **E.**   accessory
    C.   acoustic

75. Damage to CN-12 will cause the tongue to deviate in which manner?

    A.   downward   **D.**   away from the side of injury
    B.   upward   **E.**   furrow and curve upward
    C.   toward the side of injury

76. The twitching of small muscle fibers is:

    A.   spasm.   **D.**   fasciculations.
    B.   tics.   **E.**   atrophy.
    C.   tremors.

77. In cases of muscular dystrophy, the patient's muscles:

    A.   increase in size.   **D.**   decrease in strength.
    B.   decrease in size.   **E.**   both A and D
    C.   increase in strength.

78. The nerves associated with movement of the biceps and triceps are:

    A.   C2, C3, C4.   **D.**   T1, T2, T3.
    B.   C6, C7, C8.   **E.**   C8, T1, median nerve.
    C.   C8, T1, T2

79. Which of the following procedures describes the Romberg test? Have the patient:

    A.   walk heel-to-toe in a straight line.
    B.   stand with eyes closed for 20 to 30 seconds.
    C.   walk across the room and turn and walk back again.
    D.   do a shallow knee bend on each leg in turn.
    E.   walk first on his heels, then toes.

80. An area of skin innervated by a specific peripheral nerve root is a(n):

    A.   afferent region.   **D.**   dermatome.
    B.   sensory topographic region.   **E.**   both A and C
    C.   myotome.

81. The score on the muscle strength scale that describes a patient able to perform active movement against gravity is:

    A.   5.   **D.**   2.
    B.   4.   **E.**   1.
    C.   3.

82. To assess the sensory system, you must test for:

    A.   pain.   **D.**   dermatome.
    B.   light touch.   **E.**   A, B, and C
    C.   temperature.

83. Babinski's response is positive when the sole of the foot is stroked and:
- **A.** the big toe plantar flexes while other toes dorsiflex.
- **B.** the big toe plantar flexes while other toes fan out.
- **C.** the big toe dorsiflexes while other toes fan out.
- **D.** the big toe dorsiflexes while other toes plantar flex.
- **E.** all toes plantar flex.

84. In caring for the ill or injured child, it is important to be which of the following?
- **A.** confident
- **B.** direct
- **C.** honest
- **D.** calm
- **E.** all of the above

85. Which of the following is NOT recommended as part of the assessment and care for an ill or injured child?
- **A.** Separate the patient from the parents if possible.
- **B.** Give the patient a toy or object to play with.
- **C.** Elicit a parent's help in obtaining a history.
- **D.** Perform invasive procedures late in the assessment if possible.
- **E.** Provide feedback and reassurance.

86. The soft spots in the skull, called fontanelles, close at about what age?
- **A.** 6 months
- **B.** 12 months
- **C.** 18 months
- **D.** 24 months
- **E.** 30 months

87. Bulging along the sutures of the skull of a young child suggests which of the following?
- **A.** dehydration
- **B.** reduced venous pressure in the jugular veins
- **C.** decreased arterial pressure
- **D.** arterial blockage to the cerebrum
- **E.** increased intracranial pressure

89. Which of the following statements regarding the chest of an infant or small child is FALSE?
- **A.** Children have a less mobile mediastinum than adults.
- **B.** The chest is rather elastic.
- **C.** The chest is rather flexible.
- **D.** Chest fractures are less likely.
- **E.** The chest is comprised of more cartilage than the adult's.

90. Stiffness in the neck, especially when associated with fever in a child suggests:
- **A.** meningitis.
- **B.** streptococcus infection.
- **C.** epilottitis.
- **D.** imminent onset of febrile seizures.
- **E.** croup.

91. The normal respiratory rate for an infant is:
- **A.** 30 to 50 breaths per minute.
- **B.** 30 to 60 breaths per minute.
- **C.** 24 to 40 breaths per minute.
- **D.** 22 to 34 breaths per minute.
- **E.** 18 to 30 breaths per minute.

92. The normal systolic blood pressure for the newborn is:
- **A.** 60 to 90.
- **B.** 87 to 105.
- **C.** 95 to 105.
- **D.** 95 to 110.
- **E.** 112 to 128.

93. Which of the following is NOT true regarding the abdomen of the child?
- **A.** The liver is proportionally larger than the adult's.
- **B.** The spleen is proportionally larger than the adult's.
- **C.** The abdominal muscles provide less protection than the adult's.

D. The abdomen rarely bulges at the end of inspiration.
E. Inguinal hernias are common in young children.

94. Which of the following statements is true regarding the recording of examination findings?
A. The patient care report is only as good as the accuracy, detail, and depth you provide.
B. The patient chart is a legal document.
C. The absence of an expected sign in a patient may be just as important as its presence.
D. The universally accepted organization for recording patient information is SOAP.
E. all of the above

95. The patient's chief complaint is recorded under which element of the SOAP documentation format?

A.	S		**D.**	P
B.	O		**E.**	none of the above
C.	A			

True/False

96. Noticing areas of warmth during palpation might reflect an injury before significant edema and discolouration develop.
A. True
B. False

97. Dull, flat sounds during percussion are normally heard over solid organs such as the liver.
A. True
B. False

98. In general, you should auscultate before performing inspection and percussion.
A. True
B. False

99. The popliteal pulse point is located just below the inguinal ligament.
A. True
B. False

100. Normal values for blood pressure are higher in women after menopause than before menopause.
A. True
B. False

101. Kaussmaul's respirations (tachypnea and hyperpnea) may be caused by renal failure or diabetic ketoacidosis.
A. True
B. False

102. It is important to attempt to evaluate your patient's respiratory rate and volume without his being aware of it.
A. True
B. False

103. The first blood pressure reading is the diastolic blood pressure.
A. True
B. False

104. Pulse pressure is the difference between the systolic and diastolic pressures.
  A. True
  B. False

105. Shivering normally stops when the core body temperature reaches 34 degrees Celsius.
  A. True
  B. False

106. If you attempt to take a blood pressure and cannot obtain a reading, you should wait at least 5 minutes before making a second attempt.
  A. True
  B. False

107. If you obtain a pulse oximeter reading below 90% you should consider aggressive airway management or ventilatory assistance.
  A. True
  B. False

108. Hearing words transmitted clearly as you auscultate the chest with the stethoscope is a normal finding called bronchophony.
  A. True
  B. False

109. Both retractions and bulging of the intercostals spaces are normal effects of respiration.
  A. True
  B. False

110. Pleural rubs are often heard with pneumonia and pleurisy.
  A. True
  B. False

111. With pulsus paradoxus, the amplitude of pulse increases with inspiration and diminishes with expiration.
  A. True
  B. False

112. Ascitites are bulges in the flanks and across the abdomen indicating edema caused by congestive heart failure.
  A. True
  B. False

113. Bilateral edema suggests a deep vein thrombosis or venous occlusion.
  A. True
  B. False

114. Rigid muscle tone throughout movement is common in Parkinson's disease.
  A. True
  B. False

115. During your testing of a patient's muscle strength, you notice one side to be slightly stronger than the other. This is a normal finding.
  A. True
  B. False

116. When testing deep tendon reflexes, a hyperactive response suggests upper motor neuron disease.
  A. True
  B. False

117. A positive Babinski response indicates peripheral nervous system lesion.
  A. True
  B. False

_____ **118.** When assessing children, the more invasive a procedure the earlier in the assessment you should perform it.
  A. True
  B. False

_____ **119.** Because the tissue of the child's upper airway is so flexible, injuries, infections, or minor obstructions do not adversely affect it as seriously as they would an adult's.
  A. True
  B. False

_____ **120.** Because of the structure of the thoracic cage, the child is less likely to develop tension pneumothorax than the adult.
  A. True
  B. False

Matching

Pulse Points

Write the letter of the pulse point in the space provided next to the description of its location.

Pulse Point

A.	brachial	**F.**	posterior tibial
B.	carotid	**G.**	radial
C.	dorsalis pedis	**H.**	subclavian
D.	femoral	**I.**	temporal
E.	popliteal	**J.**	ulnar

Location

_____ **121.** side of the head
_____ **122.** anterior neck
_____ **123.** upper arm
_____ **124.** lower arm, on the thumb side
_____ **125.** lower arm, on the little finger side
_____ **126.** inguinal area
_____ **127.** behind the knee
_____ **128.** top of the foot
_____ **129.** inside of the lower leg, behind the ankle

Assessment terminology

Write the letter of the assessment term in the space provided next to its definition or description.

Term

  A. bradycardia
  B. bradynpnea
  C. hypertension
  D. hypotension
  E. Kortokoff sounds
  F. manometer
  G. opthalmoscope
  H. otoscope
  I. tachycardia
  J. tachypnea
  K. tidal volume

Definition

_____	**130.**	rapid breathing
_____	**131.**	pulse rate faster than 100
_____	**132.**	higher than normal blood pressure
_____	**133.**	pressure gauge with a a scale calibrated in mmHG
_____	**134.**	pulse rate slower than 60
_____	**135.**	sound of blood hitting arterial walls
_____	**136.**	lower than normal blood pressure
_____	**137.**	handheld device used to examine the interior of the ears and nose
_____	**138.**	amount of air one breathing moves into and out of the lungs
_____	**139.**	handheld device used to examine the interior of the eye
_____	**140.**	slow breathing

Chapter 7

Patient Assessment in the Field

Review of Chapter Objectives

With each chapter of the Workbook, we identify the objectives and the important elements of the text content. You should review these items and refer to the pages listed if any points are not clear.

After reading this section of the chapter, you should be able to:

1. Recognize hazards/potential hazards associated with the medical and trauma scene. pp. 343-349

During the scene assessment, you must examine the scene before you arrive at the patient's side. It is a time to evaluate and prepare for hazards including blood, fluids, airborne pathogens, and other conditions that may threaten your life or health. These conditions include the hazards of fire, structural collapse, traffic, unstable surfaces, electricity, broken glass, or jagged metal. Hazardous materials can involve chemical spills, radiation, and toxic environments. Finally, scene hazards can also include violent, disturbed, or unruly bystanders or patients. These hazards are not limited to the trauma scene but may be found at many medical scenes as well.

2. Identify unsafe scenes and describe methods for making them safe. pp. 343-349

Your responsibility at the emergency scene is to recognize hazards including fire, structural collapse, traffic, unstable surfaces, electricity, broken glass, jagged metal, and hazardous materials and then act appropriately to protect yourself, other rescuers, and your patient. Unless you are specially trained and equipped to handle a specific hazard, do not enter the scene. In most cases, you will rely on the fire department, rescue service, police department, power company, hazmat team, or other specially trained personnel to secure the scene before you enter. If there is ever a question of whether a scene is safe or unsafe, do not enter the scene.

3. Discuss common mechanisms of injury/nature of illness.   pp. 350-352

Trauma is induced by a mechanism of injury through which forces enter the body and do physical harm. Common mechanisms include blunt trauma—for example, vehicle crashes (auto, recreational, watercraft, and bicycle), pedestrian vs. vehicle impacts, falls—and penetrating trauma—for example, gunshot and knife wounds. Medical problems have a related cause called the nature of the illness. The scene can provide evidence as to the nature of the illness. Examples include the presence of nebulizers, which suggest asthma, drug paraphernalia, which suggest overdose, and medications, which suggest preexisting cardiac or other problems.

4. Predict patterns of injury based on mechanism of injury.   pp. 350-352, 363-364

Analyze the strength, direction, and nature of the forces expressed to the patient during the incident. This analysis will suggest the probable type of injury, the organs involved, and the seriousness of injury. In a vehicle crash, for example, such things as a broken windshield, a bent steering wheel, an intrusion into the passenger compartment, and the use of restraints by occupants can suggest potential injuries and their severity. Types of injuries can also be predicted for each type of vehicle crash— frontal, lateral, rear-end, rotational, and rollover. The analysis of the accident can lead to your anticipation of possible injuries, or an index of suspicion.

5. Discuss the reason for identifying the total number of patients at the scene. pp. 349-350

Determining the number of patients at a scene is important to assure that the needed resources are summoned to the scene and that every patient is cared for. At each and every scene, you should ask yourself, "Could there be others who are injured or ill?" While at the trauma scene it is common to find a patient wandering among the bystanders, the medical scene can have "hidden patients" too. The wife of a cardiac arrest patient, for example, may herself become a patient because of the emotional stress of the incident. Knowing the number of patients can help you gauge whether on-scene resources are adequate or whether you need to request that additional units and manpower be dispatched to the scene. The earlier this request is made, the quicker those resources will arrive.

6. Organize the management of a scene following assessment.　　pp. 343-349

The management of the scene following the scene assessment includes requesting both the appropriate units and personnel to manage scene hazards and the appropriate number and care levels of ambulances and personnel to treat the patients. You must also take the necessary steps to assure overall scene safety and to protect yourself, the patient, other scene personnel, and bystanders. The scene assessment also prepares you to manage the care of the patient by helping you recognize the mechanism of injury and anticipate injuries (index of suspicion) or by recognizing the nature of the illness.

7. Explain the reasons for identifying the need for additional help or assistance during the scene assessment.　pp. 343, 345-349

Multiple patients at the emergency scene can rapidly overwhelm your ability to provide effective care. If you wait until you are at a patient's side before calling for additional help, you may be distracted from making the call and delay an effective response. In cases where the number of patients far outstrips your ability to provide care, you may need to initiate a mass casualty response.

8. Summarize the reasons for forming a general impression of the patient.　　pp. 353

The initial general impression of your patient takes into account the patient's age, gender, race, and other factors that will help you determine the seriousness of the problem and establish your priorities for patient care and transport. As you learn more about the patient through the initial assessment and the focused history and physical assessment, you will refine and improve on the accuracy and depth of the general impression. As you develop your general impression of the patient early in the assessment process, you can also begin to establish a rapport with him or her, explaining why you are there, what will be happening to him or her, and giving the patient the opportunity to refuse care.

9. Discuss methods of assessing mental status/levels of consciousness in the adult, infant, and child patient.　　pp. 354-355

Initially determine the patient's mental status by categorizing him according to the AVPU system. Using this method, the patient is classified either **A**lert, responsive to **V**erbal stimuli, responsive to **P**ainful stimuli, or **U**nresponsive. You can further refine the evaluation by questioning the patient to determine orientation to place, time, and person and by differentiating his or her response to pain into purposeful and purposeless movement and decerebrate and decorticate posturing. An alert response for the infant or child is difficult to assess because of that patient's limited speech capabilities. Evaluate pediatric patients for activity and curiosity, being aware that the quiet child is often a seriously ill or injured one.

10. Discuss methods of assessing and securing the airway in the adult, child, and infant patient. pp. 355-357

The patient who is speaking clearly (or the child or infant who is crying loudly) has a patent airway. For other patients, position your head at the patient's mouth and look, listen, and feel for air moving through the airway. If you detect no movement, open the airway by using either the jaw thrust (in patients with trauma and suspected spine injury) or the head-tilt/chin-lift. Suction any fluids from the airway and remove obstructions using the Heimlich maneuver or laryngoscopy with Magill forceps. Secure the airway, as needed, with an oral or nasal airway, endotracheal intubation, or creation of a needle or surgical airway. When you have a pediatric patient, be sure to position the head and neck properly (using slight extension and padding under the shoulders), taking account of the differences in the pediatric anatomy. Also, reduce the size of the airways, laryngoscope blades, and endotracheal tubes you use with these patients.

11. State reasons for cervical spine management for the trauma patient. p. 353

The spinal cord is the major communication distribution and collection conduit for the central nervous system. It is protected by the spinal column, the bony and flexible structure that runs from the base of the skull to just below the pelvis. If the column is injured, it may become unstable and permit injury to the spinal cord. Because injuries to the cord have such serious consequences, you should immobilize the spine early in your assessment and care to protect this essential communication pathway. Its immobilization will not harm the patient, while uncontrolled movement can cause permanent spinal cord injury.

12. Analyze a scene to determine if spinal precautions are required. pp. 354-355, 363-364

Your examination of the scene and the analysis of the mechanism of injury will suggest or rule out the potential for spinal injury. The patient with a significant mechanism of injury—severe vehicle crash, fall from a height, injury causing a major long bone fracture, or any injury or mechanism of injury that suggests the body was subjected to significant trauma forces—has a likelihood of spinal fracture and requires spinal precautions.

13. Describe methods for assessing respiration in the adult, child, and infant patient. pp. 357-358

If your patient is speaking clearly (or if an infant or child patient is crying loudly) presume the airway is clear. Otherwise, listen for the sounds of airway restriction or obstruction, such as gurgling, stridor, or wheezes. If airway sounds are absent, place your ear at the patient's mouth while you listen, watch, and feel for air movement through it. If there is any doubt about airway patency, position the head with the jaw thrust or head-tilt/chin-lift. With a child, do not hyperextend the neck as this may block the airway. You may have to place padding behind the shoulders of a small child or infant to maintain proper head positioning.

14. Describe the methods used to locate and assess a pulse in the adult, child, and infant patient. pp. 358-361

Use the pads of your fingers and apply gentle, increasing pressure until you feel a strong pulsing over the radial artery in the adult and brachial artery in the small child or infant. If the radial or brachial pulse cannot be felt, check the carotid or, in the infant, the apical pulse. An adult radial pulse generally suggests a blood pressure of at least 80 mmHg, while a carotid pulse suggests a systolic blood pressure of at least 60 mmHg. Pulse rates usually decrease with age from a high of 100 to 180 in the infant to 60 to 100 in the adult. The pulse should be strong and regular.

15. Discuss the need for assessing the patient for external bleeding. p. 358

The patient with the potential for external hemorrhage must be assessed to determine both the nature and the extent of the blood loss. Any significant external hemorrhage must be halted and the amount of loss approximated to help prevent hypovolemia and to determine what effects the loss will have on the patient's body.

16. Describe normal and abnormal findings when assessing skin colour, temperature, and condition.   p. 358

Normal skin is warm, moist, and pink in colour (in light-skinned people), reflecting good perfusion. The body's compensation for shock results in vasoconstriction, which produces mottled, cyanotic, pale or ashen skin colour, and skin that is cool to the touch. Capillary refill times may exceed 3 seconds, though this may be due to a number of preexisting conditions in adults.

17. Explain the reason and process for prioritizing a patient for care and transport.   pp. 361-362

At the conclusion of the initial assessment, you must determine your patient's priority, which will indicate how to proceed with assessment, care, and transport. With a seriously ill or injured patient, perform a rapid head-to-toe assessment. With a stable medical or trauma patient, perform a focused history and secondary assessment. You will also need to determine the priority for transport—either immediate transport with care rendered en route or with most care provided at the scene followed by transport.

18. Use the findings of the initial assessment to determine the patient's perfusion status. pp. 358-361

The initial assessment provides you with a general impression of the patient, a determination of the patient's mental status, and an evaluation of the airway, breathing, and circulation. This information indicates the status of the patient's respiration/oxygenation and circulation. It also indicates the patient's level of consciousness and the perfusion of the body's most important end-organ, the brain.

19. Describe orthostatic vital signs and evaluate their usefulness in assessing a patient in shock.   p. 379

The test for orthostatic vital signs, also called the tilt test, evaluates vital signs (blood pressure and pulse rate) before and after moving the patient from the supine to the seated, then to the full standing position. If after 30 to 60 seconds either the blood pressure drops by more than 10 mmHg or the pulse rate rises by more than 10, consider the test positive and suspect hypovolemia. (Note that the change in pulse rate is the more sensitive indicator.) Do not use this test when other indicators of shock are present as it places stress on the cardiovascular system.

20. Describe the secondary assessment of the medical patient. pp. 375-379

The medical patient secondary assessment evaluates the head, ears, eyes, nose, and throat (HEENT), chest, abdomen, pelvis, extremities, posterior surface, and vital signs discretely, looking for illness or disease signs. The exam may be modified to meet the specific patient complaints of chest pain, respiratory distress, altered mental status, and acute abdomen. The medical patient exam may also include the results of pulse oximetry as well as cardiac and glucose level monitoring.

21. Differentiate between the assessment for unresponsive, altered mental status, and alert medical patients.   pp. 373-382

Responsive and unresponsive medical patients are examined in much different fashions. The **responsive patient** can provide information regarding his or her chief complaint, history of the present illness, past medical history, and current health status. This information, along with a secondary assessment focused on the areas of expected signs, provides the information necessary to make a field diagnosis.

The **unresponsive patient** cannot provide this information, and the care giver must garner it from family and bystanders and through a more intensive and comprehensive secondary assessment. The **patient with an altered mental status** is assessed like the unresponsive patient, though some information may be obtained from the patient. The information may not be reliable, hence the need for a more comprehensive secondary assessment.

22. Discuss the reasons for reconsidering the mechanism of injury. p. 363

After the initial and rapid trauma assessments or focused history and secondary assessment, you have gathered enough information about your patient to determine if the mechanism of injury (and your resulting index of suspicion for associated injuries) agree with your assessment findings. If they do, maintain your priority for care and transport. If they do not agree, reevaluate your index of suspicion and the physical findings and possibly adjust your patient's priority. If you do alter your patient's priority, always err on the side of precaution.

23. Recite examples and explain why patients should receive a rapid trauma assessment. p. 365

Every patient with a significant mechanism of injury, an altered level of consciousness, or multiple body-system traumas should receive the rapid trauma assessment. These patients are likely to have serious internal injuries and/or hemorrhage. However, the signs and symptoms of serious injury and shock are often hidden by other, more gruesome or painful injuries or by the body's compensatory mechanisms. Without maintaining a high index of suspicion for serious injury and evaluating the patient via the rapid trauma assessment, you are likely to overlook the patient with serious and life-threatening injury.

24. Describe the secondary assessment of the trauma patient. pp. 362-372

The physical assessment of the trauma patient begins during the initial assessment with the check of the ABCs and then branches to either the rapid trauma assessment or focused history and physical assessment. The patient with a serious mechanism of injury, altered mental status, or multi-system trauma receives a rapid trauma assessment, a fast, systematic physical assessment evaluating body regions where serious or life-threatening problems are likely to occur. This assessment is a rapid evaluation of the critical structures and regions of the head (HEENT), neck, chest, abdomen, pelvis, extremities, posterior body, and vital signs. The patient with isolated trauma has an assessment directed at the areas of expected injury or patient complaint.

25. Describe the elements of the rapid trauma assessment and discuss their evaluation. pp. 365-371

Each region of the body is inspected, palpated, and, as appropriate, auscultated and percussed to identify the signs of injury (DCAP-BTLS and crepitation). For each region, the specific assessment considerations include the following:

Evaluate the **head** for any signs of serious bleeding and deformity from skull fracture. Also check for discharge from the ears and nose, for the stability of the facial bones, and for the patency of the airway.

Evaluate the **neck** for lacerations involving the major blood vessels and serious hemorrhage and possible air embolism. Examine the jugular veins for abnormal distention and palpate the position and any unusual motion of the trachea. Also examine for subcutaneous emphysema and then any evidence of spinal trauma.

Evaluate the **chest** for signs of respiratory distress, including use of accessory muscles and retractions, and any signs of open wounds. Also observe the motion of the chest. Chest excursion should be bilaterally equal and symmetrical. Palpate for signs of clavicular or costal fracture and subcutaneous emphysema. Erythema may be present, but the frank ecchymotic discolouration of a contusion takes time to develop. Auscultate the lungs at the mid-axillary line for bilaterally equal breath sounds.

Evaluate the **abdomen** for exaggerated abdominal wall motion, and inspect and palpate for signs of injury, noting rigidity, guarding, tenderness, and rebound tenderness.

Evaluate the **pelvis** for signs of injury and apply pressure directed posteriorly and medially to the iliac crests and pressure directed posteriorly to the symphysis pubis to check for pelvic instability.

Evaluate the **extremities** for signs of injury, distal circulation, and innervation.

Evaluate the **posterior body** for signs of injury, and be especially watchful for potential signs of spinal injury.

Evaluate **vital signs,** first to establish a baseline, and then to obtain other readings to compare to that baseline. Evaluate direct pupil response to light during the rapid trauma assessment, but evaluate the other pupillary responses during more specific and directed evaluation.

Gather a patient **history** while you perform the rapid trauma assessment. This should include the elements of the SAMPLE assessment (**S**igns/Symptoms, **A**llergies, **M**edications, **P**ast medical history, **L**ast oral intake, and **E**vents preceding the incident).

26. Identify cases when the rapid assessment is suspended to provide patient care.   p. 365

The rapid trauma assessment is interrupted to provide patient care whenever you identify any life-threatening condition that can be quickly addressed. Just as you would suction the airway when you find it full of fluids during the initial assessment, you might provide pleural decompression during the rapid trauma assessment when you notice a developing tension pneumothorax. You might also administer oxygen to a patient who begins to display dyspnea and accessory muscle use during your chest examination. Other examples might include employing the PASG for the patient with the early signs of shock compensation and an unstable pelvic fracture found during the pelvic assessment or immediate provision of spinal immobilization upon noticing a neurologic deficit during the extremity exam.

27. Discuss the reason for performing a secondary assessment including the focused history and physical assessment.pp. 362, 374, 382

The focused history and secondary assessment is the third step (following the scene assessment and primary assessment) of the patient assessment process. It is an assessment directed at the areas where the signs of serious injury or illness are expected. It also draws upon a quick history to identify information supporting a specific diagnosis and elements critical to the continued care of the patient. The focused history and secondary assessment takes you quickly toward determining the nature of the illness or the existence of serious and specific injuries. It is performed in different ways for trauma patients with significant injuries or mechanisms of injury, trauma patients with isolated injuries, responsive medical patients, and unresponsive medical patients.

28. Describe when and why a detailed physical assessment is necessary.   p. 344

The detailed assessment is a combination of a detailed history and a comprehensive physical assessment either to identify or to learn more about the effects of an illness or injury on the body. It, in its entirety, is employed only when all other assessment and care procedures have been performed, most likely during transport to the hospital and then only for patients with serious trauma or disease. Since the seriously ill or injured patients require constant care, this assessment is rarely performed in the prehospital setting. However, portions of the detailed physical assessment are frequently employed to examine specific body regions, looking for expected signs of illness or injury.

29. Discuss the components of the secondary survey.   pp. 383-389

The secondary survey involves a comprehensive evaluation of each body region using the skills of inspection, palpation, auscultation, and percussion. It begins at the head and progresses downward to the extremities and includes the following:

Head. Inspect and palpate for any skull or facial asymmetry, deformity, instability, tenderness, unusual warmth, or crepitation. Look for the development of Battle's sign and periorbital ecchymosis.

Eyes. Carefully inspect the eye for shape, size, colouration, and foreign bodies as well as pupillary equality, light reactivity, consensual movement, and visual acuity.

Ears. Examine the external ear for signs of injury and the ear canal for hemorrhage or discharge.

Nose and sinuses. Palpate the external aspect of the nose and examine the nares for signs of injury, hemorrhage, discharge, and flaring. The nasal mucosa is rich in vasculature and may bleed heavily.

Mouth and pharynx. Examine the oral cavity for signs of injury and the potential for airway compromise. Notice any fluids or odors and examine tongue movement for signs of cranial nerve injury.

Neck. Briefly inspect the neck for signs of injury with special attention to open wounds and possible severe hemorrhage and air embolism. Palpate the trachea to identify any unusual movement and examine for jugular vein distention.

Chest and lungs. Observe the patient's breathing for symmetrical chest movement and respiratory pattern. Note any accessory muscle use, and auscultate and percuss for unusual findings. Look for signs of injury, and palpate for crepitation and tenderness.

Cardiovascular system. Look to the skin for pallor, and palpate a pulse for rate, rhythm, and strength. Auscultate for heart sounds, and locate the point of maximal impulse.

Abdomen. Inspect and palpate for signs of injury and rebound tenderness, rigidity, and guarding.

Pelvis. Observe the area, then place medial and posterior pressure on the iliac crests and posterior pressure on the symphysis pubis.

Genitalia. As needed, examine these organs for hemorrhage and, in the male, priapism.

Anus and rectum. If hemorrhage is present, inspect the anus and rectum and apply direct pressure to halt bleeding.

Peripheral vascular system. Inspect all four extremities, observing and palpating for signs of injury and skin colour, moisture, temperature, and capillary refill to assure distal circulation.

Musculoskeletal system. Palpate the musculature of the extremities, feeling for differences in muscle tone and the flexibility and the active and passive range of motion in joints.

Nervous system. Evaluate the nervous system by examining the following:

• **Mental status and speech.** Assess the patient's level of consciousness and orientation and compare these findings to earlier ones. Note speech patterns and the patient's appropriateness of dress and actions.

• **Cranial nerves.** Test the discrete cranial nerves that have not already been tested.

• **Motor system.** Inspect the patient's general body structure, positioning, muscular development, and coordination.

• **Sensory system.** Test for ability to sense pain, touch, position, temperature, and vibration over the extremities, and as necessary, the dermatomes.

• **Reflexes.** Test deep tendon reflexes with a reflex hammer, noting heightened or diminished responses. Test superficial abdominal reflexes and plantar response.

Vital signs. Repeat the evaluation of the vital signs including blood pressure, pulse, respiration, temperature, and pupillary response.

30. Explain what additional care is provided while performing the detailed secondary assessment.   pp. 383-389

Since the complete detailed secondary assessment is an elective assessment, any time a significant sign of injury or the patient's condition suggests a care step, perform that step. The same principle applies when a portion of the comprehensive secondary assessment is performed on a discrete body region after the focused history and secondary assessment.

31. Distinguish between the detailed secondary assessment that is performed on a trauma patient and that of the medical patient.   pp. 383-389

The detailed secondary assessment for the trauma patient focuses evaluation on the areas where signs of injury are expected based upon the mechanism of injury analysis or the patient's complaints (for example, examination for signs of anterior chest injury when an auto steering wheel is deformed). The detailed secondary assessment for the medical patient is directed to the areas of patient complaint as well as those areas where the signs of an expected illness might be found (for example, an examination for pitting edema in the dependent areas with the congestive heart failure patient). The history component of the assessment also differs with trauma and medical patients. With the trauma patient, you may gather an abbreviated (SAMPLE) history, while with the medical patient, you may perform a more in-depth history evaluation as described in Chapter 10, "History Taking."

32. Differentiate between patients requiring a detailed physical assessment and those who do not.   p. 383

The patients who receive a complete secondary assessment are patients with serious medical or trauma injuries. They receive the detailed secondary assessment during transport to the hospital after other important care measures have been employed. They represent a very small percentage of patients that you will treat because seriously ill or injured patients often require almost continuous care. *Portions* of the detailed exam will, however, be performed on many patients, and these portions will be directed at a body region where signs of injury or illness are expected. Patients receiving portions of the detailed exam include those with isolated injuries and those patients with stable medical problems. Seriously ill or injured patients may receive a detailed exam aimed at discovering significant signs of the pathology generally associated with cardiac, respiratory, vascular, abdominal, musculoskeletal, or nervous system problems.

33. Discuss the rationale for repeating the initial assessment as part of the ongoing assessment.   pp. 390-393

The initial assessment, with its examination of mental status and evaluation of the airway, breathing, and circulation, contains crucial elements of continuing patient assessment. These components of the initial assessment can quickly tell you when the patient is suffering from a life-threatening or serious problem and can help you monitor the patient's need for care. For this reason, these components are an integral part of any ongoing assessment.

34. Describe the components of the ongoing assessment.   pp. 390-393

The components of the ongoing assessment include reassessment of the pertinent elements of the initial assessment, focused history and secondary assessment or rapid trauma assessment, and vital signs and include:

> **Mental status.** Quickly reevaluate the patient's mental status to determine AVPU status or level of orientation.
> **Airway patency/breathing rate and quality.** Perform a quick check of airway patency and breathing rate, volume, and quality to assure respiration is adequate.
> **Pulse rate and quality.** Quickly reevaluate the pulse rate, strength, and regularity to assure they remain within normal limits.
> **Skin condition.** Quickly check the skin for moisture, temperature, and capillary refill to monitor distal perfusion.
> **Vital signs.** Reassess blood pressure and temperature (along with pulse and respiration) and compare to baseline findings to determine whether the patient's condition is improving, deteriorating, or remaining the same.
> **Focused assessment.** Quickly reevaluate the signs of injury/illness to identify any changes. This may include reevaluating pertinent negatives to rule out an evolving problem.
> **Effects of interventions.** Repeat the ongoing assessment soon after any major intervention to determine the intervention's impact on the patient's condition.
> **Transport priorities.** Based upon the findings of the ongoing assessment, either confirm or modify the patient's priority for care and transport.

35. Describe trending of assessment components.   pp. 390-393

Trending of the elements of the ongoing assessment—comparing of sequential findings—will suggest whether your patient's condition is improving, deteriorating, or remaining the same. This information prompts you to modify your priorities for patient care and transport, and may ultimately cause you to modify your field diagnosis.

36. Discuss medical identification devices and systems.   p. 372

Examine the patient's wrists, ankles, and neck for medical alert jewelry reflecting preexisting medical conditions such as diabetes, epilepsy, allergies, use of medications, and the like. Also check the wallet or purse for such information. This information may help you and the emergency department in prescribing care for the patient.

37. Given several preprogrammed and moulaged medical and trauma patients, provide the appropriate scene survey, initial assessment, focused assessment, detailed assessment, and ongoing assessments. pp. 342-393

During your classroom, clinical, and field training, you will assess real and simulated patients and develop management plans for them. Use the information presented in this text chapter, the information on patient assessment in the field presented by your instructors, and the guidance given by your clinical and field preceptors to develop good patient assessment skills. Continue to refine these skills once your training ends and you begin your career as a paramedic.

CONTENT SELF-EVALUATION

_____ **1.** Which component of the patient assessment process will be performed during patient transport for a trauma patient with an isolated injury?
- **A.** scene survey
- **B.** initial assessment
- **C.** focused history and secondary assessment
- **D.** secondary assessment
- **E.** ongoing assessment

_____ **2.** Which of the following is NOT a component of the scene assessment?
- **A.** body substance isolation
- **B.** general impression of the patient
- **C.** location of all patients
- **D.** mechanism of injury/nature of the illness analysis
- **E.** scene safety

_____ **3.** Which of the following body substance isolation devices will you employ with every patient you treat?
- **A.** latex or vinyl gloves
- **B.** protective eyewear
- **C.** face mask
- **D.** gown
- **E.** HEPA mask

_____ **4.** Whenever you plan to intubate a patient, you should wear:
- **A.** latex or vinyl gloves and a gown.
- **B.** protective eyewear, a gown, and a face mask.
- **C.** latex or vinyl gloves, protective eyewear, and a face mask.
- **D.** protective eyewear and a gown.
- **E.** latex or vinyl gloves.

_____ **5.** The intent of the safety analysis portion of the scene survey is to assure the safety of:
- **A.** the patient.
- **B.** bystanders.
- **C.** fellow responders.
- **D.** yourself.
- **E.** all of the above

_____ **6.** When called to a shooting or domestic disturbance, until the police arrive and secure the scene you should remain:
- **A.** several blocks away from the residence.
- **B.** in front of the residence.
- **C.** two buildings past the residence.

D. two buildings before the residence.

E. at the end of the block before the residence.

7. At which of the following incidents would you expect to discover more than one patient in your scene assessment?

A. a motorcycle accident

B. a carbon monoxide poisoning in a home

C. shortness of breath

D. a fall out of a tree

E. all of the above

8. Your anticipation of possible injuries based upon your analysis of the event is known as the:

A. mechanism of injury.

B. provisional diagnosis.

C. differential diagnosis.

D. index of suspicion.

E. kinetic analysis.

9. The combined strength, direction, and nature of forces that injured your patient is known as the :

A. mechanism of injury.

B. provisional diagnosis.

C. differential diagnosis.

D. index of suspicion.

E. kinetic analysis.

10. The initial assessment includes all of the following EXCEPT:

A. forming a general impression of the patient.

B. stabilizing the cervical spine as needed.

C. immobilizing of fractures.

D. assessing the airway.

E. assessing the circulation.

11. The general patient impression is:

A. your initial statement of the patient's primary problem.

B. your initial, intuitive evaluation of your patient.

C. your determination of the patient's clinical status.

D. the summary of your primary assessment findings.

E. a description of the location and position of the patient.

12. The purpose of the primary assessment is to:

A. determine the patient's primary problem.

B. establish the patient's neurological and cardiorespiratory status.

C. identify and correct immediately life-threatening patient conditions.

D. identify immediately or potentially life-threatening conditions.

E. establish the patient's clinical status.

13. If the mechanism of injury suggests the possibility of spinal injury, the cervical spine should be stabilized:

A. after the airway is established.

B. just before you attempt artificial ventilation.

C. before checking mental status.

D. after checking mental status.

E. at the end of the primary assessment.

14. The AVPU system is used to assess:

A. neurological status.

B. mental status.

C. airway status.

D. chance of brain injury.

E. cardiovascular status.

15. If you suspect spinal injury in an unconscious patient, you should:

A. open the airway using the modified jaw thrust.

B. open the airway using the head-tilt/chin-lift.

C. open the airway using the cross-over finger technique.
D. place the patient in the lateral recumbent position.
E. insert a nasopharyngeal airway.

16. A noisy airway with snoring sounds often indicates:
A. respiratory burns.
B. upper airway obstruction due to foreign body obstruction or swelling.
C. the presence of fluid in the posterior pharynx.
D. constriction of the lower bronchial tubes due to bronchospasm.
E. partial obstruction of the upper airway by the tongue or epiglottis.

17. Gurgling sounds indicate:
A. respiratory burns.
B. upper airway obstruction due to foreign body obstruction or swelling.
C. the presence of fluid in the posterior pharynx.
D. constriction of the lower bronchial tubes due to bronchospasm.
E. partial obstruction of the upper airway by the tongue or epiglottis.

18. A high-pitched screeching sound on inspiration is usually caused by:
A. lower airway obstruction due to swelling.
B. upper airway obstruction due to foreign body obstruction or swelling.
C. the presence of fluid in the posterior pharynx.
D. constriction of the lower bronchial tubes due to bronchospasm.
E. partial obstruction of the upper airway by the tongue or epiglottis.

19. For stridor that is caused by respiratory burns, the care procedure most likely to maintain the airway is:
A. suctioning.
B. blow-by oxygen and a quiet ride to the hospital.
C. a surgical airway.
D. early endotracheal intubation.
E. vasoconstrictor medications.

20. Abnormally shallow, rapid respirations, altered mental status, accessory muscle use, and cyanosis are signs of:
A. respiratory distress.   **D.** inadequate respirations.
B. respiratory arrest.   **E.** hypopneic.
C. apnea.

21. A patient with abnormally deep respirations is said to be:
A. hyperpneic.   **D.** bradypneic.
B. tachypneic.   **E.** hypopneic.
C. eupneic.

22. The presence of a radial pulse suggests that the systolic blood pressure is at least:
A. 40 mmHg.   **D.** 100 mmHg.
B. 60 mmHg.   **E.** 120 mmHg.
C. 80 mmHg.

23. The presence of a carotid pulse suggests that the systolic blood pressure is at least:
A. 40 mmHg.   **D.** 100 mmHg.
B. 60 mmHg.   **E.** 120 mmHg.
C. 80 mmHg.

24. Mottled, cyanotic, pale, ashen skin often indicates:
A. poor perfusion.   **D.** hypertension.
B. carbon monoxide poisoning.   **E.** emphysema.
C. diabetic ketoacidosis.

25. Which of the following patients would you consider stable and continue with assessment and treatment on scene?

A. 34 year-old confused woman with no peripheral pulses and a weak, irregular carotid pulse.
B. unresponsive pediatric patient with high fever who is vomiting frequently
C. 24 year-old man with multiple abrasions, found walking after a motorcycle accident at 60 kmh
D. conscious 56 year-old woman with a closed femur fracture
E. 5 year old girl who ingested several of her parents' medications with a pulse rate of 60/min.

26. The focused history and secondary assessment is conducted differently for the four different categories of patients. Which of the following is NOT one of those categories?
A. responsive medical patient
B. unresponsive medical patient
C. pediatric patient with altered consciousness
D. trauma patient with an isolated injury
E. trauma patient with a significant mechanism of injury

27. Which of the following is NOT a mechanism of injury that calls for rapid transport to the trauma center?
A. ejection from a vehicle
B. vehicle rollover
C. severe vehicle deformity in a high-speed crash
D. fall from less than 20 feet
E. bicycle collision with loss of consciousness

28. The decision to provide rapid transport of a patient to the trauma center is predicated upon either the mechanism of injury or the:
A. blood pressure reading.   D. clinical presentation.
B. patient's request.   E. none of the above
C. pulse oximetry reading.

29. Your patient was a pedestrian struck by a vehicle traveling at 65 kmh. The patient has bilateral femur fractures, one of which is compound. His radial pulse is rapid and easily felt. His breathing is a bit rapid, but full. His skin is pale, cool, and damp. You should:
A. perform a rapid trauma assessment, complete minimum stabilization, transport, and perform IV procedures en route.
B. complete minimum stabilization, transport, and perform a rapid trauma assessment and IV procedures en route.
C. perform a rapid trauma assessment, transport, stabilize fractures and perform IV procedures en route.
D. perform a rapid trauma assessment, perform IV procedures, splint fractures, then transport.
E. complete minimum stabilization, perform IV procedures, transport, and complete your rapid trauma assessment en route.

30. The rapid trauma assessment is a:
A. secondary assessment for trauma patients.
B. fast, systematic search for serious or life-threatening injuries.
C. systematic search for all injuries.
D. quick check to explore the nature of the primary problem.
E. thorough, but prioritized secondary assessment conducted once the unstable trauma patient is en route to hospital.

31. Scalp wounds tend to bleed heavily because:
A. there is a lack of a protective vasospasm mechanism.
B. hair interferes with the clotting mechanism.
C. the close proximity of the skull permits blood to flow quickly outward.
D. direct pressure is difficult to apply.
E. the scalp is a high blood pressure area.

32. Jugular vein distention in a patient placed in the semi-Fowler's position is:
   A.   normal for children, but unusual in adults.
   B.   a sign of hypertension.
   C.   a sign of hypotension.
   D.   an indication that something is inhibiting blood return to the chest.
   E.   an indication that something is inhibiting blood flow away from the heart.

33. Subcutaneous emphysema is best described as:
   A.   a grating sensation.
   B.   air trapped under the skin.
   C.   air leaking from the respiratory system.
   D.   retraction of the tissues between the ribs.
   E.   fluid accumulation just beneath the skin.

34. Suprasternal and intercostal retractions are caused by:
   A.   tension pneumothorax.   D.   flail chest.
   B.   subcutaneous emphysema.   E.   high intrathoracic pressure.
   C.   airway obstruction or restriction.

35. To assure adequate air exchange for the patient with a flail chest, you should:
   A.   perform a needle decompression.
   B.   assist ventilations with a BVM and oxygen.
   C.   apply oxygen only.
   D.   perform an endotracheal intubation.
   E.   cover the wound with an occlusive dressing.

36. When assessing the pelvis for possible fracture, you should apply:
   A.   anterior pressure on the iliac crests.
   B.   lateral pressure on the symphysis pubis.
   C.   firm pressure on the lower abdomen.
   D.   medial and posterior pressure on the iliac crests.
   E.   pressure to move the hips to the flexed position.

37. Your finding that a patient is able to move a limb, but the limb is cool, pale, and without a pulse is consistent with:
   A.   neurologic compromise.
   B.   vascular compromise.
   C.   both a vascular and neurologic compromise.
   D.   spinal injury.
   E.   peripheral nerve root injury.

38. The SAMPLE history is appropriate for:
   A.   major trauma cases only.   D.   conscious trauma patients only.
   B.   minor trauma cases only.   E.   unconscious trauma patients only.
   C.   all trauma patients.

39. With a patient who has a crushing injury to his index finger received when it was caught in a closing door, which form of patient assessment would be most reasonable?
   A.   the rapid trauma assessment and a SAMPLE history
   B.   the rapid trauma assessment and a detailed history
   C.   a detailed secondary assessment
   D.   a detailed patient history and a secondary assessment focused on the injury
   E.   a SAMPLE history and a secondary assessment focused on the injury

40. While gathering the history of a chest pain patient, you will likely:
   A.   attach a cardiac monitor.   D.   start an IV, if appropriate.
   B.   administer oxygen.   E.   all of the above
   C.   take vital signs.

41. When obtaining the History of the Present Illness from a responsive medical patient, you should use the:
- **A.** SAMPLE history.
- **B.** DCLAP-BTLS mnemonic.
- **C.** OPQRST-ASPN acronym.
- **D.** AVPU model.
- **E.** systems inquiry approach.

42. Once you have obtained the history in a responsive medical patient, you should:
- **A.** transport with further assessment en route.
- **B.** initiate definitive treatment.
- **C.** perform a detailed physical assessment.
- **D.** begin a focused secondary survey.
- **E.** transport with further treatment en route.

43. If you hear bilateral rales on inspiration when auscultating a patient's chest, you should suspect:
- **A.** congestive heart failure.
- **D.** chronic obstructive pulmonary disease.
- **B.** bronchospasm.
- **E.** all of the above
- **C.** asthma.

44. In a patient who displays hyperresonance to percussion, you should suspect:
- **A.** pleural effusion.
- **D.** emphysema.
- **B.** pulmonary edema.
- **E.** none of the above
- **C.** pneumonia.

45. Vital signs provide the paramedic with:
- **A.** a window into what is happening with the patient.
- **B.** an objective capsule of the patient's clinical status.
- **C.** possible indications of severe illness.
- **D.** possible indications of the need to intervene.
- **E.** all of the above

46. A pulse oximetry reading of 88 percent would indicate the need for:
- **A.** aggressive airway and ventilatory care.
- **B.** administration of blow-by oxygen.
- **C.** repositioning of the patient's head.
- **D.** no care at this point.
- **E.** careful monitoring of the patient for further deterioration.

47. Obtain a blood glucose reading for patients with:
- **A.** head injuries.
- **D.** an isolated medical problem.
- **B.** altered mental status.
- **E.** all patients.
- **C.** hypotension.

48. The detailed secondary assessment is most likely performed for:
- **A.** the severe trauma patient.
- **D.** the unresponsive medical patient.
- **B.** the minor trauma patient.
- **E.** both A and D
- **C.** the responsive medical patient.

49. Paramedics employ the complete secondary assessment at the scene:
- **A.** rarely.
- **B.** occasionally.
- **C.** frequently.
- **D.** rarely in trauma patients, frequently in medical patients.
- **E.** frequently in trauma patients, rarely in medical patients.

50. You should reassess your unresponsive medical patient:
- **A.** at least once en route to hospital.
- **B.** every 5 minutes.

C. every 15 minutes.
D. whenever you have time between other treatment activities.
E. upon arrival at the hospital.

True/False

_____ **51.** As a paramedic, you will certainly never perform a comprehensive history and secondary assessment in the acute setting.
A. True
B. False

_____ **52.** The goal of the primary assessment is to identify and correct immediately life-threatening conditions.
A. True
B. False

_____ **53.** You should delay the call for additional ambulances until you begin your initial assessment because you will not have enough information to determine the needs of the scene until then.
A. True
B. False

_____ **54.** The two functions that must be assumed by the first arriving EMS unit in the mass casualty situation are incident command and scene isolation.
A. True
B. False

_____ **55.** You should have a higher index of suspicion for complications to injury when dealing with the very young and the very old.
A. True
B. False

_____ **56.** If you suspect the potential for spinal injuries, you should have your partner manually stabilize the head and neck after you assess the patient's mental status.
A. True
B. False

_____ **57.** You should be conservative when extending the head and neck of infants and young children as their upper airway structures are very flexible.
A. True
B. False

_____ **58.** Tachypnea and hyperpneia are compensatory mechanisms that suggest the body is trying to rid itself of excess acids.
A. True
B. False

_____ **59.** You should consider the patient of a motor vehicle rollover incident as unstable, even if she was wearing a seatbelt.
A. True
B. False

_____ **60.** A patient with multiple injuries usually complains about the most serious injury.
A. True
B. False

_____ **61.** Because most life-threatening injuries occur to the head or thorax, the limbs of a major trauma patient should be assessed in the secondary survey, not the rapid trauma assessment.
A. True
B. False

62. If you find a depression in the skull during your rapid trauma assessment, you must carefully palpate to find the margins of the injury.
    A.   True
    B.   False

63. When comparing bilateral breath sounds on the chest of a trauma patient, unequal air movement may indicate the presence of a pneumothorax or hemothorax.
    A.   True
    B.   False

64. Young children with a lower airway obstruction often grunt in an effort to create back pressure and maintain an open airway.
    A.   True
    B.   False

65. Patients who present with wheezing will likely require bronchodilators.
    A.   True
    B.   False

66. Bruising over the umbilical area or flanks indicating intra-abdominal hemorrhage generally develops early.
    A.   True
    B.   False

67. If you cannot palpate a pulse in an injured limb, you should assess the adequacy of perfusion by checking the temperature, colour, and condition of the skin in the extremity.
    A.   True
    B.   False

68. The SAMPLE model is an abbreviated history that is particularly useful for seriously injured patients or when time is critical.
    A.   True
    B.   False

69. "Normal" values in medical tests represent the range of values found in 75% of the healthy population.
    A.   True
    B.   False

70. In most cases you will perform standard medical care authorized by standing orders before contacting online medical direction for other orders.
    A.   True
    B.   False

Matching

Write the letter of the injury or condition in the space provided next to the assessment finding to which it applies.

Injury or condition

    A. stroke or brain injury
    B. spinal injury
    C. flail chest
    D. cardiac tamponade
    E. pneumothorax
    F. tension pneumothorax
    G. airway obstruction

H. intra-abdominal hemorrhage
I. vascular compromise
J. peripheral nerve damage
J. pelvic fracture

Assessment Finding

_____ **71.** injured limb with no distal pulse and pale, ashen skin.

_____ **72.** Cullen's sign (bruising over the umbilicus).

_____ **73.** paradoxical movement.

_____ **74.** subcutaneous emphysema.

_____ **75.** absent breath sounds on one side, with diminished sounds on the other side.

_____ **76.** exaggerated abdominal wall motion.

Write the letter of the injury or condition in the space provided next to the assessment finding to which it applies.

Injury or condition

A. pulmonary edema
B. hypovolemia
C. cardiac tamponade
D. tension pneumothorax
E. upper airway obstruction
F. lower airway obstruction
G. congestive heart failure
H. asthma
I. pulmonary embolism
J. pneumonia
K. thoracic aneurysm
L. brain hypoxia
M. brain anoxia

Assessment Finding

_____ **77.** fixed, dilated pupils.

_____ **78.** dullness in percussion of the chest.

_____ **79.** unequal pulses in the upper extremities.

_____ **80.** prolonged expiratory phase.

_____ **81.** jugular vein distention in a sitting patient.

_____ **82.** localized wheeze.

_____ **83.** bilateral inspiratory rales

_____ **84.** pitting edema in the lower limbs

_____ **85.** flat jugular veins when patient is supine

Chapter 8

Communications

Review of Chapter Objectives

With each chapter of the Workbook, we identify the objectives and the important elements of the text content. You should review these items and refer to the pages listed if any points are not clear.

After reading this chapter, you should be able to:

1. Identify the role and importance of verbal, written, and electronic communications in the provision of EMS.   p. 397-402

EMS is a team endeavor that requires effective communications among the various participants in the response and patient care. This communication is between you and the emergency dispatcher, the patient, his family, bystanders, other emergency response personnel, such as police, fire, and rescue personnel, and health care professionals from physicians' offices, clinics, and emergency departments, and finally with the medical direction physician. These communications, be they oral, written, or electronic, establish the key links that assure the best patient outcome.

2. Describe the phases of communications necessary to complete a typical EMS response.

Detection and citizen access pp. 399-400
This marks the initial entry point into the emergency service system at which a party identifies that an emergency exists and then requests EMS assistance through a universal entry number such as 911 or some other mechanism.

Call taking p. 400
This is the stage of EMS response in which a call taker questions the caller about the reported emergency in order to identify its exact location, determine the nature of the call, and initiate an appropriate response.

Emergency response   p. 400
This phase includes the activities occurring from the moment a dispatcher requests a response by an EMS unit until the call concludes with the unit back in service. It includes various radio, face-to-face, and written communications among the dispatcher, emergency response crews, the patient, family and bystanders, and health care professionals, including the medical direction physician.

Prearrival instructions   pp. 400-401
These are a series of predetermined, medically approved instructions given by the dispatcher to the caller to help the caller provide some patient support until EMS personnel arrive.

Call coordination and incident recording   pp. 401

These terms refer to the interactions between the dispatcher and the responding units that assure an efficient and appropriate response. Call coordinating, for example, might involve changing the mode of response and the number and type of responding units. Incident recording refers to the logging of times associated with various response activities and the tape recording of communications associated with the call.

Discussion with medical direction   p. 401

This is the opportunity for the care provider to describe the patient he or she is caring for and to obtain approval from the medical direction physician to initiate invasive or advanced life support procedures. Communication with medical direction also permits the emergency department to prepare for the patient's arrival.

Transfer communications   p. 402

These are the communications that occur between the first responder and the paramedic or as the patient is delivered to the emergency department. They are intended to communicate the results of the assessment, the care given, and the patient's response to care prior to the arrival of the paramedic or arrival at the emergency department.

3. List factors that impede and enhance effective verbal and written communications. pp. 397-398

The factors impacting effective verbal or written communications are either semantic (dealing with the meaning of words) or technical (hardware).

In the area of semantics, the use of standard codes and plain English in verbal communications enhances good and clear communications, while use of nonstandard codes and jargon may confuse it. The same holds true for written communication. Nonstandard abbreviations and subjective, sloppy, incomplete, or illegible documentation leads to confusion and miscommunication. Complete, objective, legible, and efficient documentation leads to an efficient transfer of information. A well-designed prehospital care report makes written communication easier.

In the technical area, a well-designed and maintained radio or phone communications system will go a long way in assuring good and dependable communications. Improperly maintained or operated radios will, on the other hand, likely provide only intermittent and poor quality communication.

4. Explain the value of data collection during an EMS response.   pp. 398,406

The written call report is a record that includes the patient's name and address, scene location, agency responding, crew on board, and the times associated with response, arrival, and transport to a care facility. It also contains the results of the assessment and care of the patient. This administrative information can be used to bill for services and improve EMS system efficiency, by quality assurance/improvement committees to improve system performance, and by educators and researchers to identify what the system is doing and the impacts of its interventions. Finally, the call report becomes a legal record of the incident and the EMS care provided or offered.

5. Recognize the legal status of verbal, written, and electronic communications related to an EMS response.   pp. 397-398, 409-410

The legal guidelines that apply to verbal and written communication in emergency medical service also apply to electronic communications. The information in these communications is considered confidential and must only be released in approved circumstances. The reports must be objective and not demean, libel, or slander another person. Any such action is accountable in a court of law.

6. Identify current and new technology used to collect and exchange patient and/or scene information electronically.   pp. 403-406

Cellular phones today provide duplex communications directly from the patient's side to the emergency department. These lightweight and versatile devices enhance EMS-to-physician communications and permit excellent ECG transmission. The only disadvantages to cell phones are user fees and unreliability at peak times.

Another electronic aid to dispatch is the facsimile or fax machine. It permits dispatch to send hard copy to the responding unit's station, assuring that elements of the address and nature of the dispatch are communicated accurately.

Computers are also increasing the efficiency of the dispatch system by recording times and system action in real time and making data recovery and research much easier.

Other new technologies that may affect prehospital care include: the electronic touch pad, which allows rapid recording of patient information; the handheld computer, which uses a pen-based system to log patient information and times associated with the emergency response and care; electronic transmission of diagnostic information (including pulse oximetry, 12-lead ECG, blood sugar, and end-expiratory CO_2 monitoring) provided directly to the emergency department, which may change the degree and number of field interventions permitted. In the future, voice recognition software may make real-time narrative recording of patient evaluation and interventions at the emergency scene and during transport a reality.

7. Identify the various components of the EMS communications system and describe their function and use.   p.396,399-402

The emergency medical dispatcher (EMD) is the person who takes the call for assistance, dispatches the appropriate units, monitors the call's progress, and assures that the pertinent response data is recorded. He or she may guide the caller through initial emergency care using prearrival instructions.

The patient, his family, and bystanders are responsible for detecting the emergency, accessing the emergency response system, and relaying information about the cause and nature of the emergency to EMS system personnel. Since they are not trained in emergency medical communication, the responsibility of assuring good communications falls on the members of the EMS system. Personnel from other responding agencies such as the police, fire service, rescue, and other ambulance services are also individuals who provide information important to assuring proper EMS response, and their input must be taken into account to assure scene coordination and optimum utilization of resources.

Health care professionals (aides, nurses, physician assistants, nurse practitioners, and physicians) at clinics, physicians' offices, and emergency departments are important people in the EMS system. They can provide invaluable information about the patient and the care he or she has had or should receive.

Finally, the medical director and medical direction physicians are significant resources for the prehospital emergency care provider. They are the individuals who extend their licenses to paramedics, thereby permitting them to practice prehospital care. These physicians also represent a body of knowledge of emergency medicine that may be tapped while paramedics are at the scene, en route with a patient, or at the emergency department for guidance regarding patient care.

8. Identify and differentiate among the following communications systems:

Simplex   p. 403
This refers to a radio or communication system that uses only one frequency and allows only one unit to transmit at a time. With this type of communication, one party must wait until the speaking party completes his message before beginning to speak.

Multiplex   p. 403
This is a duplex system with an additional capability of transmitting data, like an ECG strip, simultaneously with voice.

Duplex   p. 403
This is a radio or communication system that uses two frequencies for each channel, thus permitting two units to transmit and listen at the same time. This is similar to telephone communication, where one party can interrupt the other.

Trunked systems   p. 403
These are computer-controlled systems that pool all radio frequencies and assign transmissions to unused frequencies to assure the most efficient use of available communications channels.

Digital communications systems   pp. 403-404

These systems translate analog sounds into digital code for transmissions that are less prone to interference and are more compact than analog (normal voice) communications. This type of a system can be enhanced with devices like the mobile data terminal, which displays information such as street addresses, and can prompt the responder to send information like "arrived."

Cellular telephones p. 404

These are part of a multiplex radio-telephone system tied to a computer that uses radio towers to transmit signals in regions called cells. The technology is inexpensive but can accrue substantial monthly charges; the transmissions may be interrupted by certain geographic features; and heavy use at peak times may limit access to the system.

Facsimile machines p. 404

These devices transmit and receive printed information through telephone or wireless communication systems. Such a machine might give a responding unit a print-out of the nature and street address of the call or, possibly, detailed medical information about it.

Computers p. 405

The use of these devices in EMS is expanding rapidly. They are already helping to analyze data for review of calls and dispatches. Portable input devices, such as the touch pad and handheld computer, are being developed to permit recording of emergency response events in the field. In the future, paramedics may use computers with voice recognition software to complete prehospital care reports without paper.

9. Describe the functions and responsibilities of the Federal Communications Commission.   pp. 409-410

Industry Canada controls and regulates radio communications in Canada. It assigns broadcast frequencies and has set aside several frequencies within each radio bandwidth for emergency medical services. Public safety frequencies are generally found in the VHF (very high frequency) range.

10. Describe the role of emergency medical dispatch and the importance of prearrival instructions in a typical EMS response.   pp. 399-402

The emergency medical dispatcher (EMD) is the first person in the EMS system that communicates with the scene and possibly the patient. He or she begins and coordinates the EMS response and communications and assures data regarding the call are recorded. He or she also provides prearrival instructions to callers—for example, how to perform mouth-to-mouth artificial ventilation on an apneic patient—so that emergency care can begin as early as possible, thus helping to maintain the victim until trained prehospital personnel can arrive.

11. List appropriate caller information gathered by the emergency medical dispatcher. p. 400

The information that is gathered by the EMD to determine the response priority and that is then communicated to the appropriate responding EMS service includes:
• Caller's name
• Call-back number
• Location or address of the event
• Nature of the call
• Any additional information necessary to prioritize the call

12. Describe the structure and importance of verbal patient information communication to the hospital and medical direction.   pp. 406-409

The verbal patient report to hospital personnel and the medical direction physician is essential to assure the efficient transfer and continuity of care. It consists of the following:
• Information identifying the care provider and level of training
• Patient identification information (name, age, sex, etc.)

• Subjective patient data (chief complaint, additional symptoms, past history, etc.)
• Objective patient data (vital signs, pulse oximetry readings, etc.)
• Plan for care of patient

For the trauma patient, the information and order of presentation is the same, although the subjective and objective information are modified to include mechanism of injury and suspected injuries.

13. Diagram a basic communications system. p. 397-398

Basic communication is the process of exchanging information between individuals. A model for a communications system should start with an idea, followed by the encoding of that idea into useful language, sending the encoded message via a medium (direct voice, radio, or written), having another person receive and decode the message, and ultimately, receiving feedback from the original message.

14. Given several narrative patient scenarios, organize a verbal radio report for electronic transmission to medical direction.   pp. 406-409

During your classroom, clinical, and field training, you will communicate with various elements of the EMS system, including dispatchers, patients, family members, bystanders, other EMS and scene personnel, and health care professionals, including medical direction physicians. Use the information presented in this text chapter, the information on communication presented by your instructors, and the guidance given by your clinical and field preceptors to develop good communication skills. Continue to refine these skills once your training ends and you begin your career as a paramedic.

CONTENT SELF-EVALUATION

_____ 1. Essential participants in communications within the EMS system include:
A.   the emergency medical dispatcher.
B.   the patient, his family, or bystanders.
C.   other responders, including police, fire, and other ambulance personnel.
D.   health care providers, including nurses, physicians, and medical direction physicians.
E.   all of the above

_____ 3. Because different systems have used similar codes to mean different things, a recent trend in EMS communications is to:
A.   use plain English instead of 10 codes.
B.   use plain English alongside 10 codes.
C.   standardize the use of 10 codes across the country.
D.   move to alpha-numeric code systems.
E.   use alpha-numeric codes alongside 10 codes.

_____ 3. The communication network element that receives low power transmissions and rebroadcasts them at a higher power is called a:
A.   microwave link.
B.   remote console.
C.   portable radio.
D.   repeater.
E.   base station.

_____ 4. A radio band is a:
A.   series of radios that communicate one with another.
B.   pair of radio frequencies used for multiplexing.
C.   range of radio frequencies.
D.   pair of radio frequencies used for duplexing.
E.   none of the above

5. The frequency band penetrates concrete and steel well and is preferred for urban communications is:
   A. UHF (ultra high frequency).
   B. VHF (very high frequency).
   C. HF (high frequency).
   D. LF (low frequency).
   E. VLF (very low frequency).

6. The frequency band travels farther and over varied terrain well and is preferred for rural communications is:
   A. UHF (ultra high frequency).
   B. VHF (very high frequency).
   C. HF (high frequency).
   D. LF (low frequency).
   E. VLF (very low frequency).

7. Which of the following statements about your prehospital care report (PCR) is true?
   A. Your PCR must be kept on file for at least 3 years.
   B. You must have your PCR signed on arrival at the receiving institution.
   C. Your PCR is a legal record of the call and becomes part of your patient's medical record.
   D. Your PCR is a privileged document and cannot be used in court without your permission.
   E. All of the above statements are true

8. Use of proper terminology in both written and verbal communications will:
   A. decrease the length of communications.
   B. increase the accuracy of communications.
   C. increase the clarity of communications.
   D. reduce the ambiguity in communications.
   E. all of the above

9. Features of the enhanced 911 centre include all of the following EXCEPT:
   A. display of the caller's location.
   B. display of the caller's phone number.
   C. immediate call-back ability.
   D. a system of physician/ambulance interface.
   E. both B and C.

10. The answering centre for emergency calls that then transfers them to the appropriate agency for dispatch is the:
   A. enhanced 911 centre.   **D.** Emergency Routing Centre.
   B. PSAP.   **E.** none of the above
   C. GPS.

11. The automobile computers, which provide information about the location, speed, type of collision, and suspected severity of damage are known as:
   A. GPS system.   **D.** mobile terminals.
   B. black boxes.   .   **E.** PSAP.
   C. enhanced data heads.

12. The system that uses standardized caller questioning to determine the level and type of response is:
   A. priority dispatching.   **D.** prearrival instructions packaging.
   B. system status management. **E.** dispatch triage.
   C. enhanced emergency medical dispatch.

13. The role of the modern-day emergency medical dispatcher includes:

A. priority dispatching.
B. prearrival instructions.
C. call coordinating.

D. incident recording.
E. all of the above

14. The service in which the EMD gives emergency care instructions to the caller at the scene is known as:
A. priority dispatching.
B. prearrival instructions.
C. call coordination.
D. emergency medical life support.
E. online medical direction.

15. Which of the following is NOT generally used for facilitating communication between paramedics on the scene and medical direction physicians?
A. radio
B. landline telephone
C. cellular telephone

D. facsimile machine
E. all of the above are generally used

16. The report that occurs as you transfer patient responsibilities to the emergency department staff must include:
A. chief complaint.
B. assessment findings.
C. care rendered.

D. results of care.
E. all of the above

17. A radio system that transmits and receives on the same frequency is called:
A. simplex.
B. duplex.
C. triplex.

D. multiplex.
E. trunking.

18. Which radio transmission design permits the receiver to interrupt the caller while the caller is talking?
A. simplex
B. duplex
C. multiplex

D. trunking
E. none of the above

19. A radio system that allows simultaneous two-way voice communication and data transmission is called:
A. simplex.
B. duplex.
C. triplex.

D. multiplex.
E. trunking.

20. The radio system that uses a computer to determine and assign available frequencies is called:
A. simplex.
B. duplex.
C. multiplex.

D. trunking.
E. none of the above

21. Mobile data terminals are devices that:
A. provide dispatch with geographic location and speed on all ambulances.
B. provide basic digital communications between emergency vehicles and dispatch.
C. record a digital patient care record at the scene.
D. record vehicle use data such as speed, acceleration, braking, and rotational forces.
E. transmit patient data such as ECG, pulse, and blood pressure from the field to the base hospital.

22. Advantages of cellular communications in EMS include all of the following EXCEPT:
A. duplex capability.
B. allowing direct physician/patient communication.
C. inability of people with scanners to monitor calls.

D. reduced on-line times.
E. transmission of better ECG signals.

23. All of the following are appropriate for good EMS communications EXCEPT:
A. speaking close to the microphone.
B. speaking across or directly into the microphone.
C. talking in a normal tone of voice.
D. speaking without emotion.
E. taking time to explain everything in detail.

24. If the portable radio you are using is unable to transmit well from your location, attempt to:
A. move to higher ground.
B. touch the antenna to something metal.
C. tilt the antenna to a 45 degree angle.
D. hold the transmit button down for two seconds before beginning to speak.
E. change to an alternate channel that may have better reception.

25. Radio communications in Canada are regulated by:
A. Industry Canada and the Spectrum Management branch.
B. Department of Communications.
C. Canadian Radio-television and Telecommunications Commission.
D. Federal Communications Commission.
E. various provincial and territorial communications regulatory bodies.

True/False

26. In general, the use of codes decreases the radio time and increases the recipient's understanding of the message, which has led many EMS systems to adopt extensive use of codes for their communications.
A. True
B. False

27. Priority dispatch refers to the process of prioritizing resources within an EMS based on the severity of the call and distance to the scene.
A. True
B. False

28. An EMS system should record any communications between paramedics on the scene and online medical personnel.
A. True
B. False

29. Your ability to transmit clear, concise, controlled reports is key to helping medical directors develop trust in your judgment and decisions.
A. True
B. False

30. If the receiving nurse or physician is unable to receive your verbal report, it is appropriate to give your completed patient care report and clear the hospital.
A. True
B. False

31. Many EMS systems require the receiving physician or medical director to sign the PCR for any medications administered by paramedics.
A. True
B. False

32. Duplex radio systems encourage a much freer discussion and consultation between paramedics and physicians.
   A.   True
   B.   False

33. Digital data and voice transmission is much faster and much more accurate than analog transmission.
   A.   True
   B.   False

34. You should use the same format and provide the same type of information when transmitting patient reports about medical or trauma patients.
   A.   True
   B.   False

35. Using the echo procedure when receiving directions from a dispatcher or orders from a physician helps ensure that the relayed information is accurately understood.
   A.   True
   B.   False

Matching

Write the letter of the appropriate definition in the space provided next to the radio code or term to which it applies.

Definition

A. Meet with
B. Listen carefully to this
C. I understand
D. Please wait
E. We cannot find this incident/patient

F.   End of transmission
G.   Landing zone
H.   Wait before entering the scene
I.   Estimated time of arrival
J.   Please repeat what you said

Term

_____   **36.** stand by

_____   **37.** be advised

_____   **38.** stage

_____   **39.** copy

_____   **40.** clear

_____   **41.** say again

_____   **42.** LZ

_____   **43.** clear

_____   **44.** ETA

_____   **45.** rendezvous

Chapter 9

Documentation

Review of Chapter Objectives

With each chapter of the Workbook, we identify the objectives and the important elements of the text content. You should review these items and refer to the pages listed if any points are not clear.

After reading this chapter, you should be able to:

1. Identify the general principles regarding the importance of EMS documentation and ways in which documents are used. pp. 412-414

The principal EMS document, the prehospital care report (PCR), is the sole permanent written documentation of the response, assessment, care, and transport offered during an emergency call. It is a medical document conveying details of medical care and patient history that remains a part of the patient record as well as a legal document that may be reviewed in a court of law. The PCR may also be reviewed by medical direction to determine the appropriateness of your actions during the call and used by your service to bill the patient for services. Lastly, the PCR may be used by researchers to determine the effectiveness of care measures in improving patient outcomes.

2. Identify and properly use medical terminology, medical abbreviations, and acronyms. pp. 415, 417-420

Medical terminology is the very precise and exact wording used to describe the human body and injuries or illnesses. Proper use of this terminology turns the PCR into a medical document. However, if terms are misspelled or misused, they may distract from the document and confuse the reader about the patient's condition and the care he either has had or should receive. Carry a pocket dictionary, and only use words when you are sure of both their spelling and usage. The same holds true of medical abbreviations. They must be applied properly and have the same meaning to both the writer and reader. EMS systems should use a standardized set of abbreviations and acronyms to assure good and efficient documentation.

3. Explain the role of documentation in agency reimbursement. p. 413

Good documentation is essential for ambulance agencies that bill for services they provide. The PCR provides the name and address of the patient as well as the nature and circumstances of injury and illness. It also includes the care and transport provided. Without this information, the service may not be able to obtain reimbursement for services rendered and, ultimately, to afford to provide the vehicle, equipment, and personnel necessary to provide prehospital emergency care.

4. Identify and eliminate extraneous or nonprofessional information. p. 425

The ambulance call should be documented in a brief and professional way. The PCR describing it may be scrutinized by hospital staff, the medical direction physician, quality improvement committees, supervisors, lawyers, and the news media. Any derogatory comments, jargon, slang, biased statements, irrelevant opinions, or libelous statements will distract from the seriousness of the document and from acceptance of the preparer's professionalism.

5. Describe the differences between subjective and objective elements of documentation. pp. 425-427

Subjective information is information that you obtain from others or is your opinion that is not based on observable facts. It includes the patient's, family's, or bystander's description of the chief complaint and symptoms, medical history, and nature of the illness or mechanism of injury. **Objective information** is information you obtain through direct observation, palpation, auscultation, percussion, or diagnostic evaluation of your patient. It includes the vital signs and the results of the physical exam, including such things as glucose level determination and ECG monitor and pulse oximeter readings.

6. Evaluate a finished document for errors and omissions and proper use and spelling of abbreviations and acronyms.   pp. 422, 424-425

The PCR must contain all information obtainable and necessary for describing the patient's condition recorded in a clearly legible way. The report must be written so that another health care provider can easily understand what is being said and can mentally picture the scene, the patient presentation, the care rendered, and the transport offered by the initial providers. In many cases, what to include in the PCR is a judgment decision made by the care provider, though the report must contain an accurate description of the patient's medical or trauma problem and an accurate and complete history. Correct spelling and use of medical terms is essential and reflects the knowledge of the care provider. Proper use of abbreviations and acronyms can help make the PCR more concise; their improper use, however, may produce ambiguity, confusion, and misunderstanding in readers. Reread the finished PCR and check it carefully before submitting it.

7. Evaluate the confidential nature of an EMS report.   p. 435

Confidentiality is a patient right and breaching it can result in severe consequences. Do not discuss or share patient or call information with anyone not involved in the care of the patient. The only exceptions—as necessary—are administration, which may need information for billing; police agencies carrying out a criminal investigation; requests for the information under subpoena from a court; and quality assurance committees that may need the information (with the patient's name blocked out) for system review and improvement or for research.

8. Describe the potential consequences of illegible, incomplete, or inaccurate documentation. pp. 422, 424-425

A legible, complete, and accurate PCR is essential to call documentation. The information in it must be easy to read thanks to both good penmanship and conscientious attention to detail. The report must describe all the pertinent information gathered at the scene and en route to the hospital as well as all actions taken by you and others in the care of the patient. Failure to create a thorough, readable PCR reduces the information available to other care givers and may reduce their ability to provide effective care. The document you produce also reflects on your ability to provide assessment and care and your professionalism in general.

9. Describe the special documentation considerations concerning patient refusal of care and/or transport. pp. 431-432

Be careful in the documentation of a patient who refuses care and/or transport. While a conscious and mentally competent patient has the right to refuse care, his doing so may pose legal problems for care providers. Document the nature and severity of the patient's injuries, any care you offered, any care he refused, and document carefully the assessment criteria you used to determine the patient was capable of making the decision to refuse care or transport. Also document the patient's reasons for refusing care and your efforts to convince him to change his mind. If possible, have the refusal of care and your explanation to the patient of the consequences of care refusal signed by the patient and witnessed by family or bystanders or police. Advise the patient to seek other medical help, like his family physician, and to call EMS again if he changes his mind or his condition worsens.

10. Demonstrate how properly to record direct patient or bystander comments.   p. 421

Direct statements by patients and bystanders must be recorded exactly as they were made and the key phrases placed in quotation marks. Treating the information this way is highly important because it identifies that the information is directly from the source, not an interpretation. Identify clearly the source of any quotation you include in a PCR.

11. Describe the special considerations concerning mass casualty incident documentation. p. 433

Often a mass casualty situation calls for an atypical EMS response and unusual documentation procedures. Care providers rarely stay with a patient from the beginning to the end of prehospital care, and the time spent at a patient's side is very much at a premium. Hence documentation must be efficient and incremental. Document your assessment findings and any interventions you perform at the patient's side quickly and clearly. Many agencies or systems have their own forms such as triage tags that simplify the documentation procedure.

12. Demonstrate proper document revision and correction.   p. 424

Everyone makes mistakes during a health care career and during the process of care documentation. When this happens, it is essential to make corrections in such a way that there is no appearance of impropriety. If an error is made, draw a single line through the error and enter the correction and your initials. If the error is noted after the report is turned in, write a narrative addendum explaining both the nature of the error and the needed correction and assure that the addendum is included with all copies of the PCR. Correct errors as soon as possible after they are discovered.

13. Identify the types and describe the key elements of other professional correspondence. p. 434-435

Professional correspondence includes your patient care report, personal notebooks, occurrence reports, accident investigation reports, and illness/injury forms. Administrative correspondence includes payroll forms, personnel records, and scheduling documents. In addition, you may be required to write letters, reports, proposals, articles for local papers or journals, and other forms of correspondence. All well-written documents have a beginning, middle, and end. Well written documents are planned, concisely written, followed established formats, and are edited for spelling, grammar, and language.

13. Given a prehospital care report form and a narrative patient care scenario, record all pertinent administrative information using a consistent format, identify and record the pertinent reportable clinical data for each patient, correct errors and omissions using proper procedures, and note and record "pertinent negative" clinical findings.   pp. 412-435

During your classroom, clinical, and field training, you will complete various reports, including prehospital care reports, on the real and simulated patients you attend. Use the information presented in this text chapter, the information on documentation presented by your instructors, and the guidance given by your clinical and field preceptors to develop good documentation skills. Continue to refine these skills once your training ends and you begin your career as a paramedic.

CONTENT SELF-EVALUATION

_____   **1.** The prehospital care report is likely to be reviewed by which of the following?

A.	researchers	D.	medical professionals
B.	EMS administrators	E.	all of the above
C.	lawyers		

2. Which of the following is NOT an appropriate purpose for reviewing a prehospital care report?
   A. identify a chronological account of the patient's mental status
   B. learn about what calls other paramedics had
   C. help detect patient improvement or deterioration
   D. identify what bystanders and family may have said at the scene
   E. determine baseline assessment findings

3. Your best defense against a plaintiff's attempting to find inconsistencies and ambiguities in your account is:
   A. your partner's recollection.
   B. additional information from your personal notebook.
   C. a complete, accurate, and objective prehospital care record.
   D. substantiation of your assessment findings in the receiving hospital's records.
   E. dispatch tapes and records.

4. The prehospital care report should contain all of the following EXCEPT:
   A. a description of your patient's condition when you arrived.
   B. your opinions about the patient's attitude or social/economic situation.
   C. a description of your patient's condition after interventions.
   D. the medical status of your patient upon arrival at the emergency department.
   E. response time to the call.

5. A well-written prehospital care record avoids using:
   A. the patient's words.
   B. the oral statements of friends or family members.
   C. findings that rule out conditions that are not the cause of the patient's primary problem.
   D. abbreviations and acronyms due to their subjective nature.
   E. information that does not relate to the call or presenting problem.

6. Which of the following is NOT a time commonly recorded on the prehospital care report?

A.	call received	D.	arrival at the scene
B.	dispatch time	E.	departure from the scene
C.	arrival at the patient's side		

7. Which of the following is NOT an example of a pertinent negative?
   A. no shortness of breath in a myocardial infarction patient
   B. no history of epilepsy in a patient having seizures
   C. clear breath sounds in a congestive heart failure patient
   D. a blood pressure of 90/60
   E. no jugular vein distention in a congestive heart failure patient

8. The recommended way of indicating the exact words spoken by a patient or bystander is to:
   A. underline the passage.
   B. draw one line through the center of the word or passage.
   C. begin and end the passage with quotation marks.
   D. place the passage in parentheses.
   E. none of the above

9. The benefit of check boxes on a prehospital care report is that they:
   A. assure common information is recorded for every call.
   B. eliminate the need for a patient narrative.
   C. address every chief complaint.

D. speed the completion of the narrative.
E. all of the above

10. When should the prehospital care report be completed?
   A. at the end of the day
   B. at the end of your duty shift
   C. once back at quarters
   D. shortly after leaving the hospital
   E. immediately after completing the emergency call

11. If you make an error while writing your prehospital care report, you should:
   A. start a new record and shred the initial record.
   B. block the error out with multiple strike-through lines.
   C. simply cross through the error with one line and initial it.
   D. leave the error in place, but add the correction following the error.
   E. any of these are acceptable alternatives

12. What is the best way to add additional information to the prehospital care report after it has been submitted to the hospital?
   A. Search and make changes on all copies.
   B. Change only the original report.
   C. Create an addendum and add it to all reports.
   D. Never add additional material to the report once distributed.
   E. Send a memorandum to medical control.

13. Which of the following is the best example of a subjective and possibly libelous statement?
   A. "The patient smelled of beer."
   B. "The patient walked with a staggering gait."
   C. "The patient used abusive language and spoke with slurred speech."
   D. "The patient was drunk and obnoxious."
   E. None of the above is a potentially libelous statement.

14. Which of the following is a part of the subjective patient information?
   A. chief complaint
   B. patient's medications
   C. trends in vital signs
   D. head to toe (physical examination) findings
   E. all of the above

15. The portion of your narrative report that contains your general impression of the patient is the:
   A. subjective narrative.   **D.** SOAP plan.
   B. objective narrative.   **E.** none of the above
   C. assessment/management plan.

16. Which of the following is true about the body systems method of assessment?
   A. It focuses on general body areas.
   B. It is best suited to screening and preadmission assessments requiring comprehensive assessment of all body systems.
   C. It is best suited to medical patients with critical conditions.
   D. It is a comprehensive approach that is well suited to any unstable patient.
   E. It should not be used if the patient's primary problem involves only a single system.

17. SOAP and CHART are two common methods of:
   A. obtaining a critical history.
   B. ensuring that all critical interventions in the primary assessment are complete.

C. performing a physical assessment.
D. organizing a narrative report.
E. requesting additional orders from an online physician.

18. The management portion of your documentation should include which of the following?
    A. any interventions
    B. the results of ongoing assessments
    C. any changes in the patient's condition
    D. the patient's condition when care is transferred at the emergency department
    E. all of the above

19. Which of the following is NOT a part of the subjective information recorded on the PCR?
    A. vital signs
    B. past medical history
    C. review of systems
    D. chief complaint
    E. none of the above

20. Which of the following are elements of the objective information recorded on the PCR?
    A. family history
    B. history of the present illness
    C. the results of the physical exam
    D. diagnostic tests
    E. all of the above

21. SOAP and CHART are used because they:
    A. provide common information in a consistent and well organized format.
    B. allow the reader to focus on the critical actions taken during a critical call.
    C. provide a chronological account of your assessment.
    D. emphasize the mechanism of injury or history of the present illness.
    E. take a body-systems approach to documenting your findings.

22. The most significant feature of the patient management format of documentation is that it:
    A. focuses on the chief complaint.
    B. focuses exclusively on assessment findings.
    C. uses a free-flowing narrative style.
    D. is most frequently used for patients with minor injuries/problems.
    E. documents the chronological sequence of events and actions.

23. The call incident format for documenting an emergency response is best suited for:
    A. the unresponsive medical patient.
    B. the responsive medical patient.
    C. the trauma patient with no significant mechanism of injury.
    D. the trauma patient with a significant mechanism of injury.
    E. the trauma patient with an isolated injury.

24. If your patient refuses service against medical advice, it is important to:
    A. obtain the signature of the patient releasing the crew from liability.
    B. obtain the signature of the patient and at least two unbiased observers indicating that the patient refused care against advice.
    C. clearly document that the patient has an adequate mental status and understands your diagnosis, suggested treatments, and possible consequences of refusing care.
    D. consult with the patient's personal physician before allowing the patient to refuse.
    E. obtain the assistance of law enforcement officials to bring the patient to hospital.

25. When creating a report or other form of professional correspondence, you present and develop your ideas in the:
    A. introduction.
    B. body of the document.
    C. executive summary.

    D.   conclusion.

    E.   abstract.

True/False

_____ **26.** The PCR is the most comprehensive and reliable record of an ambulance call.

    A.   True

    B.   False

_____ **27.** The prehospital care report may yield information that the quality improvement committee may use to identify problems with individual paramedics or with the EMS system.

    A.   True

    B.   False

_____ **28.** Response time is the measure of elapsed time between when a unit is dispatched and when the crew arrives at the patient's side..

    A.   True

    B.   False

_____ **29.** Medical abbreviations and acronyms allow you to increase the amount of information that you can supply in your written reports.

    A.   True

    B.   False

_____ **30.** Since your watch, the dispatch clock, and other timing devices are not often synchronized, it is important to record all times on the PCR care report from one clock or watch when possible or to indicate when different clocks are used.

    A.   True

    B.   False

_____ **31.** During documentation of the physical exam, you do not have to record findings which are normal.

    A.   True

    B.   False

_____ **32.** It is better to quote the patient directly rather than paraphrasing or summarizing his or her words..

    A.   True

    B.   False

_____ **33.** On a layered response call or when an air-medical crew transports your patient, you must still document your assessment and treatment up to the point you transferred care.

    A.   True

    B.   False

_____ **34.** You should document a pediatric assessment in head-to-toe order, even though you may have performed it from toe-to-head.

    A.   True

    B.   False

_____ **35.** In a mass casualty situation you are still responsible for documenting a complete prehospital care record for all patients that you treat or transport.

    A.   True

    B.   False

Matching

Write the letter of the word or phrase in the space provided next to the appropriate abbreviation.

Phrase

A. shortness of breath
B. acute myocardial infarction
C. positive end-expiratory pressure
D. litres per minute
E. nausea/vomiting
F. do not resuscitate
G. breath sounds/blood sugar
H. cubic centimeter
I. not applicable
J. nitroglycerin
K. intraosseous
L. weight
M. sexually transmitted disease

N. against medical advice
O. congestive heart failure
P. chief complaint
Q. left lower quadrant
R. electrocardiogram
S. to keep open
T. central nervous system
U. intracranial pressure
V. jugular vein distention
W. treatment
X. motor vehicle collision
Y. year old

Abbreviation

_____ 36. CC

_____ 37. y/o

_____ 38. wt

_____ 39. CNS

_____ 40. SOB

_____ 41. n/v

_____ 42. AMI

_____ 43. CHF

_____ 44. ICP

_____ 45. MVC

_____ 46. STD

_____ 47. NTG

_____ 48. LLQ

_____ 49. BS

_____ 50. ECG

_____ 51. JVD

_____ 52. n/a

_____ 53. AMA

_____ 54. DNR

_____ 55. PEEP

_____ 56. Tx

_____ 57. IO

_____ 58. TKO

_____ 59. LPM

_____ 60. CC

Chapter 10

Clinical Decision Making

Review of Chapter Objectives

With each chapter of the Workbook, we identify the objectives and the important elements of the text content. You should review these items and refer to the pages listed if any points are not clear.

After reading this chapter, you should be able to:

1. **Compare the factors influencing medical care in the out-of-hospital environment to other medical settings.   p. 438**

   Most health care providers function in very controlled and supportive environments. The paramedic carries out the skills of other health care providers, but often does so in hostile and adverse conditions. Paramedics perform assessments, form field diagnoses, and devise and employ patient management plans at the scenes of emergencies in spite of poor weather, limited ambient light, limited diagnostic equipment, and few support personnel. The paramedic also must perform these skills under extreme constraints of time and often without on-scene consultation and supervision.

2. **Differentiate between critical life-threatening, potentially life-threatening, and non-life-threatening patient presentations.   pp. 438-439**

   Critical life-threatening presentations include major multi-system trauma, devastating single system trauma, end-stage disease presentations, and acute presentations of chronic disease. These patients may present with airway, breathing, neurological, or circulatory (shock) problems and demand aggressive resuscitation.

   Potential life-threatening presentations include serious multi-system trauma and multiple disease etiologies. Patient presentation generally includes moderate to serious distress. The care required is sometimes invasive but generally supportive.

   Non-life-threatening presentations are isolated and uncomplicated minor injuries or illness. The patient is stable without serious signs or symptoms or the need for aggressive intervention.

3. **Evaluate the benefits and shortfalls of protocols, standing orders, and patient care algorithms.   pp. 439, 440**

   Protocols are written guidelines identifying the specific management of various medical and trauma patient problems. They may also be developed for special situations such as physician-on-the-scene, radio failure, and termination of resuscitation. They provide a standard care approach for patients with "classical" presentations. They do not apply to all patients or to patients who present with multiple problems and should not be adhered to so rigidly as to limit performance in unusual circumstances.

   Standing orders are protocols that a paramedic can perform before direct on-line communication with a medical direction physician. They speed emergency care but may not address the atypical patient.

Patient care algorithms use flow-charts with lines, arrows, and boxes to outline appropriate care measures based on patient presentation or response to care. They are generally useful guides and encourage uniform patient care, but again, they do not adequately address the atypical patient.

4. **Define the components, stages, and sequences of the critical-thinking process for paramedics. pp. 439-443**

   Components of critical thinking include the following:

   ### Knowledge and Abilities
   Knowledge and abilities comprise the first component of critical thinking. Your knowledge of prehospital emergency care is the basis for your decisions in the field. This knowledge comes from your classroom, clinical, and field experience. It is used to sort out your patient's presentation to determine the likely cause of the problem and to select the appropriate care skills. Your abilities are the technical skills you employ to assess or care for a patient.

   ### Useful Thinking Styles
   • **Reflective vs. Impulsive Situation Analysis.** Reflective analysis refers to taking time to deliberately and analytically contemplate possible patient care, as might occur with unknown medical illness. Impulsive analysis refers to the immediate response that you must provide in a life-threatening situation, as might be required with decompensating shock or cardiac arrest.
   • **Divergent vs. Convergent Data Processing.** Divergent data processing considers all aspects of a situation before arriving at a solution and is most useful with complex situations. Convergent data processing focuses narrowly on the most important aspects of a situation and is best suited for uncomplicated situations that require little reflection.
   • **Anticipatory vs. Reactive Decision Making.** With anticipatory decision making, you respond to what you think may happen to your patient. With reactive decision making, you provide a care modality once the patient presents with a symptom.

   ### Thinking under Pressure
   Thinking under pressure is a difficult but frequent challenge of prehospital emergency medicine. The "fight or flight" response may diminish your ability to think critically to such an extent that you are only able to respond at the pseudo-instinctive level, with preplanned and practiced responses (like the mental checklist) that are performed almost without thought. One example of a mental checklist includes the following steps:
   Scan the situation by standing back and looking for subtle clues to the patient's complaint or problem.
   Stop and think of both the possible benefits and side effects of each of your care interventions.
   Decide and act by executing your chosen care plan with confidence and authority.
   Maintain control of the scene, patient care, and your own emotions, even under the stress of a chaotic scene.
   Reevaluate your patient's signs and symptoms and your associated care plan and make changes as the situation changes.

5. **Apply the fundamental elements of critical thinking for paramedics. pp. 445-447**
   Form a concept. Gather enough information from your first view of the patient and scene size-up to form a general impression of the patient's condition and the likely cause.
   Interpret the data. Perform the patient assessment and analyze the results in light of your previous assessment and care experience. Form a field diagnosis.
   Apply the principles. With the field diagnosis in mind, devise a management plan to care for the patient according to your protocols, standing orders, and patient care algorithms.
   Evaluate. Through frequent ongoing assessments, reassess the patient's condition and the effects of your interventions.
   Reflect. After the call, critique your call with the emergency department staff and your crew to determine what steps might be improved and add this call to your experience base.

6. **Describe the effects of the "fight or flight" response and its positive and negative effects on a paramedic's decision making.** p. 444

The "fight or flight" response is the intense activation of the sympathetic branch of the autonomic nervous system. Secretion of the system's major hormone, epinephrine, causes an increase in heart rate and cardiac output. It raises respiratory rate and volume, directs blood to the skeletal muscles, dilates the pupils (for distant vision), and increases hearing perception. However, the increased epinephrine may diminish critical thinking ability and concentration, impairing your ability to perform well in an emergency unless you raise your assessment and care skills to a pseudo-instinctive level, at which point acting under the pressure of an emergency becomes second nature.

7. **Summarize the "six Rs" of putting it all together.** p. 447

Read the scene. Observe the scene or general environment for clues to the mechanism of injury or nature of the illness.

Read the patient. Observe, palpate, auscultate, smell, and listen to the patient for signs and symptoms. Assure the ABCs and obtain a set of vital signs.

React. Address the priorities of care from the ABCs to other critical, then serious, then minor problems and care priorities.

Reevaluate. Conduct frequent ongoing assessments to identify any changes caused either by the disease or by your interventions.

Revise the management plan. Based on the ongoing assessments, revise your management plan to best serve your patient's changing condition.

Review performance. At the end of every response, critique the performance of your crew and identify ways to improve future responses.

8. **Given several preprogrammed and moulaged trauma and medical patients, demonstrate clinical decision making.** pp. 437-447

With your classroom, clinical, and field experience, you will assess and develop a management plan for the real and simulated patients you attend. Use the information presented in this text chapter, the information on clinical decision making presented by your instructors, and the guidance given by your clinical and field preceptors to develop good clinical decision-making skills. Continue to refine these skills once your training ends and you begin your career as a paramedic.

CONTENT SELF-EVALUATION

_____ 1. Which of the following terms best describes the first paramedics of the 1970s?
   A. field technician
   B. prehospital emergency care practitioner
   C. orderly
   D. field attendant
   E. field aide

_____ 2. Using your knowledge and experience to make critical decisions regarding patient care is known as:
   A. critical decision-making.   D. patient assessment.
   B. clinical judgment.   E. field assessment.
   C. making a provisional diagnosis.

_____ 3. The preliminary list of possible causes for your patient's problem is known as the:
   A. field diagnosis.   D. improvisation.
   B. differential diagnosis.   E. standing order.
   C. chief complaint.

_____ 4. The term describing the severity of a patient's condition is:

A. multiparity.
B. epiphysis.
C. tonicity.

D. acuity.
E. declivity.

5. The paramedic's final determination of the patient's most likely primary problem is known as the:
A. field diagnosis.
B. differential field diagnosis.
C. chief complaint.

D. improvisation.
E. standing order.

6. Which of the following situations is most likely to require a high level of critical thinking or clinical judgment?
A. closed femur fracture
B. pedestrian struck with multiple fractures and internal bleeding
C. 58 year-old male in cardiac arrest
D. syncope and chest pain in a 40 year-old woman with a history of diabetes
E. all of these patient require a high level of critical thinking.

7. A policy of administering nitroglycerin to a cardiac chest pain patient is an example of a(n):
A. protocol.
B. standing order.
C. algorithm.

D. special care enhancement.
E. proviso.

8. A policy by which nitroglycerin can be administered to a cardiac chest pain patient without a physician's order is an example of a(n):
A. protocol.
B. standing order.
C. algorithm.

D. special enhancement.
E. proviso.

9. Which of the following terms represents a flow chart of patient care procedures?
A. protocol
B. standing order
C. algorithm

D. special care enhancement
E. proviso

10. The major disadvantage to the use of protocols and standing orders is that they:
A. apply only to atypical patients.
B. often do not permit the paramedic to adapt to a patient's unique presentation.
C. only cover multiple disease etiologies.
D. address only patients with vague presentations.
E. restrict the options that paramedics have for creating a management plan.

11. When confronted with a complex emergency scene, you must:
A. be disciplined, stay focused, and follow your standard assessment process.
B. anticipate the most likely cause of your patient's problem and modify your standard assessment pattern to confirm your initial impression.
C. focus on the primary problem and do not allow potential complications to distract you.
D. consult with online medical direction early in the process.
E. be prepared to modify your protocols to meet the unique needs of the patient at hand.

12. The style of situation analysis that focuses on the most important aspect of a critical situation is:
A. reflective.
B. impulsive.
C. divergent.

D. convergent.
E. anticipatory.

13. The style of situation analysis that causes you to respond instinctively to a situation rather than to think about it is:

A.   reflective.   D.   convergent.
B.   impulsive.   E.   anticipatory.
C.   divergent.

14. The style of situation analysis that takes into account all aspects of a complex situation is:
A.   reflective.   D.   convergent.
B.   impulsive.   E.   anticipatory.
C.   divergent.

15. The style of situation analysis where you act thoughtfully, deliberately, and analytically is:
A.   reflective.   D.   convergent.
B.   impulsive.   E.   anticipatory.
C.   divergent.

16. The style of situation analysis that involves proactively considering possible ramifications of your actions is:
A.   reactive.   D.   convergent.
B.   impulsive.   E.   anticipatory.
C.   divergent.

17. The style of situation analysis where you deal with issues and events as they occur is:
A.   reactive.   D.   convergent.
B.   impulsive.   E.   anticipatory.
C.   divergent.

18. Involuntary actions, such as the "fight or flight" response are controlled by the:
A.   parasympathetic nervous system.   D.   somatic nervous system.
B.   autonomic nervous system.   E.   central nervous system.
C.   peripheral nervous system.

19. The term pseudo-instinctive refers to:
A.   an innate ability to recognize the correct course of action in a specific situation.
B.   the learned ability to recognize the correct course of action in a specific situation.
C.   learned actions that have been practiced until they can be done without thinking.
D.   innate responses that are performed without thinking.
E.   proactive responses to situations that are potentially life-threatening.

20. "Scanning the situation" is a strategy that helps you:
A.   avoid focusing too narrowly on one aspect of your patient's situation.
B.   consider the ramifications of your potential actions.
C.   act in a confident and decisive manner.
D.   be aware of your own responses and control yourself in a stressful situation.
E.   anticipate your patient's response to your proposed management plan.

21. Which of the following is NOT a step in the critical decision-making process?
A.   forming a concept   D.   summarizing the result
B.   interpreting the data   E.   evaluating the interventions
C.   applying the principles

22. Observing the patient's general appearance, taking vital signs, and exploring the chief complaint are part of which step in the critical decision-making process?
A.   forming a concept   D.   summarizing the result
B.   interpreting the data   E.   evaluating the interventions
C.   applying the principles

23. When interpreting the data, which of the following best describes the method you should use for determining the differential field diagnosis?
A.   consider the most serious condition that fits your patient's situation.
B.   consider all possible causes of your patient's signs and symptoms.

C. consider the most common and statistically probable conditions that fit your patient's presentation.

D. choose the most common condition that fits your patient's signs and symptoms.

E. choose the condition that your experience leads you to feel is the most likely cause of your patient's primary problem.

24. Observing the patient's response to your interventions and adapting you management plan is part of which step in the critical decision-making process?

A. reflecting	D. summarizing
B. interpreting the data	E. evaluating
C. applying the principles	

25. Which of the following is NOT an element of the six "Rs" of critical decision making?

A. reading the scene	D. reading the patient
B. researching the management plan	E. reevaluating
C. reacting	

True/False

26. In most cases, contact your medical direction physician after your assessment, but before developing a management plan.
A. True
B. False

27. The major difference between clinical decision-making for paramedics and other clinicians is that paramedics must work in uncontrolled and unpredictable environments under circumstances that do not exist in other clinical settings.
A. True
B. False

28. Calls involving cardiac arrest or major trauma generally require fewer critical decisions because caring for them is largely rote and standardized.
A. True
B. False

29. Patients who fall between minor medical and life-threatening on the acuity spectrum pose the greatest challenge to your critical thinking abilities.
A. True
B. False

30. In the case where a particular protocol does not seem to fit the patient presentation, you should contact the medical direction physician for advice and direction regarding your patient's care.
A. True
B. False

31. When faced with a patient with non-specific or confusing symptoms, you should focus your assessment on the primary body system involved in the patient's chief complaint.
A. True
B. False

32. When you focus your assessment based on your differential field diagnosis and determine a likely cause for you patient's condition, you are developing your clinical diagnosis.
A. True
B. False

33. Facilitating behaviours for encouraging critical thinking include staying calm, planning for the worst, and working systematically.
  A. True
  B. False

34. One way to remain in control in otherwise extremely stressful situations is to learn to perform technical skills at a pseudo-instinctive level.
  A. True
  B. False

35. The best method for developing clinical judgment is to broaden and deepen your knowledge of anatomy, physiology, and pathophysiology.
  A. True
  B. False

Matching

Write the letter of the step in the critical decision-making process in the space provided next to the emergency response action appropriate for that step.

A. Form a concept
B. Interpret the data
C. Apply the principles
D. Evaluate
E. Reflect

_____   **36.** Form a field diagnosis

_____   **37.** Provide ongoing assessment

_____   **38.** Perform the focused physical exam

_____   **39.** Pulse oximetry

_____   **40.** Follow standing orders

_____   **41.** Differential diagnosis

_____   **42.** Assess MS-ABCs

_____   **43.** Employ protocols

_____   **44.** Determine if treatment is improving the patient's condition

_____   **45.** Compare field diagnosis with receiving physician's diagnosis

Chapter 11

Assessment-Based Management

Review of Chapter Objectives

With each chapter of the Workbook, we identify the objectives and the important elements of the text content. You should review these items and refer to the pages listed if any points are not clear.

After reading this chapter, you should be able to:

1. Explain how effective assessment is critical to clinical decision making.   **pp. 451-453**

Assessment forms the foundation for patient care. You can't treat or report a problem that is not found or identified. To find a problem, you must gather, evaluate, and synthesize information. Based on this process, you can then make a decision and take the appropriate actions to formulate a management plan and determine the priorities for patient care.

A paramedic is entrusted with a great deal of independent judgment and responsibility for performing correct actions for each individual patient, including such advanced skills as ECG interpretation, rapid sequence intubation, and medication administration. Additionally, the medical director and hospital staff must rely on your experience and expertise as you describe the patient's condition and your conclusions about it. Consequently, the ability to reason and to reach a field diagnosis is critical to paramedic practice.

2. Explain how the paramedic's attitude and uncooperative patients affect assessment and decision making.   pp. 453-455

Attitude
Your attitude is one of the most critical factors in performing an effective assessment. You must be as nonjudgmental as possible to avoid "short-circuiting" accurate data collection and pattern recognition by leaping to conclusions before completing a thorough assessment. Remember the popular computer mnemonic GIGO—garbage in/garbage out. You can't reach valid conclusions about your patient based on hasty or incomplete assessment. Seek to identify any preconceived notions that you may have about a group and then work to eliminate them.

Uncooperative patients
Admittedly, uncooperative patients make it difficult to perform good assessments. However, you must remember that there are many possible causes for patient belligerence. Whenever you assess an uncooperative or a restless patient, consider medical causes for the behaviour—hypoxia, hypovolemia, hypoglycemia, or a head injury. Be careful not to jump to the conclusion that the patient is "just another drunk" or a "frequent flyer." The frequent flier that you have transported for alcoholic behaviour in the past may, this time, be suffering from trauma or a medical emergency.

In addition, cultural and ethnic barriers—as well as prior negative experiences—may cause a patient to lack confidence in the rescuers. Such situations make it difficult for you to be effective at the scene, and the patient in fact may refuse to provide express consent for treatment or transport. However, it is your job to increase patient confidence. Become familiar with the cultural customs of any large ethnic populations in your area. Find out about available translation services. Above all, don't permit yourself to make snap judgments about the patient.

3. Explain strategies to prevent labeling, tunnel vision, and decrease environmental distractions.　　pp. 453-456

A number of factors—both internal (for example, your personal attitudes) and external (for example, the patient's attitude, distracting injuries, or environmental factors at the scene)—can affect your assessment of the patient and ultimately your decisions on how to manage treatment.

Labeling and tunnel vision

The dangers of labeling have been discussed in objective 2. However, another internal factor that can negatively affect your assessment is tunnel vision. Do not focus on distracting injuries, such as scalp lacerations, that look worse than they really are. Instead, resist the temptation to form a field diagnosis too early. Always take a systematic approach to patient assessment to avoid distractions and to find and prioritize care for all of the patient's injuries and conditions. In general, follow an inverted pyramid format that progresses from a differential diagnosis to a narrowing process to your field diagnosis. (For more information on the inverted pyramid format, see the diagram on page 451 of your textbook.)

Environmental distractions

You've probably already experienced some of the environmental factors that can affect patient assessment and care—scene chaos, violent or dangerous situations, high noise levels, crowds of bystanders, or even crowds of responders. Limit these distractions through the careful staging of personnel (see objectives 4 and 5). In the case of a large number of rescuers, you might assign crowd control tasks to some of them or stage them nearby. They can then be brought to the scene when and if necessary. Finally, you might change environments completely. Sometimes the best way to deal with excessive environmental noise and distractions is to rapidly load the patient into the ambulance and leave the scene. You can always pull over for further assessment in a quieter environment.

4. Describe how personnel considerations and staffing configurations affect assessment and decision making.　　pp. 455-456

As a rule, assessment is best achieved by one rescuer. A single paramedic can gather information and provide treatment sequentially. In the case of two paramedics, one paramedic can assess the patient, while the other provides simultaneous treatment. With multiple responders, however, assessment and history may take place entirely by "committee," which often leads to disorganized management. It can also be difficult to manage a patient if the responders are all at the same professional level and have no clear direction. Therefore, it is important to plan for these events so that personnel can have pre-designated roles. These roles may be rotated among team members so no one is left out, but there must be a plan to avoid "freelancing." If there is only one paramedic, then that person must assume all advanced care roles.

5. Synthesize and apply concepts of scene management and choreography to simulated emergency calls.　　p. 455-456

Points in the textbook and direction by your instructors and clinical or field preceptors will help you to manage and choreograph simulated emergency calls. When approaching these practice sessions, remember the importance of an effective preplan. In the case of a two-person team, the roles of team care leader and patient care provider can be assigned on an alternating basis. Paramedics who work together regularly may develop their own plan, but a universally understood plan allows for other rescuers to participate in a rescue without interrupting the flow. While the dynamics of field situations may necessitate changes in plans, a general "game plan" can go a long way toward preventing chaos. If field dynamics dictate a change in the preplanned roles, you are still working from a solid base.

6. Explain the roles of the team leader and the patient care person.   pp. 455-456

In setting up a two-person team, keep in mind the general tasks performed by the team leader and patient care provider as outlined below.

Roles of Team Leader	Roles of Patient Care Provider
Establishes patient contact	Provides "scene cover"
Obtains history	Gathers scene information
Performs physical exam	Talks to relatives/bystanders
Presents patient	Obtains vital signs
Handles documentation	Performs interventions
Acts as EMS commander	Acts as triage group leader

7. List and explain the rationale for bringing the essential care items to the patient.   pp. 456-457

Having the right equipment at the patient's side is essential. As a paramedic, you must be prepared to manage many conditions and injuries or changes in the patient's condition. Assessment and management must usually be done simultaneously. If you do not have the right equipment readily available, then you have compromised patient care and, in fact, the patient may die.

8. When given a simulated call, list the appropriate equipment to be taken to the patient.   pp. 456-457

Think of your equipment as items in a backpack. Just like backpacking, you must downsize your equipment to minimum weight and bulk to facilitate rapid movement. At the same time, you need certain essential items to ensure survival—in this case, patient survival. The following is a list of the essential equipment for paramedic management of life-threatening conditions. You must bring these items to the side of every patient, regardless of what you initially think you may need.

• **Infection Control**
—Infection control supplies—e.g., gloves, eye shields
• **Airway Control**
—Oral airways
—Nasal airways
—Suction (electric or manual)
—Rigid tonsil-tip and flexible suction catheters
—Laryngoscope and blades
—Endotracheal tubes, stylettes, syringes, tape
• **Breathing**
—Pocket mask
—Manual ventilation bag-valve mask
—Spare masks in various sizes
—Oxygen masks, cannulas, and extension tubing
—Occlusive dressings
—Large-bore IV catheter for thoracic decompression
• **Circulation**
—Dressings
—Bandages and tape
—Sphygmomanometer, stethoscope
—Note pad and pen or pencil
• **Disability**
—Rigid collars
—Flashlights
• **Dysrhythmia**
—Cardiac monitor/defibrillator
• **Exposure and Protection**

—Scissors

—Space blankets or something to cover the patient

You may also pack some optional "take in" equipment, such as drug therapy and venous access supplies. The method by which these supplies are carried may depend upon how your system is designed—e.g., paramedic ambulances versus paramedics in non-transporting vehicles. It may also depend upon local protocols, flexibility of standing orders, the number of paramedic responders in your area, and the difficulty of accessing patients because of terrain or some other problem.

9. Explain the general approach to the emergency patient.   pp. 457-461

In addition to having the right equipment, you need to have the essential demeanor to calm or reassure the patient. You must look and act the professional, while exhibiting the compassion and understanding associated with an effective "bedside manner." While patients may not have the ability to rate your medical performance, they can certainly rate your people skills and service. Be aware of your body language and the messages it sends, either intentionally or unintentionally. Think carefully about what you say and how you say it—this includes your conversations with other members of the EMS team and anyone else on the scene.

Once again, it helps to preplan your general approach to the patient. This will prevent confusion and improve the accuracy of your assessment. One team member should engage in an active, concerned dialogue with the patient. This same person should also demonstrate the listening skills needed to collect information and to convey a caring attitude. Taking notes may prevent asking the same question repeatedly as well as ensuring that you acquire and pass on accurate data.

10. Explain the general approach, patient assessment differentials, and management priorities for patients with various types of emergencies that may be experienced in prehospital care. pp. 457-461

Scene Size-Up
Before approaching the patient (see objective 9), you must carefully size up the scene. The scene size-up has the following components: body substance isolation, ensuring scene safety, locating all patients, and identifying the mechanism of injury or the nature of the illness.

Initial assessment
After you size up the scene, you quickly begin the initial assessment for the purpose of detecting and treating immediate life threats. The components of the initial assessment are:
• Forming a general impression
• Determining mental status (AVPU)
• Assessing airway, breathing, and circulation
• Determining the patient's priority for further on-scene care or immediate transport

Depending upon your findings during initial assessment, you might take either the contemplative or the resuscitative approach to patient care. You might also decide to immediately transport the patient.

Contemplative approach. In general, use the contemplative approach when immediate intervention is not necessary. In such situations, the focused history and physical exam, followed by any required interventions can be performed at the scene, before transport to the hospital.

Resuscitative approach. Use the resuscitative approach whenever you suspect a life-threatening problem, including:

• Cardiac or respiratory arrest
• Respiratory distress or failure
• Unstable dysrhythmias
• Status epilepticus
• Coma or altered mental status
• Shock or hypotension

• Major trauma
• Possible C-spine injury

In these cases, you must take immediate resuscitative action (such as CPR, defibrillation, or ventilation) or other critical action (such as supplemental oxygen, control of major bleeding, or C-spine immobilization). Additional assessment and care can be performed after resuscitation and the rapid trauma assessment and/or en route to the hospital.

Immediate evacuation. In some cases, you will need to immediately evacuate the patient to the ambulance. For example, a patient with severe internal bleeding requires life-saving interventions beyond a paramedic's skills. You might also resort to immediate evacuation if the scene is too chaotic for rational assessment or if it is too unsafe or unstable.

Focused history and physical exam
Following the initial assessment, you will perform the focused history and physical exam. Based on the patient's chief complaint and the information gathered during the initial assessment, you should consider your patient to belong to one of the following four categories:
• Trauma patient with a significant mechanism of injury or altered mental status
• Trauma patient with an isolated injury
• Medical patient who is unresponsive
• Medical patient who is responsive

For a trauma patient with a significant MOI or altered mental status or for an unresponsive medical patient, perform a rapid trauma assessment for the trauma patient; perform a rapid medical assessment for the medical patient. For a trauma patient with an isolated injury or for a responsive medical patient, perform a secondary assessment focused on body systems related to the chief complaint.

Ongoing assessment and detailed secondary assessment
The ongoing assessment must be performed on all patients to monitor and to observe trends in the person's condition—every 5 minutes if the patient is unstable, every 15 minutes if the patient is stable. Ongoing assessments must be performed until the patient is transferred to the care of hospital personnel. The ongoing assessment includes evaluation of the following:
• Mental status
• Airway, breathing, and circulation
• Transport priorities
• Vital signs
• Focused assessment of any problem areas or conditions
• Effectiveness of interventions
• Management plans

The secondary assessment is similar to but more thorough than the rapid trauma assessment. It is generally performed only on trauma patients and only if time and the patient's condition permit.

Identification of life-threatening problems
At all stages of the assessment, from initial assessment through ongoing assessments, from the scene to the ambulance to arrival at the hospital, you must actively and continuously look for and manage any life-threatening problems. Basically your role as a paramedic is to rapidly and accurately assess the patient and then to treat for the worst-case scenario. This is the underlying principle of assessment-based management—your guide to providing effective medical care.

11. Describe how to effectively communicate patient information face to face, over the telephone, by radio, and in writing.   pp. 461–462

The ability to communicate effectively is the key to transferring patient information, whether in an out-of-hospital setting or within the hospital itself. Although neither primary nor advanced care interventions may be required for every patient, a skill that will be used on every single patient is that of presentation, whether it is over the radio or telephone, in writing, or in face-to-face transfers at the receiving facility.

Effective presentation and communication skills help establish a paramedic's credibility. They also inspire trust and confidence in patients. If you present your assessment, your findings, and your treatment in a clear, concise manner, you give the impression of a job well done. A poor presentation, on the other hand, implies poor assessment and poor patient care.

Special Considerations/Operations

The most effective oral presentations usually meet these guidelines:
• Last less than one minute
• Are very concise and clear
• Avoid excessive use of medical jargon
• Follow a basic format, usually the SOAP format or some variation
• Include both pertinent findings and pertinent negatives
• Conclude with specific actions, requests, or questions related to the plan

An ideal presentation should include the following:
• Patient identification, age, sex, and degree of distress
• Chief complaint
• Present illness/injury
—Pertinent details about the present problem
—Pertinent negatives
• Past medical history
—Allergies
—Medications
—Pertinent medical history
• Physical signs
—Vital signs
—Pertinent positive findings
—Pertinent negative findings
• Assessment
—Paramedic impression
• Plan
—What has been done
—Orders requested

12. Given various preprogrammed and moulaged patients, provide the appropriate scene size-up, initial assessment, focused assessment, and detailed assessment, then provide the appropriate care, ongoing assessments, and patient transport. pp. 450-463

In order to develop as an entry-level practitioner at the paramedic level, it is important to participate in scenario-based reviews of commonly encountered complaints. Laboratory-based simulations require you to assess a preprogrammed patient or mannequin. Use the information presented in the textbook, the information on assessment-based management provided by your instructors, and the guidance given by your clinical and field preceptors to develop good assessment-based management skills. Remember—the chance to practice does not stop at the classroom. While a paramedic student or the new member of a team, take advantage of every opportunity to practice your new skills.

CONTENT SELF-EVALUATION

_____   **1.** The process of keeping an open mind on approach to a call, then narrowing your focus can be described as:

A. tunnel vision.
B. an inverted pyramid.
C. patient assessment.
D. clinical judgment.
E. assessment triangle.

2. Which of the following gives the correct order of steps in the clinical decision making of the inverted pyramid?
A. field diagnosis, differential diagnosis, narrowing process
B. narrowing process, field diagnosis, differential diagnosis
C. field diagnosis, narrowing process, differential diagnosis
D. differential diagnosis, field diagnosis, narrowing process
E. differential diagnosis, narrowing process, field diagnosis

3. The foundation of patient care is:
A. the detailed physical exam.
B. PCP protocols.
C. assessment.
D. medication administration.
E. ACP protocols.

4. The most significant factor that physicians often consider in their diagnosis is:
A. the detailed physical exam.
B. your patient care record.
C. your field diagnosis.
D. history.
E. trends in vital signs.

5. All of the following are examples of external factors that can affect assessment EXCEPT:
A. the attitude of family members.
B. an uncooperative patient.
C. distracting injuries.
D. scene chaos.
E. personal attitudes.

6. Protocols and standing orders do not replace:
A. good history taking.
B. a good attitude.
C. good judgment.
D. the team approach.
E. pattern recognition.

7. When dealing with a "frequent flyer" who is uncooperative or hostile, a paramedic should consider which of the following conditions:
A. head injury.
B. hypoglycemia.
C. alcohol intoxication.
D. subdural hematoma.
E. all of the above

8. The team leader is generally the care provider who:
A. first contacts the patient.
B. is the senior crew member.
C. will accompany the patient to the hospital.
D. has the most experience.
E. is most familiar with the patient.

9. A team leader's roles include all of the following EXCEPT:
A. obtains a history.
B. performs the physical exam.
C. handles documentation.
D. triages patients.
E. performs a detailed exam.

10. Roles of a patient care provider include:
A. talking to bystanders.
B. obtaining vital signs.
C. gathering scene information.
D. providing scene cover.
E. completing documentation.

11. Emergency medical responders may include:
A. police and firefighters.
B. industrial first aid attendants.
C. life guards.
D. community volunteers.
E. all of the above

12. Which of the following personnel should delegate tasks regarding patient care in a multiple agency response?

A.	scene commander	**D.**	first arriving agency
B.	EMS team leader	**E.**	senior member on scene
C.	EMS patient care provider		

13. Which of the following is probably optional "take in" equipment carried by paramedics?

A.	rigid collars	**D.**	space blankets
B.	infection control supplies	**E.**	sphygmomanometer
C.	drug therapy		

14. Body substance isolation should be initiated:

A. during scene assessment.
B. during the Primary Survey.
C. once you have initiated contact with the patient.
D. if potentially communicable diseases are identified.
E. after ensuring all hazards are controlled.

15. Components of the initial assessment include all of the following EXCEPT:

A.	obtaining baseline vital signs.	**D.**	determining the patient's priority.
B.	assessing ABCs.	**E.**	assessing mental status.
C.	assessing the scene.		

16. A patient with severe internal bleeding is a candidate for:

A.	the resuscitative approach.	**D.**	a divergent approach.
B.	the contemplative approach.	**E.**	a convergent approach.
C.	immediate evacuation.		

17. A patient with stable chest pain is a candidate for:

A.	the resuscitative approach.	**D.**	a divergent approach.
B.	the contemplative approach.	**E.**	a convergent approach.
C.	immediate evacuation.		

18. When faced with a chaotic scene in which you are unable to perform a rational assessment, you should:

A.	use the resuscitative approach.	**D.**	take a divergent approach.
B.	use the contemplative approach.	**E.**	take a convergent approach.
C.	prepare for immediate evacuation.		

19. A patient in status epilepticus is a candidate for:

A.	the resuscitative approach.	**D.**	a divergent approach.
B.	the contemplative approach.	**E.**	a convergent approach.
C.	immediate evacuation.		

19. A patient in status epilepticus is a candidate for:

A.	the resuscitative approach.	**D.**	a divergent approach.
B.	the contemplative approach.	**E.**	a convergent approach.
C.	immediate evacuation.		

20. A patient with a mild allergic reaction is a candidate for:

A.	the resuscitative approach.	**D.**	detailed physical exam.
B.	the contemplative approach.	**E.**	both B and D
C.	immediate evacuation.		

21. If you must transport an unstable trauma patient, you should:

A. place the patient on an immobilization device and continue with further assessment and treatment en route.
B. place the patient on an immobilization device, apply a hard collar, and continue with further assessment and treatment en route.
C. transport, then apply a hard collar and stabilize injuries en route.
D. splint major fractures, initiate IV access, apply a hard collar, then transport.
E. splint major fractures, transport apply a hard collar, and initiate IV access en route.

_____ **22.** You should perform a rapid trauma assessment for:
  - **A.** all trauma patients.
  - **B.** trauma patients with a single-system injury.
  - **C.** unresponsive trauma patients.
  - **D.** trauma patients with a significant mechanism of injury or an altered mental status.
  - **E.** trauma patients with a significant mechanism of injury who can provide a coherent history.

_____ **23.** You should remain on scene to perform a secondary assessment focused on the body systems related to the patient's chief complaint for:
  - **A.** all medical patients.
  - **B.** unresponsive medical patients.
  - **C.** responsive medical patients or trauma patients with isolated injuries.
  - **D.** trauma patients with a single system injury.
  - **E.** all medical and trauma patients.

_____ **24.** You must look for and manage life-threatening problems:
  - **A.** during the scene assessment and primary survey.
  - **B.** during the primary survey.
  - **C.** during the primary and secondary survey.
  - **D.** during your focused secondary survey.
  - **E.** at all stages of the call.

_____ **25.** The most effective patient presentations will:
  - **A.** use medical jargon.
  - **B.** follow the SOAP format.
  - **C.** be done in writing.
  - **D.** last 5 to 10 minutes.
  - **E.** exclude subjective findings.

True/False

_____ **26.** In a medical patient, the physical exam takes precedence over the history.
  - **A.** True
  - **B.** False

_____ **27.** In a trauma patient, the physical exam takes precedence over the history.
  - **A.** True
  - **B.** False

_____ **28.** The ability to recognize patterns is to constantly research and review medical literature.
  - **A.** True
  - **B.** False

_____ **29.** Sometimes your field diagnosis will be based on a combination of pattern recognition and intuition.
  - **A.** True
  - **B.** False

_____ **30.** You should treat a "frequent flier" just like you would any other patient.
  - **A.** True
  - **B.** False

_____ **31.** You should form your field diagnosis as early as possible in your assessment.
  - **A.** True
  - **B.** False

_____ **32.** Patient assessment is best performed by two paramedics rather than just one.
  - **A.** True
  - **B.** False

33. If possible, you should monitor and reassess unstable patients every 5 minutes and stable patients every 15 minutes.

    A.   True

    B.   False

34. In critical patients, a detailed physical exam is more important than continuing ongoing assessments.

    A.   True

    B.   False

35. The location of pain is not a reliable indicator of its source when dealing with visceral pain.

    A.   True

    B.   False

Matching

Write the letter of the team member in the space provided next to the actions that member would generally perform on a call.

A.   team leader

B.   patient care provider

36. obtain history

37. obtain vital signs

38. handle documentation

39. gather scene information

40. perform interventions

Chapter 12

Anatomy and Physiology

Part 1: The Cell and the Cellular Environment

Review of Chapter Objectives

Because Chapter 12 is lengthy, it has been divided into parts to aid your study. Read the assigned textbook pages, then progress through the objectives and self-evaluation materials as you would with other chapters. When you feel secure in your grasp of the content, proceed to the next part.

After reading this part of the chapter, you should be able to:

1. Describe the structure and function of the normal cell.   pp. 466-470

The cell is the basic unit of life and structured like a self-sustaining city. The cell is bound by a membrane that permits certain substances to pass to maintain electrolyte balance and permit the movement of nutrients and waste products. The fluid filling the cell is cytoplasm while small structures, called organelles, perform specific functions within the cell. All cells have the same basic structure but differentiate into ones that perform differing functions. Muscle cells cause movement, nervous cells transmit impulses. Cells of the digestive system permit absorption; gland cells secrete substances such as hormones, mucus, sweat, and saliva; all cells also excrete wastes; and respiration is the process by which they transform oxygen and nutrients into energy. Cells also enlarge and divide in a process called reproduction. Cells are organized into tissues, tissues into organs, organs into organ systems, and organ systems into an organism.

2. List the types of tissue.   p. 470

Epithelial tissue lines internal and external body surfaces. It provides protection and specialized functions such as secretion, absorption, diffusion, and filtration. Major examples are the skin and the lining of the digestive tract.

Muscle tissue has the capability to contract when stimulated. It is of three types: cardiac muscle, found only in the heart; skeletal muscle, which is under voluntary control; and smooth muscle, found in the intestines and blood vessels, which is not under voluntary control.

Connective tissue is the most abundant tissue in the body and provides support, connection, and insulation. Connective tissue includes bone, cartilage, and fat. Blood may also be classified as connective tissue.

Nerve tissue is specialized tissue capable of transmitting electrical impulses throughout the body and makes up the brain, spinal cord, and peripheral nerves.

3. Define organs, organ systems, the organism, and system integration.   **pp. 470-474**

Organs are groups of tissue that function together to provide a specific or many specific functions. Examples include the heart, brain, kidneys, or lungs. Groups of organs also function together, in organ systems, to provide functions for the human body. Such organ systems include the cardiovascular system, the respiratory system, the gastrointestinal system, the genitourinary system, the reproductive system, the nervous system, the endocrine system, the lymphatic system, the muscular system, and the skeletal system. The sum of all cells, tissues, organs, and organ systems is the organism. System integration is the dynamic organization of the cells, tissues, organs, and organ systems that provides and maintains the internal environment, homeostasis.

4. Describe the cellular environment (fluids and electrolytes), including osmosis and diffusion.   **pp. 474-483**

The body goes to great lengths to maintain a constant internal and cellular environment (homeostasis). Major factors of this environment include hydration, the movement of substances into and out of the cell, and acid/base balance.
• **Hydration.** Water composes about 60 percent of the total body weight and plays a very important role in the body's internal environment. Some 75 percent of the body's water is contained within the cells (intracellular fluid), while 7.5 percent is contained within the vascular system (intravascular fluid). The remaining water is found between cells (interstitial fluid) and in other spaces within the body. An abnormal decrease in body hydration (dehydration) may be caused by increased gastrointestinal losses, sweating, internal (third space) losses, plasma losses, or other types of losses. An abnormal increase in body water is called overhydration.
• **Electrolytes.** Electrolytes are molecules that dissociate into negatively and positively charged particles (called ions) when dissolved in water. The normal distribution of body water is dependent on the distribution of electrolytes among the body spaces (intravascular, interstitial, and intracellular).
• **Osmosis and diffusion.** Diffusion is the movement of molecules from an area of higher concentration to one of lower concentration. Osmosis is the movement of a solvent (like water) through a membrane to equalize the concentration of electrolytes on each side of the membrane. The body also moves electrolytes through cell membranes (against the osmotic gradient) by active transport and facilitated diffusion. These processes are responsible for maintaining a fluid electrolyte balance among the intravascular, interstitial, and intracellular spaces.

5. Discuss acid-base balance and pH.   **pp. 483-486**

The concentration of free hydrogen ions in a fluid reflects its acidity and is noted as a logarithmic value called pH. A pH of 1 is extremely acidic, while a pH of 14 is without hydrogen ions and extremely basic (or alkalotic). The body maintains a slightly alkalotic environment by regulating the quantity of free hydrogen ions. Normal body pH ranges from 7.35 to 7.45. The body maintains its pH through a bicarbonate buffer system, the respiratory system, and the kidneys.

CONTENT SELF-EVALUATION

1. The fundamental unit of life is:
   A.   the cell.
   B.   tissue.
   C.   the organ.
   D.   the organism.
   E.   DNA.

2. One of the three main elements of a typical cell is the:
   A.   cell membrane.
   B.   cilia.
   C.   leukocyte.
   D.   eosinophil.
   E.   basophil.

3. The characteristic ability of a cell membrane to selectively permit material to pass through it is called:

    A. diffusiveness.

    B. imperviousness.

    C. semipermeability.

    D. cytoplasmicism.

    E. isotonicism.

4. The thick viscous fluid that fills the cell and gives it shape is called:

    A. ribosome.

    B. lysosome.

    C. cytoplasm.

    D. protoplasm.

    E. either C or D

5. The structure that contains the genetic material including the cell's DNA is the:

    A. endoplasmic reticulum.

    B. Golgi apparatus.

    C. nucleus.

    D. mitochondria.

    E. cytokine.

6. The compound that provides the cell with most of its energy is:

    A. DNA.

    B. phosgene.

    C. carbon dioxide.

    D. ATP.

    E. carbohydrate.

7. The tissue type that covers the internal and external body surfaces is:

    A. epithelial.

    B. smooth muscle.

    C. nerve.

    D. connective.

    E. skeletal muscle.

8. The tissue type that is mostly under voluntary control is:

    A. epithelial.

    B. cardiac muscle.

    C. nerve.

    D. connective.

    E. skeletal muscle.

9. The tissue type that provides support and insulation is:

    A. epithelial.

    B. cardiac muscle.

    C. nerve.

    D. connective.

    E. skeletal muscle.

10. The body organ system that produces most body heat is the:

    A. muscular system.

    B. gastrointestinal system.

    C. genitourinary system.

    D. endocrine system.

    E. lymphatic system.

11. The body organ system that is important in fighting disease and filtration is the:

    A. muscular system.

    B. gastrointestinal system.

    C. genitourinary system.

    D. endocrine system.

    E. lymphatic system.

12. The term that is applied to the building up and tearing down of biochemical substances to produce energy is:

    A. anatomy.

    B. physiology.

    C. catabolism.

    D. anabolism.

    E. metabolism.

13. Medications given by paramedics act on specialized receptors known as:

    A. chemorecptors.

    B. endocrine glands.

    C. synaptic receptors.

    D. baroreceptors.

    E. post synaptic receptors.

14. The natural tendency of the body to maintain a constant internal environment is:

    A. cellular equilibrium.

    B. homeostasis.

    C. metabolism.

    D. physiology.

    E. paracrine signaling.

15. The body's major baroreceptors are located in the:

A. arch of the aorta.
D. inner ears.
B. brainstem.
E. medulla oblongata.
C. lung tissue.

16. Chemoreceptors in the brain that trigger increased rate and depth of respirations are monitoring:

A. carbon dioxide in the blood.
B. carbon dioxide in the cerebrospinal fluid.
C. cabon monoxide in the blood.
D. oxygen in the blood.
E. oxygen in the cerebrospinal fluid.

17. The feedback system that decreases stimulation as the target organ responds is the:

A. positive feedback loop.
D. beta adrenergic system.
B. negative feedback loop.
E. cholinergic loop.
C. decompensation system.

18. Extracellular fluid accounts for what percentage of total body water?

A. 75 percent
D. 17.5 percent
B. 60 percent
E. 7.5 percent
C. 25 percent

19. A fluid that dissolves other substances is a(n):

A. solute.
D. solvent.
B. electrolyte.
E. anhydrous.
C. hydrate.

20. Which of the following is a source of body fluid loss and dehydration?

A. diarrhea
D. poor nutritional states
B. hyperventilation
E. all of the above
C. pancreatitis

21. The term *turgor* refers to:

A. intense thirst.
D. sunken fontanelles.
B. skin tension.
E. extreme obesity.
C. highly concentrated urine.

22. Which element is most common in the human body?

A. hydrogen
D. nitrogen
B. oxygen
E. sodium
C. carbon

23. A positively charged ion is a(n):

A. anion.
D. dissociated element.
B. cation.
E. reagent.
C. electrolyte.

24. The most prevalent cation in the human body is:

A. magnesium.
D. bicarbonate.
B. chloride.
E. sodium.
C. potassium.

25. Which of the following ions is responsible for buffering the acid concentrations in the body?

A. magnesium
D. bicarbonate
B. chloride
E. sodium
C. potassium

26. A solution that contains more solute concentration on one side of a semipermeable membrane than on the other is said to be:

    A.   hypertonic.   **D.**   osmotic.

    B.   isotonic.   **E.**   diffused.

    C.   hypotonic.

27. When an isotonic solution is placed in the human bloodstream, water moves in which direction?

    A.   into the vascular space   **D.**   in both directions

    B.   does not move   **E.**   none of the above

    C.   out of the vascular space

28. When a hypertonic solution is placed in the human bloodstream, water moves in which direction?

    A.   into the vascular space   **D.**   in both directions

    B.   does not move   **E.**   none of the above

    C.   out of the vascular space

29. The movement of a solvent from an area of higher concentration through a semipermeable membrane to an area of lower concentration is termed:

    A.   diffusion.   **D.**   facilitated transport.

    B.   osmosis.   **E.**   oncosis.

    C.   active transport.

30. The pressure that draws water into the blood because of the proteins there is called:

    A.   osmolarity.   **D.**   oncotic force.

    B.   osmotic pressure.   **E.**   filtration.

    C.   hydrostatic pressure.

31. The movement of water out of the plasma across the capillary membrane into the interstitial space is:

    A.   osmolarity.   **D.**   oncotic force.

    B.   osmotic pressure.   **E.**   filtration.

    C.   hydrostatic pressure.

32. The normal pH range in the human body is:

    A.   6.9 to 7.35.   **D.**   6.9 to 7.8.

    B.   7.35 to 7.45.   **E.**   none of the above

    C.   7.45 to 7.8.

33. Which of the following would be considered alkalosis in the human?

    A.   6.9 to 7.35   **D.**   6.4 to 6.9

    B.   7.35 to 7.45   **E.**   none of the above

    C.   7.45 to 7.8

34. A decrease in pH of 1 would reflect which change in the concentration of hydrogen ions?

    A.   100 times as great   **D.**   1/100th as great

    B.   10 times as great   **E.**   a doubling

    C.   1/10th as great

35. The body system that responds most rapidly to a change in the pH is the:

    A.   respiratory system.   **D.**   buffer system.

    B.   cardiovascular system.   **E.**   genitourinary system.

    C.   digestive system.

True/False

36. The role of the endoplasmic reticulum is to synthesize and package secretions such as mucous and enzymes.

A. True
B. False

_____ **37.** Differentiation is the process by which cells with the same general structure and genetic material become specialized.
A. True
B. False

_____ **38.** Ductless or endocrine glands secrete directly into the circulatory system.
A. True
B. False

_____ **39.** Most of the input affecting body organs and homeostasis occurs via the positive feedback loop.
A. True
B. False

_____ **40.** The fluid space found between the vascular and cellular compartments is the extracellular compartment.
A. True
B. False

_____ **41.** Intracellular fluid makes up 25% of the total body water in an adult..
A. True
B. False

_____ **42.** The movement of water out of and then back into the capillary as it travels through the capillary is regulated by the protein concentration within the blood and the pressure as the blood is pushed through the capillary.
A. True
B. False

_____ **43.** The higher the pH value, the lower the concentration of hydrogen ions.
A. True
B. False

_____ **44.** The cellular environment of the human body is slightly acidic.
A. True
B. False

_____ **45.** The addition of hydrogen ions to the bloodstream will result in an increase in carbon dioxide.
A. True
B. False

Matching

Write the letter of the term in the space provided next to the description or definition to which it applies.

Term

A. cytoplasm
B. cytoskeleton
C. cytosol
D. cytotoxin
E. erythrocyte

F. granulocyte
G. leukocyte
H. lymphocyte
I. monocyte
J. phagocyte

Description

_____ **46.** Cell with the ability to ingest other cells and substances such as cell debris and bacteria

_____ **47.** Clear liquid portion of the cytoplasm in a cell

_____ **48.** Red blood cell

_____ **49.** Structure of protein filaments that supports the internal structure of a cell

_____ **50.** Substance that is toxic to cells

_____ **51.** Thick fluid that fills a cell

_____ **52.** Type of leukocyte that attacks foreign substances

_____ **53.** White blood cell

_____ **54.** White blood cell with a single nucleus

_____ **55.** White blood cell with multiple nuclei

Chapter 12

Anatomy and Physiology

Part 2: Body Systems

Review of Chapter Objectives

After reading this part of the chapter, you should be able to:

Introduction to Advanced Prehospital Care

1. **Describe the anatomy and physiology of the integumentary system, including the skin, hair, and nails.   pp. 486-489**

    The integumentary system is the largest body organ, accounting for about 16 percent of weight. It provides the outer barrier for the body and protects it against environmental extremes, fluid loss, and pathogen invasion. The three-layer structure consists of:
    • **Epidermis**
    The epidermis is the most superficial layer of the skin and consists of numerous layers of dead or dying cells. The epidermis provides a flexible covering for the skin and a barrier to fluid loss, absorption, and the entrance of pathogens.
    • **Dermis**
    The dermis is the true skin. It is made up of connective tissue and houses the sensory nerve endings; many of the specialized skin cells that produce sweat, oil, etc.; and the upper-level capillary beds that allow for the conduction of heat to the body's surface.
    • **Subcutaneous tissue**
    The subcutaneous layer, although not a true part of the skin, works in concert with the skin to insulate the body from heat loss and the effects of trauma. It consists of connective and adipose (fatty) tissues. Hair grows from follicles nourished by capillary beds and grows as either vellus hair (peach fuzz) or terminal (normal) hair. Arrector muscles attach to the follicle and with contraction cause the hairs to stand erect. With age the growth of hair decreases, it turns gray with decreased pigmentation, and some of the hair turns from terminal to vellus hair.
    Nails are found on the distal ends of the fingers and toes and are mainly for protection. They grow from the nail root towards the tip of the digit and cover a highly vascular nail bed that gives the nail its pink colour. As we age, growth decreases with decreased distal circulation, resulting in hard, thick brittle and yellowish nails.

2. Describe the anatomy and physiology of the hematopoietic system, including components of the blood, and discuss hemostasis, the hematocrit, and hemoglobin.   pp. 489-500

The components of the hematopoietic system include the blood, bone marrow, liver, spleen, and kidneys. The process of hematopoiesis forms the cellular components of blood. In the fetus, this first takes place outside the bone marrow in the liver, spleen, lymph nodes, and thymus. By the fourth month of gestation, the bone marrow begins to produce blood cells. After birth and across the span of life, bone marrow continues to fulfill this critical function, barring the development of some pathological process.

In hematopoiesis, the stem cell reproduces to maintain a constant population of cells. Some stem cells further differentiate into myeloid multipotent stem cells that, in turn, differentiate into unipotent progenitors, which ultimately mature into the formed elements of blood: red blood cells, white blood cells, and platelets. Pluripotent stem cells may also differentiate into common lymphoid stem cells, ultimately becoming lymphocytes. Erythropoietin, the hormone responsible for red blood cell production, is produced by the kidneys and, to a lesser extent, the liver. The liver also removes toxins from the blood and produces many of the clotting factors and proteins in plasma. The spleen plays an important role in the immune system with its cells that scavenge abnormal blood cells and bacteria.

The components of the blood include the white blood cells, platelets, red blood cells, and plasma. White blood cells originate in the bone marrow from undifferentiated stem cells. Leukopoiesis is the process by which stem cells differentiate into the various immature forms of the white blood cell (leukocyte). These immature forms known as -blasts mature to become granulocytes, monocytes, or lymphocytes. While leukocytes provide protection from foreign invasion, each type of white blood cell has its own unique function. Healthy people have between 5,000 and 9,000 white blood cells per milliliter of blood, but the presence of an infection can cause that number to rise to greater than 16,000.

Granulocytic white blood cells are of three types: basophils, eosinophils, and neutrophils. The basophils' primary function is in allergic reactions as they are storage sites for all of the body's circulating histamine. When stimulated, they degranulate and release histamine. Eosinophils can inactivate the chemical mediators of acute allergic response, thus modulating the anaphylactic response. The neutrophils' primary function is to fight infection.

Monocytes, another of the specialized WBCs, serve as the body's trash collectors, moving throughout the body to engulf both foreign invaders and dead neutrophils. Some monocytes remain in circulation, while others migrate to other sites to further mature into macrophages. Monocytes and macrophages also secrete growth factors to stimulate the formation of red blood cells and granulocytes. Some macrophages become fixed within tissues of the liver, spleen, lungs, and lymphatic system, becoming part of the reticuloendothelial system and having the capability to stimulate lymphocyte production in an immune response.

Lymphocytes, the primary cells of the body's immune response, can be found in the circulating blood, as well as in the lymph fluid and nodes, bone marrow, spleen, liver, lungs, skin, and intestine. These highly specialized cells contain surface receptor sites specific to a single antigen and initiate an immune response in order to rid the body of such agents.

Platelets or thrombocytes function to form a plug at an initial bleeding site and secrete several factors important to clotting. The normal number of platelets ranges from 150,000 to 450,000 per milliliter. Derived from megakaryocytes that arise from an undifferentiated stem cell in the bone marrow, platelets survive from 7 to 10 days and are removed from circulation by the spleen.

Erythropoiesis, the process of RBC production, is stimulated by erythropoietin that is secreted by the kidneys when the renal cells sense hypoxia. In turn, this stimulates the bone marrow to increase red cell production resulting in increased RBC mass and thus effectively, albeit slowly, increasing the oxygen-carrying capacity of the blood.

The life span of a red blood cell is approximately 4 months, although hemorrhage, hemolysis (RBC destruction), or sequestration by the liver or spleen may significantly reduce its life span. The spleen and liver contain macrophages (a specialized type of scavenger white blood cell) that can remove damaged or abnormal cells from circulation.

Plasma is the fluid portion of the blood and is a thick, pale yellow fluid that is 90 to 92 percent water and 6 to 7 percent proteins. It also contains electrolytes, fats, carbohydrates, gases, and chemical messengers. It transports nutrients and waste products to and from the body's cells and maintains the blood's oncotic pressure. The proteins with the plasma also assist in the clotting mechanisms and buffering the bloods pH balance.

Hemostasis involves three mechanisms that work to prevent or control blood loss, including vascular spasms that reduce the size of a vascular tear, platelet plugs (an aggregate of platelets that adheres to collagen), and lastly the formation of stable fibrin clots (coagulation).

Damage to cells or to the tunica intima (innermost lining of the blood vessels) triggers the clotting or coagulation cascade. This sequence of events (cascade) can be activated by either an intrinsic pathway (trauma to blood cells from turbulence) or an extrinsic pathway (damage to vessels).

Following the intrinsic pathway: platelets release substances that lead to the formation of prothrombin activator, which in the presence of calcium converts prothrombin to thrombin. Thrombin converts fibrinogen to stable fibrin, again in the presence of calcium, which then traps blood cells and more platelets to form a clot.

The extrinsic pathway is triggered with the development of a tear in a blood vessel. When this occurs, the smooth muscle fibers in the tunica media (middle lining of the blood vessels) contract and the resultant vasoconstriction reduces the size of the injury. This action reduces blood flow through the area, effectively limiting blood loss and allowing platelet aggregation (formation of a platelet plug) and the subsequent conversion of prothrombin activator.

Clotting factors or proteins are primarily produced in the liver and circulate in an inactive state. Prothrombin and fibrinogen are the best known of these factors. Damaged cells send out a chemical message that activates a specific clotting factor. This activates each protein in sequence until a stable clot is formed.

An enzyme on the surface of the platelet membrane makes it sticky. It is this stickiness that allows platelet aggregation to occur.

Hematocrit is the packed cell volume of red blood cells per unit of blood. This measurement is obtained by spinning a sample of blood in a centrifuge to separate the cellular elements from the plasma. Red cells are by far the heaviest component of the blood, due to their carrying the iron-containing hemoglobin and settle to the bottom of the tube. Immediately above the RBCs are the white blood cells and on top is the plasma layer. The height of the RBCs in the column is divided by the total height of the tube's contents (cellular component + plasma) and is reported as a percentage. The normal range is from 40 to 52 percent, although women tend to have slightly lower levels.

Oxygen diffuses to the blood and is transported on the hemoglobin molecule. Hemoglobin is a very efficient transporter of oxygen, and each gram holds 1.34 mL of oxygen when fully saturated. As blood passes by well-oxygenated alveoli, between 98 and 100 percent of the hemoglobin is fully saturated and carries 97 percent of the oxygen in the blood. The remaining oxygen is dissolved in the blood plasma. As the oxygenated blood reaches the tissue capillaries, hemoglobin releases the oxygen. The oxygen then diffuses through the capillary wall, into the interstitial space, and then through the cell membrane.

3. Describe the anatomy and physiology of the musculoskeletal system, including bones, joints, skeletal organization, and muscular tissue and structure.   pp. 500-522

The skeletal system is a living body system that protects vital organs, acts as a storehouse for body salts and other materials needed for metabolism, produces erythrocytes, permits us to have an upright stature, and permits us to move with relative ease through the environment. The skeletal system consists of the axial and appendicular skeletons.

The common long bone consists of a diaphysis, metaphysis, and epiphysis. The diaphysis is the hollow skeletal shaft of the long bone and contains the yellow bone marrow. It is covered by the periosteum, which contains sensory nerve fibers and initiates the bone repair cycle. The metaphysis is the transitional region between the diaphysis and the epiphysis. In this region, the thin layer of compact bone of the diaphysis shaft becomes the honeycomb of the weight-bearing epiphyseal region. The epiphysis is the articular end of the bone. Through the widening of the metaphysis and the cancellous bone underneath, the weight-bearing, articular surface distributes support over a large surface area.

Bones join at an area called a joint, where they move together to permit articulation. The actual surface of movement is the articular surface and is covered with cartilage, a smooth, shock-absorbing surface that allows free movement between the two ends of the adjoining bones. It is the actual joint surface. The joint is held together with ligaments, which are bands of connective tissue attaching bones to each other. These bands encapsulate the joint and allow some stretch, while holding the articulating bones firmly together.

The skeletal system is organized into the axial and appendicular skeletons. The axial skeleton consists of the skull, thorax, and pelvis and the cervical, thoracic, lumbar, sacral, and coccygeal spine. The appendicular skeleton consists of the upper extremity (the humerus, radius and ulna, carpals, metacarpals, and phalanges) and the lower extremity (femur, tibia and fibula, tarsals, metatarsals, and phalanges).

Muscles make up most of the body's mass, are the driving power behind body motion, and also provide most of the body's heat energy. They only have the ability to contract with force, hence are usually paired with one opposing the motion of the other. Muscles are usually attached by strong connective tissue called tendons. The point of attachment that remains stationary with muscle contraction is the origin, while the point of attachment that moves is the insertion.

4. Describe the anatomy and physiology of the head, face, and neck and their relation to the physiology of the central nervous system.   pp. 532-536

Several layers of soft, connective, and skeletal tissues protect the brain. These include the scalp, the cranium, and the meninges. The scalp is a thick and vascular layer of tissue that is strong and flexible and able to absorb tremendous kinetic energy. Beneath it are several layers of connective and muscular fascia that further protect the skull and its contents and that are only connected to the skull on a limited basis. This permits the scalp to move with glancing blows and further protects the cranium.

The skull consists of numerous bones, fused together at fixed joints called sutures. These bones form a container for the brain called the cranium. The cranium is made up of three layers of bone, two thin layers of compact bone separated by a layer of cancellous bone. This construction makes the cranium both light and very strong. This vault for the brain is fixed in volume and does not accommodate any expansion of its contents. However, in the newborn and infant, the skull is more cartilaginous and more flexible, with two open areas, the anterior and posterior fontanelles. These spaces close by 18 months.

The meninges are three layers of tissue—the dura mater, the arachnoid, and the pia mater—that provide further protection for the brain. The dura mater is a tough, fibrous layer that lines the interior of the skull and spinal foramen and is continuous with the inner periosteum of the cranium. The pia mater is a delicate membrane covering the convolutions of the brain and spinal cord. The arachnoid is a web-like structure between the dura mater and pia mater. The cerebrospinal fluid fills the subarachnoid space and "floats" the brain and spinal cord to help absorb the energy of trauma.

The brain occupies about 80 percent of the volume of the cranium and is made up of the cerebrum, cerebellum, and brainstem. The cerebrum occupies most of the cranial vault and is the center of consciousness, personality, speech, motor control, and perception. It is separated into right and left hemispheres by the falx cerebri, extending inward from the anterior, superior, and posterior central skull. The cerebellum sits beneath the posterior half of the cerebrum and is responsible for fine-tuning muscular control and for balance and muscle tone. It is separated from the cerebrum by the tentorium cerebelli, a fibrous sheath that runs transverse to the falx cerebri along the base of the cerebrum. The brainstem runs anterior to the cerebellum and central and inferior to the cerebrum. It consists of the hypothalamus, thalamus, pons, and medulla oblongata. The brainstem controls the endocrine system and most primary body functions including respiration, cardiac activity, temperature, and blood pressure.

The face, consisting of several bones covered with soft tissue, protects the special sense organs of sight, smell, hearing, balance, and taste and forms and protects the upper airway and the beginning of the alimentary canal. The brow ridge (a portion of the frontal bone), the nasal bones, and the zygoma form the eye sockets and protect the eyes. The upper jaw (the maxilla) and the moveable lower jaw (mandible) provide the skeletal structures that form the opening of the mouth. Cavities within this region (sinuses) help to provide shape to the face without increasing the weight of the head. The nasal cavity provides an extended surface to warm, humidify, and cleanse incoming air. The oral cavity houses the tongue and teeth and accommodates the early physical and chemical breakdown of food.

The neck supports the neck through the structure of the cervical spine and the massive muscles of the region. It is also an important region through which many important structures traverse. The airway travels through this region, and its components include the larynx and trachea.

Posterior to the trachea is the esophagus with the carotid artery and jugular vein pairs just lateral to this airway structure.

5. Describe the anatomy and physiology of the spine, including: **pp. 536-542**

Cervical spine
The cervical spine is the vertebral column between the cranium and the thorax. It consists of seven irregular bones held firmly together by ligaments that both support the weight of the head and permit its motion while protecting the delicate spinal cord that runs through the central portion of these bones.

Thoracic spine
The thoracic vertebral column consists of 12 thoracic vertebrae, one corresponding to each rib pair. Like the cervical spine, it consists of irregular bones held firmly together by ligaments that support the weight of the head and neck and permit its motion, while protecting the delicate spinal cord that runs through the central portion of these bones.

Lumbar spine
The lumbar spine consists of five lumbar vertebrae with massive vertebral bodies to support the weight of the head, neck, and thorax. Here the spinal cord ends at the juncture between L-1 and L-2, and nerve roots fill the spinal foramen from L-2 into the sacral spine.

Sacral spine
The sacral spine consists of five sacral vertebrae that are fused into a single plate that forms the posterior portion of the pelvis. The upper body balances on the sacrum, which articulates with the pelvis at a fixed joint, the sacroiliac joint.

Coccyx

The coccygeal region of the spine consists of three to five fused vertebrae that form the remnant of a tail.

6. Describe the anatomy and physiology of the thorax, including its skeletal and muscular structure and the organs and vessels contained within it.   pp. 542-547

The ribs, thoracic spine, sternum, and diaphragm define the structure of the thoracic cage. The skeletal components allow the cage to expand as the ribs are lifted upward and outward by contraction of the intercostal muscles, and the intrathoracic volume further expands as the diaphragm contracts and moves downward. The net action of this muscle movement is to increase the volume of the thoracic cage and to reduce its internal pressure. Air from the environment moves through the airway into the alveoli to equalize this pressure, and inspiration occurs. The intercostal muscles relax and the thorax settles, while the diaphragm rises back into the thorax, and the volume of the cavity decreases. This increases the intrathoracic pressure, and air rushes out to equalize with the environment. This is expiration. The pleura, two serous membranes, seal the lungs to the interior of the thoracic cage during this action and ensure that the lungs expand and contract with the changing volume of the thoracic cavity. The lungs have exceptional circulation, with capillary beds surrounding the alveoli to ensure a free exchange of oxygen and carbon dioxide between the alveolar air and the bloodstream.

The lungs fill all but the central portion of the chest cavity and are found on either side of the central structure, called the mediastinum. The mediastinum contains the heart, trachea, esophagus, major blood vessels, and several nerve pathways. The heart is located in the left central chest and is the major pumping element of the cardiovascular system. The inferior and superior vena cavae collect blood from the lower extremities and abdomen and the upper extremities, head, and neck, respectively, and return it to the heart. The pulmonary arteries and veins carry blood to and from the lungs respectively, and the aorta distributes the cardiac output to the systemic circulation. The trachea enters the mediastinum just beneath the manubrium and bifurcates at the carina into the left and right mainstem bronchi. The esophagus enters the mediastinum just behind the trachea and exits through the diaphragm.

7. Describe the anatomy and physiology of the nervous system, including the neuron, the central nervous system (brain and spine), and the peripheral nervous system (somatic, autonomic, sympathetic, and parasympathetic divisions).   pp. 547-565

The nervous system is the body's chief control for virtually every major function. It is divided physically into the central nervous system (CNS) and peripheral nervous system (PNS). The CNS consists of the brain and spinal cord. If the body were visualized as a computer, the CNS would be the central processing unit. Basic functions, such as continuance of heartbeat and respiration, and complex functions, such as listening to Mozart and anticipating a musical passage you particularly like, are controlled by cells in the brain. Messages within the CNS, as well as those that connect it with the rest of the body, travel as nerve impulses. The complex network of nerves outside the CNS makes up the peripheral nervous system.

The messages that carry information regarding critical body functions such as respiration pass through a part of the PNS called the autonomic nervous system; these functions do not require any conscious effort to maintain them. In contrast, messages that involve voluntary, or conscious, actions and thoughts travel through the other part of the PNS, the somatic nervous system. Both the autonomic and somatic nervous systems have two parallel tracks: one of nerves that carry messages to the brain, and another that carries messages from the brain. In terms of the computer analogy, the PNS carries the various input and output messages that run between the brain and spinal cord and the rest of the body. The autonomic nervous system is also structurally and functionally broken into two parts: the sympathetic and parasympathetic nervous systems. These two parts work together to make sure the net balance of stimulatory and inhibitory messages from the brain keep body functions such as blood pressure within normal limits.

The basic structural and functional unit is the neuron, or nerve cell. Nerve cells have a body that contains the essential cell machinery of nucleus, mitochondria, etc. Nerve processes (usually there are many) that are capable of receiving impulses from other neurons or body cells are called dendrites. An impulse that is picked up by a dendrite travels toward the cell body. Another process, the axon, carries the impulse away from the cell body. Axons may have multiple tips, which means the neuron has the capacity to send the impulse onward to more than one other nerve or other cell. Dendrites associated with neurons of the major sense organs (such as the eye or ear) convert an environmental stimulus into a nerve impulse that can be forwarded via the axon to other nerves, and eventually the brain. Dendrites associated with neurons that monitor internal conditions such as PaO_2 also convert that information into an impulse and send it to the brain. Eventually all such information is analyzed by neurons in the brain, and response impulses travel back through the PNS. These impulses eventually affect a motor neuron, causing a muscle cell to contract, or affect another type of cell such as one in a gland. Messages cannot pass directly from an axon to a dendrite because there is a tiny physical gap, called a synapse, between each pair of neurons. As the wave of electrical depolarization (due to ion fluxes of potassium rapidly leaving the neuron and sodium rapidly entering) reaches the axon tip, it causes a chemical called a neurotransmitter to be released into the synapse. (There are multiple neurotransmitters within the body. Either acetylcholine or norepinephrine is found in the neurons of the PNS. Neurotransmitters within the CNS include dopamine and serotonin.) When the neurotransmitter crosses the synapse and is taken up by the dendrite on the other side, a wave of depolarization is started in that dendrite, and the nerve impulse is then carried toward the cell body.

Most of the CNS is protected by the bones of the cranium and spine. The spinal column is made up of 33 vertebrae running from the neck to the junction with the pelvis. There is also an inner shock-absorbing, cushioning protection system. The cells of the brain and spinal cord are bathed in cerebrospinal fluid, and there are three layers of protective membranes between the neural surface and the outer, protective bone. These meninges are called the dura mater, arachnoid membrane, and pia mater (in outer-to-inner sequence). As you look at a human brain, it has six obvious structural regions: the cerebrum, the diencephalon, the mesencephalon (or midbrain), the pons, the medulla oblongata, and the cerebellum. Sometimes, this is simplified into the terminology of the forebrain (cerebrum and diencephalon), the midbrain (mesencephalon), and the hindbrain (the brainstem—pons and medulla oblongata—and the cerebellum). The largest part of the brain, with its characteristic folded outer surfaces, is the cerebrum. The cerebrum has left and right sides, or hemispheres, which are connected physically and functionally by tissue called the corpus callosum. The cerebrum is responsible for intelligence, learning, memory, and language, as well as analysis and response to sensory and motor activities. The diencephalon is covered by the cerebrum, and it is made up of a number of vital structures: the thalamus, hypothalamus, and the limbic system. This primal part of the brain is responsible for many involuntary functions such as temperature regulation, sleep, water balance, stress response, and emotion. It also has an important role in regulating the autonomic nervous system. The brainstem consists of the mesencephalon, pons, and medulla oblongata. The mesencephalon is located between the diencephalon and the pons, and it plays a role in motor coordination. It is the major region controlling eye movement. The pons is a major connection point between the upper portions of the brain and the medulla and cerebellum. The medulla oblongata itself marks the division between the brain and the spinal cord. The major centers for control of respiration, cardiac activity, and vasomotor activity are located here. The cerebellum is located in the posterior fossa of the cranium, and it also has two hemispheres, which are closely coordinated to the brainstem and higher centers. The cerebellum coordinates fine motor movement, posture, equilibrium, and muscle tone.

The hemispheres of the cerebrum do not contain identical centers. Rather, the functional responsibilities of the cerebrum have been mapped as a whole. Important centers with clinical implications in cases such as stroke or trauma include the following: (1) speech, which is located in the temporal lobe, (2) vision, which is located in the occipital lobe, (3) personality, which is located in the frontal lobes, (4) sensory, which is located in the parietal lobes, and (5) motor, which is located in the frontal lobes. As noted previously, balance and coordination are located in the cerebellum. A last important center is called the reticular activating system (RAS), which operates in the lateral portion of the medulla, pons, and especially the mesencephalon. The RAS sends impulses to and receives messages from the cerebral cortex (the outer portion of the cerebrum). This diffuse system of interlaced cells is responsible for maintaining consciousness and the ability to respond to external stimuli.

The brain receives about 20 percent of the body's total blood flow per minute. Vascular supply to the brain is provided by two systems, a physical arrangement that provides secondary supply if one system is occluded or severed. The anterior system is the carotid, and the posterior system is the vertebrobasilar. They join at the circle of Willis before entering the structures of the brain itself. Venous drainage is via the venous sinuses and the internal jugular veins. As previously noted, there is also cerebrospinal fluid (CSF) bathing the tissues of the brain and spinal cord. Most of the intracranial CSF is found in the ventricles.

The spinal cord is 17 to 18 inches long on average in adults. It leaves the brain at the medulla and passes through an opening in the skull called the foramen magnum to enter the spinal canal. The spinal cord, which ends near the level of the first lumbar vertebra (the reason why spinal taps are done below that level), conducts impulses to and from the peripheral nervous system and locally for motor reflexes. Thirty-one pairs of nerves exit the spinal cord between adjacent vertebrae. The dorsal nerve roots carry afferent fibers, ones carrying impulses to the brain. The ventral roots carry efferent fibers, which carry impulses from the brain to the periphery. Each nerve root has a corresponding area of skin called a dermatome, to which it supplies sensation. In the field, you may be able to correlate sensory deficits to the level of a spinal cord problem. The reason why our protective motor reflexes are so fast and effective lies in the fact that the afferent and efferent impulses are coordinated in the spinal cord—they do not travel the whole way to the brain before coming back. However, because they are mediated in the spinal cord, they lack fine motor control.

The peripheral nervous system (PNS) contains 12 pairs of cranial nerves, which extend directly from the lower surface of the brain and exit through small holes in the skull, and the peripheral nerves, which exit from the spinal cord as noted previously. The nerves of the PNS control both voluntary and involuntary activities. The cranial nerves supply nervous control for the head, neck, and certain thoracic and abdominal organs. The peripheral nerves can be divided into four classes: (1) somatic sensory, afferent nerves that carry impulses concerned with touch, pressure, pain, temperature, and position, (2) somatic motor, efferent nerves that carry impulses to the skeletal (voluntary) muscles, (3) visceral (autonomic) sensory, afferent nerves that carry impulses of sensation from the visceral organs (examples being fullness in the bladder or distension of the rectum), and (4) visceral (autonomic) motor, efferent nerves that serve the involuntary cardiac muscle and the smooth muscle of the viscera and the glands.

The involuntary division of the PNS is called the autonomic nervous system, and it has two components: the sympathetic nervous system and the parasympathetic nervous system. The sympathetic system is associated with the primitive "fight or flight" response to sensory stimuli. Its major nerve roots are located near the thoracic and lumbar part of the spinal cord. Stimulation causes increased heart rate and blood pressure, pupillary dilation, rise in blood sugar, as well as bronchodilation, all responses that ready the body for stress. The neurotransmitters norepinephrine and epinephrine mediate the sympathetic nervous system's actions. Sympathetic activity is also closely correlated to activity in the adrenal medulla, tissue that is of nervous system origin and that also relies on norepinephrine and epinephrine. The parasympathetic nervous system is responsible for controlling vegetative functions such as normal heart rate and blood pressure. It is associated with the cranial nerves and the sacral plexus of nerves, and it is mediated by the neurotransmitter acetylcholine. When stimulated, it causes a decrease in heart rate, an increase in digestive activity, pupillary constriction, and a reduction in blood sugar.

8. Describe the anatomy and physiology of the endocrine system, including the glands and other organs with endocrine activity. pp. 565-576

There are eight major structures associated with the endocrine system located throughout the body: the hypothalamus, pituitary gland, thyroid gland, parathyroid glands, thymus, pancreas, adrenal glands, and gonads. The pineal gland is also part of the endocrine system.

The hypothalamus, located deep within the cerebrum of the brain, is the junction between the endocrine system and the central nervous system. About the size of a pea, the pituitary gland is located adjacent to the hypothalamus within the cerebrum. The pineal gland is also located adjacent to the hypothalamus. The double-lobed thyroid gland is located in the neck anterior to and just below the cartilage of the larynx. The parathyroid glands are very small and are found on the posterior lateral surface of the thyroid gland. The thymus is located in the mediastinum just behind the sternum. The pancreas is located in the upper abdomen behind the stomach and between the duodenum and the spleen. The adrenal glands are somewhat triangular in shape and are located on the superior surface of the kidneys. Gonads can be found in the lower pelvis in women, with each ovary resembling an almond in size and shape. In men, the gonads are located in the scrotum.

The endocrine system is closely linked to the nervous system and plays a critical role in our ability to maintain life by regulating many bodily functions through chemical substances called hormones. The endocrine system is made up of ductless glands, which manufacture and secrete hormones that act in adjacent tissues or travel via the bloodstream to target organs or other endocrine glands to produce specific or generalized effects. Hormones regulate metabolic activity, growth and development, as well as mediate chemical reactions, maintain homeostatic balance, and initiate our adaptive response to stress.

9. Describe the anatomy and physiology of the cardiovascular system, including the heart and the circulatory system   pp. 576-590

The adult heart is roughly the size of a clenched fist, and it lies in the center of the mediastinum posterior to the sternum and anterior to the spine. Roughly two-thirds of the heart lies to the left of midline, with roughly one-third to the right. The bottom of the heart, the apex, lies just above the diaphragm, whereas the top of the heart, or base, lies at roughly the level of the second rib. The heart's connections with the great vessels are at the base. The heart is made up of three tissue layers: The innermost is the endocardium, which has the same type of cells as the endothelial lining of blood vessels and is continuous with the linings of the vessels entering and leaving the heart. The thickest layer is the middle layer of muscle cells, the myocardium. These unique muscle cells physically resemble skeletal muscle but have electrical properties similar to smooth muscle cells. The outermost layer of the heart is the pericardium, a protective sac made of connective tissue arranged in two layers, the visceral pericardium (also called the epicardium) and the parietal pericardium. Normally, about 25 mL of pericardial fluid is contained between the two layers of pericardium, and the heart moves freely within the pericardial sac.

The heart is made up of two side-by-side pumps, the left side and the right side. Each side has an upper chamber, the atrium, which receives blood, and a lower chamber, the ventricle, which pumps blood into other blood vessels. The atria are separated by an interatrial septum, and the ventricles are separated by an interventricular septum. The atrial walls are thin in contrast with the ventricular walls, and almost all of the heart's pumping force is generated by the ventricles. The left ventricle, which pumps blood into the aorta, has a much thicker wall than the right ventricle, which pumps blood into the pulmonary artery.

The heart contains two sets of valves that help to keep blood flowing properly through the chambers and into the aorta and pulmonary artery: The atrioventricular valves lie between each atrium and ventricle. The left atrioventricular valve is called the mitral valve, and it has two characteristic leaflets. The right atrioventricular valve is called the tricuspid valve, and it has three characteristic leaflets. When the papillary muscles that connect the valves to the walls of the heart relax, the leaflets open and blood flows from the atria into the ventricles. Special fibers called the chordae tendoneae connect the leaflets of a valve to the papillary muscles, and these fibers prevent the leaflets from prolapsing back into the atrium when the valve is open. The semilunar valves lie between the ventricles and the artery into which each empties. The left semilunar valve, or aortic valve, lies between the left ventricle and the aorta. The right semilunar valve, or pulmonic valve, lies between the right ventricle and the pulmonary artery. When these valves open, blood flows in a one-way path from the ventricles into the arteries, and backflow into the ventricles is prevented.

The superior and inferior vena cavae carry deoxygenated blood from the body to the right atrium.

Blood flows through the right atrium and ventricle before entering the pulmonary artery, which carries it to the lungs. Oxygenated blood leaves the lungs through the pulmonary veins and enters the left atrium. The left ventricle pumps the blood into the aorta, which feeds the oxygenated blood into peripheral arteries to flow to the rest of the body. Pressure within the heart is markedly higher on the left than on the right because resistance to flow is higher in the peripheral circulation than it is in the pulmonary circulation. Consequently, the myocardium of the left ventricle thickens as an infant ages to the point that the adult left ventricle is markedly thicker than the right.

The circulatory system consists of two sub-systems. In pulmonary circulation, blood enters the lungs via the pulmonary arteries and their smaller branches, the arterioles. It eventually flows through capillaries that form networks over alveoli, and gas exchange (movement of oxygen into the blood and carbon dioxide from the blood) takes place here. The oxygenated blood then flows into the pulmonary venules and larger pulmonary veins and enters the left atrium. The peripheral circulation begins with the aorta, which receives oxygenated blood from the left ventricle. The aorta has numerous branches. These arteries and the smaller arterioles ensure that oxygenated blood flows to all parts of the body. Oxygenated blood eventually enters capillary beds, and oxygen exchange between blood and tissues occurs. Deoxygenated blood enters smaller venules, which empty into the larger veins that return blood to the right atrium. Gas exchange occurs in capillaries because their walls are only one cell thick. This same cell layer, the endothelium, is the innermost layer of arteries and veins.

10. Describe the physiology of perfusion.   pp. 590-596

Perfusion is the process by which oxygen and nutrients and waste products and carbon dioxide are brought to and take from the body cells. It is essential to life, and its breakdown is the process we call shock. To ensure adequate perfusion the body requires a pump, fluid volume, and a container. The pump is the heart and for proper cardiac output, the heart must receive an adequate supply of blood (preload), have an adequate contractile force, and a proper rate of contractions. The systems fluid, blood, must be in adequate supply and fill the container, the vascular system. Additionally, the container must maintain an adequate pressure so it is able to direct blood to the tissues in need. It maintains this pressure by constricting or dilating the arterioles to maintain blood pressure. Baroreceptors monitor blood pressure and control it by changing the heart rate, strength of contraction, size of the vascular container, or the number and degree of arterioles in constriction or dilation.

11. Describe the anatomy of the respiratory system (upper and lower airway and pediatric airway) and the physiology of the respiratory system (respiration and ventilation and measures of respiratory function).   pp. 596-610

The mouth, or oral cavity, is a single cavity that serves as an auxiliary air passage. The posterior upper surface is the soft palate, which moves upward and closes off the passages from the nose to the pharynx during swallowing. The nasal cavity is a hollow two-sided chamber lined with mucous membranes that warms, filters, and humidifies air as it enters the respiratory system. Its anterior openings are the nares, or nostrils. The nasal and oral cavities empty into the pharynx, or throat. The pharynx is a muscular tube that functions as the transitional area for food and air between the nose and mouth and between the esophagus and larynx.

The larynx is the tubular structure that begins the lower airway. It consists of the thyroid and cricoid cartilages, the vocal cords, the arytenoid folds, and the upper portion of the trachea. It is the "Adam's apple" located in the anterior neck. The epiglottis is a flap-like structure covering the opening of the trachea, the glottis. It closes during swallowing to prevent food or fluids from entering the trachea and respiratory system. The vallecula is a fold formed by the epiglottis and base of the tongue. The larynx opens into the trachea, a series of cartilaginous C-shaped structures that hold the airway open. The trachea divides into two mainstem bronchi at the carina. The bronchi subdivide, finally reaching the respiratory bronchioles, the alveolar ducts, and, finally, the alveoli. The alveoli are the primary exchange structures between the respiratory system and the pulmonary capillaries of the cardiovascular system for oxygen and carbon dioxide.

The gross anatomy of the pediatric airway is very similar to that of the adult but is smaller in size with smaller airway clearances and a greater proportion of soft tissue. The larynx is more superior and anterior than in the adult, and the smallest clearance of the airway is the cricoid cartilage rather than the glottis as it is in the adult. The child's tongue is proportionally larger and more easily obstructs the airway. Because of the smaller lumen size, the soft tissue of the airway may swell more quickly to cause obstruction.

Respiration is the exchange of gases between a living organism and its environment. The volume of the thorax expands as the diaphragm contracts and displaces downward. The intercostal muscles contract, pulling the rib cage upward and outward. The muscles of the neck enhance this action as they lift the sternum. The lungs expand with the chest as the pleural seal secures the exterior of the lung to the interior of the thorax. The expansion of the lungs reduces the air pressure within them, and air flows into the alveoli. Gravity and the intrinsic elasticity of the lungs then cause the thorax to settle, the pressure within the lungs to increase, and air to be exhaled.

The air brought into the lungs contains 21 percent oxygen and very little carbon dioxide. Oxygen diffuses through the alveolar and capillary walls and is bound to the hemoglobin, while carbon dioxide diffuses in the opposite direction. The air exhaled contains about 14 percent oxygen and 5 percent carbon dioxide. The oxygen from inspired air diffuses from the alveolar space through the alveolar wall and the pulmonary capillary membrane, where it attaches to the hemoglobin of the blood. Carbon dioxide, mostly transported as bicarbonate, diffuses from the blood plasma across the capillary membrane and through the alveolar wall.

The measures of respiratory function include:
• **Total Lung Capacity (TLC)** is the volume of air in the lungs after a maximal inspiration, about 6 liters in the adult male.
• **Tidal Volume (V_T)** is the average volume of air inspired (or expired) with each breath, about 500 mL in the adult male.
• **Dead Space Volume (V_D)** is the portion of the tidal volume that does not reach the alveoli and is unavailable for gas exchange, about 150 mL.
• **Alveolar Volume (V_A)** is the amount of air that reaches the alveoli with each breath, about 350 mL.
• **Minute Volume (V_{min})** is the amount of air moved in and out of the respiratory system in one minute (minute volume = tidal volume 3 respiratory rate).
• **Alveolar Minute Volume (V_{A-min})** is the amount of gas that reaches the alveoli per minute.
• **Inspiratory Reserve Volume (IRV)** is the amount of air that can be inspired after a normal inspiration.
• **Expiratory Reserve Volume (ERV)** is the amount of air that can be exhaled after a normal exhalation.
• **Residual Volume (RV)** is the amount of air in the lungs after a maximal exhalation.
• **Functional Residual Capacity (FRC)** is the amount of air remaining in the lungs after a normal expiration.
• **Forced Expiratory Volume (FV)** is the amount of air a person can exhale after a maximal inhalation, about 4,500 mL in an adult male.

12. Describe the anatomy and physiology of the abdomen, including its divisions and the organs and vessels contained within it.   pp. 610-613

The abdomen is one of the body's largest cavities, bounded superiorly by the diaphragm, laterally by the flank muscles, inferiorly by the pelvis, posteriorly by the spine and back muscles, and anteriorly by the abdominal muscles. Since most of its border is soft tissue, it is rather unprotected from injury. The abdomen contains the continuous, muscular tube of digestion, the alimentary canal. It enters the abdomen through the hiatus of the diaphragm as the esophagus. It joins the stomach, an organ that physically mixes the food with gastric juices and then sends it out and into the small bowel. The first portion of the bowel, the duodenum, mixes the digesting food with bile (a byproduct of the liver) and pancreatic juices and then begins the process of absorption. The remainder of the small bowel draws the nutrients from the food.

As the digesting food enters the large bowel it is mixed with bacteria, releasing water and any remaining nutrients. They are absorbed, and the material is pushed by peristalsis to the rectum, awaiting defecation. The bowel is a thin and vascular tube that drains its blood supply through the liver for detoxification, where some nutrients are stored and others are added to the circulation. The liver is a large, solid organ found in the right upper quadrant, just below the diaphragm. The pancreas is a delicate organ found in the lower aspect of the upper left quadrant with a portion of it extending into the right upper quadrant. In addition to digestive juices, it manufactures insulin and glucagon. The kidneys are found deep within the flanks and filter blood to remove excess water and electrolytes. They are very vascular organs that excrete urine into the ureters through which the urine then travels to the bladder. The bladder (in the central pelvic space) rids the body of urine through the urethra. The spleen is an organ of the immune system and is very delicate and vascular, residing in the left upper quadrant.

The abdominal cavity is lined with a serous membrane, the peritoneum. It covers the anterior abdominal organs, and a double-layer sheath of it forms the omentum, which covers the anterior surface of the abdomen. The bowel is slung from the posterior wall of the abdomen by connective tissue called the mesentery that also provides perfusion to the bowel. The abdominal aorta and inferior vena cava run along the spinal column and branch frequently to serve the abdominal organs.

13. Describe the anatomy and physiology of the digestive system, including the digestive track and the accessory organs of digestion, and also the spleen. pp. 613-616

The GI tract is a long tube that extends from the mouth to the anus and is divided structurally and functionally into different parts. In general, the GI system is divided into the upper and lower GI tracts. The upper GI tract includes the mouth, esophagus, stomach, and duodenum, whereas the lower GI tract includes the remainder of the small intestine and the large intestine, rectum, and anus. In the upper GI tract, food is ingested, and preliminary physical and chemical digestion is begun. In the lower GI tract, digestion of food is completed, nutrients are absorbed into the body, and remaining fiber, intestinal bacteria, and other materials are eliminated through the anus as feces. In addition, three additional organs, the liver, gallbladder, and pancreas, are intimately associated with the GI system both structurally (through connections with the duodenum) and functionally. The vermiform appendix, a blind sac found at the junction of the small and large intestines, does not have any apparent physiologic role in GI function but is important to you because of the inflammatory condition called appendicitis, which you will see in patients in the field.

The spleen is a structure within the immune system and sits in the left upper quadrant, just behind the stomach. It is the most fragile abdominal organ and stores a great amount of blood, hence its injury can lead to significant hemorrhage.

14. Describe the anatomy and physiology of the urinary system, including the kidneys, ureters, urinary bladder, and urethra.   pp. 616-622

The two major organs of the urinary system are the kidneys and the urinary bladder. Two major structures are the ureters and the urethra. The kidney is the critical organ of the urinary system. The kidneys perform the vital functions of the urinary system, which include:

• Maintenance of blood volume with proper balance of water, electrolytes, and pH
• Retention of key substances such as glucose and removal of toxic wastes such as urea
• Major role in regulation of arterial blood pressure
• Control of the development of red blood cells

The first two roles are achieved through the production of urine in the kidneys. The kidneys' role in regulation of blood pressure is achieved in part through control of the body's fluid volume. In addition, they produce an enzyme called renin, which acts to activate a hormone (chemical messenger) called angiotensin, which is part of a hormonal pathway that acts to retain water in the body (increase blood pressure).

The structural and functional unit within the kidney is the nephron, and each kidney contains about one million nephrons, establishing the functional reserve that most people take for granted. Blood is filtered into the first part of the nephron, the glomerulus, and then moves through a length of specialized tubule. As the fluid moves through the parts of the tubule, movement of water and some materials out of the tubule and into the blood occurs (reabsorption), as does movement of some materials out of the blood and into the tubule (secretion). The kidneys can maintain an exquisitely fine control over the relative activity of reabsorption and secretion for virtually every substance that is filtered into the glomerulus. The ability of the kidney to retain glucose, excrete wastes such as urea, and thus perform all of its vital roles is extraordinary, and life depends upon it. When kidney function is too low or nonexistent, an individual will die unless the function is replaced through artificial dialysis or through kidney transplantation. The final role of the kidney, control over development of red blood cells, is achieved through production and release of a hormone called erythropoietin, which stimulates red blood cell synthesis in the bone marrow.

Each ureter runs from a kidney to the bladder, and urine moves out of the kidney through them to reach the bladder. Because ureters are very small in internal diameter, they can become blocked by internal objects such as kidney stones. The bladder is a muscular sac that expands to hold urine. During urination, stored urine is eliminated from the bladder (and the body) through the tube called the urethra.

15. Describe the anatomy and physiology of the female reproductive system, the menstrual cycle, and the pregnant uterus.   pp. 623-629

The most important female reproductive structures are located within the pelvic cavity. Essential to reproduction, these structures include the ovaries, which store eggs until maturation (once per month); the fallopian tubes, which direct the egg to the uterus; the uterus, which is a hollow chamber where the egg is fertilized and then is nurtured through the vascular uterine wall; and the vagina or birth canal. The external genitalia have accessory functions, in that they protect body openings and play an important role in sexual functioning.

A monthly hormonal cycle prepares the uterus to receive a fertilized egg. The first 2 weeks of the cycle (known as the proliferative phase) are dominated by estrogen, causing the uterine lining to thicken. In response to a surge of luteinizing hormone, ovulation takes place and an egg is released from the ovary. The secretory phase is the stage of the menstrual cycle immediately surrounding ovulation. If the egg is not fertilized, the woman's estrogen level drops sharply while the progesterone level dominates. Uterine vascularity increases in anticipation of implantation. If fertilization does not occur, estrogen and progesterone levels fall, triggering vascular changes that leave the endometrium ischemic. The ischemic endometrium is shed during the menstrual phase (menstruation), along with a discharge of blood, mucus, and cellular debris. Menstrual flow usually lasts 3 to 5 days, with an average blood loss of 50 mL.

The pregnant uterus undergoes rapid growth to support the developing fetus. Its growth displaces upward most of the contents of the abdomen and by the 32nd week of gestation fills the abdominal cavity to the lower rib margin. The uterus is a very muscular and vascular hollow organ that protects the fetus. Within it is the amniotic sac, filled with fluid that distributes the impact of trauma and protects the developing infant very well.

16. Describe the anatomy and physiology of the male reproductive system.   pp. 629-630

The genitourinary system of men includes some specifically reproductive organs and structures: the testes (the primary male reproductive organs, which produce testosterone and sperm cells) and tubing called the epididymis and vas deferens, through which sperm cells leave the testes and move toward the urethra. Sperm leaves the vas deferens to enter the urethra as it passes through the substance of the other male reproductive organ, the prostate gland, which produces fluid that mixes with sperm to produce semen, the male reproductive fluid.

CONTENT SELF-EVALUATION

1. The outermost layer of the skin is the:
- **A.** epidermis.
- **B.** subcutaneous tissue.
- **C.** cutical.
- **D.** dermis.
- **E.** sebum.

2. Which of the following glands secrete sweat?
- **A.** sudoriferous glands
- **B.** sebaceous glands
- **C.** subcutaneous glands
- **D.** adrenal glands
- **E.** none of the above

3. Which of the following types of cells are found in the dermis?
- **A.** lymphocytes
- **B.** macrophages
- **C.** mast cells
- **D.** fibroblasts
- **E.** all of the above

4. The type of hair that is short, fine, and lacks pigment is called:
- **A.** terminal.
- **B.** formative.
- **C.** scalioned.
- **D.** vellus.
- **E.** none of the above

5. All of the following are components of the adult hematopoietic system EXCEPT the:
- **A.** blood.
- **B.** bone marrow.
- **C.** thymus.
- **D.** liver.
- **E.** spleen.

6. The major determinants of blood volume are red cell mass and:
- **A.** erythropoietin levels.
- **B.** plasma volume.
- **C.** total body water.
- **D.** stem cell percentage.
- **E.** bone marrow volume.

7. The component of the red blood cell that is responsible for transporting oxygen is the:
- **A.** basophil.
- **B.** granulocyte.
- **C.** hemoglobin.
- **D.** neutrophil.
- **E.** lymphocyte.

8. All of the following will cause a right shift of the oxyhemoglobin dissociation curve and thus increase the rate that oxygen is released to the tissues EXCEPT:
- **A.** increased carbon dioxide.
- **B.** increased temperature.
- **C.** decreased pH.
- **D.** decreased activity.
- **E.** increased activity.

9. The term for the packed cell volume of red cells per unit of blood volume is:
- **A.** hematocrit.
- **B.** hemoglobin.
- **C.** red blood cell count.
- **D.** blood type.
- **E.** white blood count.

10. White blood cells that primarily function in allergic reactions to release histamine are called:
- **A.** lymphocytes.
- **B.** neutrophils.
- **C.** eosinophils.
- **D.** monocytes.
- **E.** basophils.

11. White blood cells that primarily function to fight infection are called:
   A. lymphocytes.
   B. neutrophils.
   C. eosinophils.
   D. monocytes.
   E. basophils.

12. T cells and B cells, which play critical roles in immunity, are types of white cells called:
   A. lymphocytes.
   B. neutrophils.
   C. eosinophils.
   D. monocytes.
   E. basophils.

13. The condition that occurs when the body develops antibodies against itself is called:
   A. acquired immunodeficiency.
   B. autoimmune disease.
   C. rejection.
   D. chemotaxis.
   E. inherited immunodeficiency.

14. Causes of the inflammatory process include all of the following EXCEPT:
   A. infectious agents.
   B. chemical agents.
   C. trauma.
   D. immunologic agents.
   E. genetics.

15. The formed blood cell components responsible for blood clotting are:
   A. red blood cells.
   B. white blood cells.
   C. lymphocytes.
   D. platelets.
   E. monocytes.

16. Which of the following is NOT a function performed by the musculoskeletal system?
   A. vital organ protection
   B. a portion of the immune response
   C. storage of material necessary for metabolism
   D. hemopoietic activities
   E. efficient movement against gravity

17. The bone cell responsible for maintaining bone tissue is the:
   A. osteoblast.
   B. osteoclast.
   C. osteocyte.
   D. osteocrit.
   E. none of the above

18. The bone cell responsible for dissolving bone tissue is the:
   A. osteoblast.
   B. osteoclast.
   C. osteocyte.
   D. osteocrit.
   E. none of the above

19. The central portion of a long bone is called the:
   A. diaphysis.
   B. epiphysis.
   C. metaphysis.
   D. cancellous bone.
   E. compact bone.

20. The transitional area between the end and central portion of the long bone is called the:
   A. diaphysis.
   B. epiphysis.
   C. metaphysis.
   D. cancellous bone.
   E. compact bone.

21. The type of bone tissue filling the end of the long bone is called the:
   A. diaphysis.
   B. epiphysis.
   C. metaphysis.
   D. cancellous bone.
   E. compact bone.

22. The covering of the shaft of the long bones that initiates the bone repair cycle is the:
   A. periosteum.
   B. peritoneum.
   C. perforating canal.
   D. osteocyte.
   E. epiphysis.

23. Immovable joints such as those of the skull are termed:

    A.   synovial.
    B.   synarthroses.
    C.   amphiarthroses.
    D.   diarthroses.
    E.   A or D

24. The elbow is an example of which type of joint?

    A.   monaxial
    B.   biaxial
    C.   triaxial
    D.   synarthrosis
    E.   amphiarthrosis

25. Bands of strong material that stretch and hold the joint together while permitting movement are the:

    A.   bursae.
    B.   tendons.
    C.   ligaments.
    D.   cartilage.
    E.   metaphyses.

26. The small sacs filled with synovial fluid that reduce friction and absorb shock are the:

    A.   bursae.
    B.   tendons.
    C.   ligaments.
    D.   cartilage.
    E.   metaphyses.

27. Skeletal maturity is reached by age:

    A.   6.
    B.   10.
    C.   20.
    D.   40.
    E.   45.

28. The muscular system consists of about how many muscle groups?

    A.   100
    B.   200
    C.   300
    D.   500
    E.   600

29. The muscle attachment to the bone that moves when the muscle mass contracts is the:

    A.   flexor.
    B.   extensor.
    C.   origin.
    D.   insertion.
    E.   articulation.

30. Which of the following is a layer of the scalp?

    A.   the skin
    B.   occipitalis muscle
    C.   galea aponeurotica
    D.   areolar tissue
    E.   all of the above

31. Which of the following is NOT a bone of the cranium?

    A.   frontal
    B.   mandible
    C.   parietal
    D.   sphenoid
    E.   ethmoid

32. The largest opening in the cranium is the:

    A.   auditory canal.
    B.   orbit of the eye.
    C.   foramen magnum.
    D.   tentorium.
    E.   transverse foramen.

33. Place the following layers of the meninges as they occur from the cerebrum to the skull.

    A.   dura mater, pia mater, arachnoid
    B.   dura mater, arachnoid, pia mater
    C.   arachnoid, pia mater, dura mater
    D.   arachnoid, dura mater, pia mater
    E.   pia mater, arachnoid, dura mater

34. The layer of the meninges that is strong and lines the interior of the cranium is the:

    A.   pia mater.
    B.   falx cerebri.
    C.   arachnoid.
    D.   dura mater.
    E.   tentorium.

35. The structure that divides the cerebrum into left and right halves is the:

A.   pia mater.   D.   dura mater.
B.   falx cerebri.   E.   tentorium.
C.   arachnoid.

36. Which of the following is a function of the hypothalamus?

A.   body temperature control
B.   control of the ascending reticular activating system
C.   control of respiration
D.   responsibility for sleeping
E.   maintaining balance

37. Which of the following is a function of the medulla oblongata?

A.   body temperature control
B.   control of the ascending reticular activating system
C.   control of respiration
D.   responsibility for sleeping
E.   maintaining balance

38. The normal intracranial pressure is:

A.   120 mmHg.   D.   25 mmHg.
B.   90 mmHg.   E.   less than 10 mmHg.
C.   50 mmHg.

39. The reflex that increases the systemic blood pressure to maintain cerebral blood flow is called:

A.   the ascending reticular activating system.
B.   the descending reticular activating system.
C.   autoregulation.
D.   Cushing's reflex.
E.   mean arterial pressure.

40. Which of the following nerves is responsible for voluntary movement of the tongue?

A.   CN-I   D.   CN-X
B.   CN-III   E.   CN-XII
C.   CN-VIII

41. Which of the following is the lower and moveable jaw bone?

A.   maxilla   D.   stapes
B.   mandible   E.   pinna
C.   zygoma

42. Which of the following is the bone of the cheek?

A.   the maxilla   D.   the stapes
B.   the mandible   E.   the pinna
C.   the zygoma

43. The structure responsible for our positional sense is the:

A.   ossicle.   D.   sinuses.
B.   cochlea.   E.   vitreous humor.
C.   semicircular canals.

44. Which of the following is the opening through which light travels to contact the light-sensing tissue in the eye?

A.   retina   D.   pupil
B.   aqueous humor   E.   iris
C.   vitreous humor

45. Which of the following is the light-sensing tissue in the eye?
- **A.** retina
- **B.** aqueous humor
- **C.** vitreous humor
- **D.** pupil
- **E.** iris

46. The white of the eye is the:
- **A.** sclera.
- **B.** conjunctiva.
- **C.** cornea.
- **D.** aqueous humor.
- **E.** vitreous humor.

47. The delicate, clear tissue covering the pupil and iris is the:
- **A.** sclera.
- **B.** conjunctiva.
- **C.** cornea.
- **D.** aqueous humor.
- **E.** vitreous humor.

48. The vertebral column is made up of how many vertebrae?
- **A.** 24
- **B.** 33
- **C.** 43
- **D.** 45
- **E.** 54

49. The major weight-bearing component of the vertebral column is the:
- **A.** spinous process.
- **B.** transverse process.
- **C.** vertebral body.
- **D.** spinal foramen.
- **E.** lamina.

50. The region of the vertebral column that has 12 vertebrae is the:
- **A.** cervical.
- **B.** thoracic.
- **C.** lumbar.
- **D.** sacral.
- **E.** coccygeal.

51. The region of the vertebral column that permits the greatest movement is the:
- **A.** cervical.
- **B.** thoracic.
- **C.** lumbar.
- **D.** sacral.
- **E.** coccygeal.

52. The region of the vertebral column that has five separate vertebrae is the:
- **A.** cervical.
- **B.** thoracic
- **C.** lumbar.
- **D.** sacral.
- **E.** coccygeal.

53. At its distal end, the spinal cord is attached to the:
- **A.** foramen magnum.
- **B.** peripheral nerve roots.
- **C.** sacral ligament.
- **D.** lumbar process.
- **E.** coccygeal ligament.

54. The region of the spine with the closest tolerance between the spinal cord and the interior of the spinal foramen is the:
- **A.** cervical spine.
- **B.** thoracic spine.
- **C.** lumbar spine.
- **D.** sacral spine.
- **E.** coccygeal spine.

55. Which of the following is located within the thorax?
- **A.** the heart
- **B.** both lungs
- **C.** the esophagus
- **D.** the trachea
- **E.** all of the above

56. How many rib pairs are floating ribs?
- **A.** 1
- **B.** 2
- **C.** 3
- **D.** 6
- **E.** 8

57. Which of the following lines is used to describe position on the chest wall?
- **A.** posterior axillary line
- **B.** anterior axillary line
- **C.** medial axillary line
- **D.** midclavicular line
- **E.** all of the above

58. How high does the diaphragm rise in the chest during a maximum expiration?
- **A.** to the 2nd intercostal space posteriorly
- **B.** to the 4th intercostal space posteriorly
- **C.** to the 6th intercostal space posteriorly
- **D.** to the 8th intercostal space posteriorly
- **E.** to the manubrium anteriorly

59. The muscle(s) of respiration responsible for reducing the distance between ribs and helping lift the thorax is(are) the:
- **A.** intercostal muscles.
- **B.** diaphragm.
- **C.** sternocleidomastoid muscles.
- **D.** scalene.
- **E.** rectus abdominis.

60. The structure that separates the chest cavity from the abdominal cavity is the:
- **A.** mediastinum.
- **B.** peritoneum.
- **C.** perineum.
- **D.** diaphragm.
- **E.** vena cava.

61. At the beginning of and during most of expiration, the pressure within the thorax is:
- **A.** less than the environmental pressure
- **B.** more than the environmental pressure.
- **C.** equal to the environmental pressure.
- **D.** first lower than and then higher than the environmental pressure.
- **E.** first higher than and then lower than the environmental pressure.

62. Which structures enter or exit the lungs at the pulmonary hilum?
- **A.** right mainstem bronchus
- **B.** thoracic duct
- **C.** pulmonary artery
- **D.** pulmonary veins
- **E.** all except B

63. The serous structure that ensures that the lungs expand with the thoracic cage wall and diaphragm is the:
- **A.** pleura.
- **B.** hilum.
- **C.** ligamentum arteriosum.
- **D.** lobular attachment.
- **E.** mediastinum.

64. Which of the following structures is NOT located within the mediastinum?
- **A.** thoracic duct
- **B.** phrenic nerve
- **C.** pulmonary hilum
- **D.** vagus nerve
- **E.** esophagus

65. The intercostal arteries and nerves run:
- **A.** behind the ribs.
- **B.** above the ribs.
- **C.** in front of the ribs.
- **D.** under the ribs.
- **E.** both A and D

66. The somatic nervous system primarily innervates the:
- **A.** cardiac muscle.
- **B.** glands.
- **C.** skeletal muscle.
- **D.** smooth muscle.
- **E.** respiratory system.

67. The space between the pia mater and the arachnoid membrane is the:
- **A.** epiarachnoid space.
- **B.** epidural space.
- **C.** subarachnoid space.
- **D.** subdural space.
- **E.** cerebral space.

68. This portion of the brain connects the two hemispheres of the cerebrum:
- **A.** cerebellum.
- **B.** cerebral cortex.
- **C.** corpus callosum.
- **D.** midbrain.
- **E.** diencephalon.

69. The area of the brain responsible for emotions, hormone production, and autonomic functions is the:
- **A.** hypothalamus.
- **B.** pituitary gland.
- **C.** pons.
- **D.** thalamus.
- **E.** medulla oblongata.

70. This portion of the brain regulates cardiovascular, respiratory, and digestive system activities:
- **A.** cerebellum.
- **B.** hypothalamus.
- **C.** pons.
- **D.** thalamus.
- **E.** medulla oblongata.

71. The _____ lobe of the brain is responsible for speech.
- **A.** frontal
- **B.** occipital
- **C.** parietal
- **D.** temporal
- **E.** semiparietal

72. The _____ system is responsible for consciousness and stimuli response.
- **A.** carotid
- **B.** limbic
- **C.** vertebrobasilar
- **D.** reticular activating
- **E.** cephalic

73. Which efferent fibers carry impulses to the skeletal muscles?
- **A.** somatic motor
- **B.** somatic sensory
- **C.** visceral motor
- **D.** visceral sensory
- **E.** visceral lymphatic

74. The _____ nervous system is mediated by epinephrine and norepinephrine.
- **A.** afferent
- **B.** parasympathetic
- **C.** somatic
- **D.** sympathetic
- **E.** central

75. Acetylcholine is the neurotransmitter of which nervous system?
- **A.** adrenergic
- **B.** afferent
- **C.** parasympathetic
- **D.** sympathetic
- **E.** central

76. The gland that is the connection between the endocrine system and the central nervous system is the:
- **A.** pituitary.
- **B.** hypothalamus.
- **C.** thymus.
- **D.** pineal.
- **E.** thyroid.

77. All of the following are hormones secreted by the anterior pituitary gland EXCEPT:
- **A.** growth hormone.
- **B.** oxytocin.
- **C.** prolactin.
- **D.** adrenocorticotropic hormone.
- **E.** thyroid-stimulating hormone.

78. In children, the thymus secretes a hormone that is critical to the maturation of T-lymphocytes, which play a significant role in:
- **A.** maintaining blood calcium levels.
- **B.** cell-mediated immunity.
- **C.** cellular metabolism.
- **D.** carbohydrate metabolism.
- **E.** gluconeogenesis.

79. All of the following are pancreatic hormones EXCEPT:
- **A.** polypeptide.
- **B.** glucagon.
- **C.** somatostatin.
- **D.** cortisol.
- **E.** insulin.

80. Homeostasis of blood glucose is controlled by insulin and:
- **A.** polypeptide.
- **B.** glucagon.
- **C.** somatostatin.
- **D.** cortisol.
- **E.** thymosin.

81. The substance that the alpha cells of the pancreas secrete when blood glucose levels fall is:
- **A.** polypeptide.
- **B.** glucagon.
- **C.** somatostatin.
- **D.** cortisol.
- **E.** insulin.

82. The substance secreted by the beta cells of the pancreas when blood glucose levels rise is:
- **A.** polypeptide.
- **B.** glucagon.
- **C.** somatostatin.
- **D.** cortisol.
- **E.** insulin.

83. Insulin's primary function is to:
- **A.** metabolize glucose at the cellular level.
- **B.** free glucose from muscle storage sites.

- **C.** transport glucose across the cell membrane.
- **D.** store glucose at the cellular level.
- **E.** enhance the function of glucagon.

84. The production of glucose by the processes of glycogenolysis and gluconeogenesis is triggered by:
- **A.** polypeptide.
- **B.** glucagon.
- **C.** somatostatin.
- **D.** cortisol.
- **E.** insulin.

85. All of the following are hormones secreted by the adrenal glands EXCEPT:
- **A.** epinephrine.
- **B.** cortiso .
- **C.** somatostatin.
- **D.** norepinephrine.
- **E.** aldosterone.

86. Glucocorticoids play a role in maintaining blood glucose levels by promoting gluconeogenesis and:
- **A.** decreasing glucose utilization.
- **B.** increasing glucose utilization.
- **C.** promoting salt and fluid retention.
- **D.** decreasing salt and fluid retention.
- **E.** potentiating the effects of catecholamines.

87. The primary function of aldosterone is to:
- **A.** regulate sodium and potassium excretion.
- **B.** regulate calcium and magnesium excretion.
- **C.** promote gluconeogenesis.
- **D.** inhibit gluconeogenesis.
- **E.** stimulate glucocorticoid production.

88. From innermost to outermost, the three tissue layers of the heart are:
- **A.** the endocardium, the pericardium, and the myocardium.
- **B.** the endocardium, the myocardium, and the syncytium.
- **C.** the endocardium, the myocardium, and the pericardium.

D.   the myocardium, the epicardium, and the pericardium.

E.   the epicardium, the myocardium, and the endocardium.

89. The small, specialized fibers that connect to the heart valve leaflets and prevent the valves from prolapsing are called:

A.	atrial strictures.	**D.**	semilunar structures.
B.	chordae tendoneae.	**E.**	none of the above
C.	papillary muscles.		

90. The blood vessel that returns blood to the atria from the body is the:

A.	aorta.	**D.**	pulmonary vein.
B.	inferior vena cava.	**E.**	both B and C
C.	superior vena cava.		

91. The blood supply to the left ventricle, interventricular septum, part of the right ventricle, and the heart's conduction system comes from the two branches of the left coronary artery, which are the:

A.   anterior descending artery and the circumflex artery.

B.   anterior descending artery and the posterior descending artery.

C.   circumflex artery and the posterior descending artery.

D.   circumflex artery and the marginal artery.

E.   marginal artery and the posterior descending artery.

92.   Stimulation of the heart by the sympathetic nervous system results in:

A.   negative inotropic and chronotropic effects.

B.   negative chronotropic and dromotropic effects.

C.   positive chronotropic and dromotropic effects.

D.   positive inotropic and chronotropic effects.

E.   positive inotropic and dromotropic effects.

93. The difference between the charge of the inside of a myocardial cell and its exterior before contraction is termed:

A.	action potential.	**D.**	resting potential.
B.	depolarization.	**E.**	none of the above
C.	sodium/potassium balance.		

94. The myocardial property that permits the heart cells to depolarize on their own is called:

A.	depolarization.	**D.**	automaticity.
B.	conductivity.	**E.**	conductivity.
C.	excitability.		

95. The inner layer of the blood vessels are which of the following?

A.	lumen	**D.**	tunica adventitia
B.	tunica intima	**E.**	Purkinje
C.	tunica media		

96. An inadequate delivery of oxygenated blood to body cells is:

A.	hypoxia.	**D.**	ischemia.
B.	anoxia.	**E.**	infarction.
C.	hypoperfusion.		

97. The normal cardiac stroke volume is about:

A.	50 mL	**D.**	100 mL
B.	60 mL	**E.**	120 mL
C.	70 mL		

98. Which of the following affects the cardiac output?

A.	preload	**D.**	cardiac rate
B.	afterload	**E.**	all of the above
C.	cardiac contractile force		

99. The arteriole has the ability to change its internal diameter by as much as:

A.	twice.	D.	fivefold.
B.	three times.	E.	seven times.
C.	fourfold.		

100. Which of the following blood vessel(s) have (has) the greatest effect on blood pressure?

A.	aorta	D.	arterioles
B.	the major arteries	E.	venules
C.	the veins		

101. The nasal cavity is responsible for all of the functions listed below EXCEPT:

A.	warming the air.	D.	cleansing the air.
B.	deoxygenating the air.	E.	the sense of smell.
C.	humidifying the air.		

102. The space located between the base of the tongue and the epiglottis is called the:

A.	vallecula.	D.	epiglottic fossa.
B.	cricoid.	E.	glottic opening.
C.	arytenoid fold.		

103. Which of the following is the only bone in the axial skeleton that does not articulate with another bone?

A.	the mandible	D.	the thyroid
B.	the maxilla	E.	the zygomatic bone
C.	the hyoid bone		

104. Which of the following correctly lists the order in which air passes through airway structures during inspiration?

A. trachea, larynx, laryngopharynx, nasopharynx, nares
B. nares, nasopharynx, trachea, laryngopharynx, larynx
C. nares, nasopharynx, laryngopharynx, larynx, trachea
D. laryngopharynx, nares, nasopharynx, larynx, trachea
E. trachea, nares, laryngopharynx, larynx, nasopharynx

105. The point at which the trachea divides into the two mainstem bronchi is called the:

A.	hilum.	D.	carina.
B.	parenchyma.	E.	pleura.
C.	vallecula.		

106. The tissue covering each lung and the interior of the thorax is the:

A.	hilum.	D.	carina.
B.	parenchyma.	E.	pleura.
C.	vallecula.		

107. Which of the following is NOT one of the differences in respiration between pediatric patients and adults?

A. The pediatric airway is smaller in all aspects.
B. Pediatric ribs are softer and contribute less to respiration than those of adults.
C. Children rely more on their diaphragms for breathing than adults do.
D. The glottis is the narrowest point of the pediatric airway, while the cricoid cartilage is the narrowest point in adults.
E. Children's teeth are softer and more prone to damage than those of adults.

108. Internal respiration occurs in the:

A.	peripheral capillaries.	D.	pulmonary capillaries.
B.	airway.	E.	both C and D
C.	alveoli.		

109. Which aspect of the respiratory cycle is passive?
- **A.** inspiration
- **B.** expiration
- **C.** neither A nor B
- **D.** both A and B
- **E.** both A and B, but only during stress

110. The oxygenated circulation that provides perfusion for the lung tissue itself flows through the:
- **A.** pulmonary arteries.
- **B.** pulmonary veins.
- **C.** bronchial arteries.
- **D.** bronchial veins.
- **E.** none of the above

111. The amount of nitrogen in the air is approximately:
- **A.** 79 percent.
- **B.** 4 percent.
- **C.** 0.4 percent.
- **D.** 0.04 percent.
- **E.** 0.10 percent.

112. The normal oxygen saturation of hemoglobin in blood as it leaves the lungs is about:
- **A.** 75 percent.
- **B.** 85 percent.
- **C.** 90 percent.
- **D.** 95 percent.
- **E.** 97 percent.

113. The majority of the carbon dioxide carried by the blood is:
- **A.** carried by the hemoglobin.
- **B.** dissolved in the plasma.
- **C.** transported as bicarbonate.
- **D.** found as free gas in the blood.
- **E.** carried as free radicals.

114. Which of the following will reduce the carbon dioxide levels in the blood?
- **A.** administration of bicarbonate
- **B.** administration of antacids
- **C.** hyperventilation
- **D.** high-flow oxygen
- **E.** hypoventilation

115. Which of the following would NOT increase the production of carbon dioxide?
- **A.** fever
- **B.** airway obstruction
- **C.** shivering
- **D.** metabolic acids
- **E.** exercise

116. The primary center controlling respiration is located in the:
- **A.** medulla.
- **B.** pons.
- **C.** spinal cord.
- **D.** cerebrum.
- **E.** cerebellum.

117. Which of the following is the secondary or backup stimulus that causes respiration to occur?
- **A.** an increase in pH of the blood
- **B.** a decrease in pH of the blood
- **C.** an increase in pH of the cerebrospinal fluid
- **D.** a decrease in pH of the cerebrospinal fluid
- **E.** reduced oxygen levels in the blood

118. The amount of air moved with one normal respiratory cycle is called:
- **A.** minute volume.
- **B.** alveolar air.
- **C.** tidal volume.
- **D.** dead air space.
- **E.** total lung capacity.

119. The volume of air contained in a normal inspiration is about:
- **A.** 150 mL.
- **B.** 350 mL.
- **C.** 500 mL.
- **D.** 6,000 mL.
- **E.** none of the above

120. Which of the following abdominal organs is found in the left upper quadrant?

- **A.** spleen
- **B.** gallbladder
- **C.** appendix
- **D.** sigmoid colon
- **E.** liver

121. Which of the following abdominal organs is found in the right lower quadrant?

- **A.** spleen
- **B.** gallbladder
- **C.** appendix
- **D.** sigmoid colon
- **E.** liver

122. Which of the following abdominal organs is found in all of the abdominal quadrants?

- **A.** pancreas
- **B.** gallbladder
- **C.** appendix
- **D.** sigmoid colon
- **E.** small bowel

123. Which of the following statements is TRUE regarding the digestive tract?

- **A.** It is a 25-foot-long hollow tube.
- **B.** It churns food.
- **C.** It introduces digestive juices.
- **D.** It moves food via peristalsis.
- **E.** all of the above

124. In what order does digesting food pass through the digestive tract?

- **A.** duodenum, ileum, jejunum, colon
- **B.** duodenum, jejunum, ileum, colon
- **C.** jejunum, ileum, colon, duodenum
- **D.** ileum, jejunum, colon, duodenum
- **E.** colon, jejunum, ileum, duodenum

125. The movement of digesting material through the digestive system occurs through a process called:

- **A.** peristalsis.
- **B.** chyme.
- **C.** peritonitis.
- **D.** emulsification.
- **E.** evisceration.

126. The largest solid organ of the abdomen is the:

- **A.** spleen.
- **B.** small bowel.
- **C.** pancreas.
- **D.** gallbladder.
- **E.** liver.

127. The delicate vascular organ that performs some immune functions is the:

- **A.** spleen.
- **B.** small bowel.
- **C.** pancreas.
- **D.** gallbladder.
- **E.** liver.

128. The major functions of the urinary system include all EXCEPT:

- **A.** maintenance of blood volume.
- **B.** control of development of white blood cells.
- **C.** regulation of arterial blood pressure.
- **D.** maintenance of the balance of electrolytes and blood pH.
- **E.** removal of many toxic wastes from the blood.

129. The enzyme that is produced by the kidney and is part of the physiologic response to low blood pressure is called:

- **A.** aldosterone.
- **B.** angiotensin.
- **C.** erythropoietin.
- **D.** renin.
- **E.** progesterone.

130. Which of the following structures is part of the external female genitalia?
- **A.** ovary
- **B.** perineum
- **C.** uterus
- **D.** vagina
- **E.** fallopian tube

131. An elastic canal that connects the internal and external female genitalia is the:
- **A.** ureter.
- **B.** urethra.
- **C.** vagina.
- **D.** vulva.
- **E.** fallopian tube.

132. The layer of the uterine wall where the fertilized egg implants is the:
- **A.** dermametrium.
- **B.** cyclometrium.
- **C.** myometrium.
- **D.** perimetrium.
- **E.** endometrium.

133. Which of the following hormones is released by the ovaries?
- **A.** estrogen
- **B.** follicle-stimulating hormone
- **C.** gonadotropin
- **D.** luteinizing hormone
- **E.** thymosin

134. The menstrual cycle generally lasts:
- **A.** 2 weeks.
- **B.** 28 days.
- **C.** 7 days.
- **D.** 9 months.
- **E.** 3 weeks.

135. The onset of ovulation that establishes female sexual maturity is known as:
- **A.** menarche.
- **B.** menopause.
- **C.** menses.
- **D.** menstruation.
- **E.** menacme.

136. The _____ phase of the menstrual cycle terminates with ovulation.
- **A.** ischemic
- **B.** menstrual
- **C.** proliferative
- **D.** secretory
- **E.** fallow

137. Which process occurs during the proliferative phase of the menstrual cycle?
- **A.** drop in estrogen level
- **B.** rupture of small endometrial blood vessels
- **C.** shedding of the endometrium
- **D.** thickening of the endometrium
- **E.** the endometrium becomes pale

138. The age range in which menopause generally occurs is:
- **A.** 35–40 years.
- **B.** 40–55 years.
- **C.** 45–55 years.
- **D.** 50–60 years.
- **E.** 60–65 years.

139. During pregnancy, a woman's circulatory volume increases by about::
- **A.** 15%.
- **B.** 25%.
- **C.** 30%.
- **D.** 45%.
- **E.** 75%..

140. Sperm cells are eliminated from a man's body after they move out of the testicles and pass through the following structures in first-to-last sequence:
- **A.** vas deferens, epididymis, urethra.
- **B.** ureter, epididymis, vas deferens, urethra.
- **C.** epididymis, vas deferens, urethra.
- **D.** epididymis, vas deferens, prostate gland, urethra.
- **E.** vas deferens, epididymis, prostate gland, urethra.

True/False

_____ **141.** The macrophages and lymphocytes begin the inflammation response by killing invading bodies and triggering a call for other, similar cells.
  A.   True
  B.   False

_____ **142.** The Bohr effect describes the relationship between pH and oxygen delivery in that the more acidic the blood, the more readily oxygen is released to the tissues.
  A.   True
  B.   False

_____ **143.** More than half the energy created by muscle motion is in the form of heat energy.
  A.   True
  B.   False

_____ **144.** The cerebellum is the center of conscious thought and perception.
  A.   True
  B.   False

_____ **145.** While the brain accounts for only 2 percent of the total body weight, it requires 15 percent of the cardiac output and 20 percent of the body's oxygen supply.
  A.   True
  B.   False

_____ **146.** The capillaries serving the brain are thicker and less permeable than those in the rest of the body.
  A.   True
  B.   False

_____ **147.** The structure of the meninges of the spinal column is similar to the structure of the meninges of the cranium.
  A.   True
  B.   False

_____ **148.** The right lung has only two lobes because the heart's greatest mass is on the right.
  A.   True
  B.   False

_____ **149.** Antidiuretic hormone plays a role in maintaining fluid balance by increasing water reabsorption.
  A.   True
  B.   False

_____ **150.** Catecholamines such as epinephrine and norepinephrine are hormones secreted by the adrenal medulla.

A.   True
B.   False

_____ **151.** The relaxation phase of the cardiac cycle is called dyastole.
  A.   True
  B.   False

_____ **152.** Specialized myocardial structures called intercalated discs enable the atria to act as an electrophysiologic syncytium and the ventricles to act as another one.
  A.   True
  B.   False

_____ **153.** The sinuses help trap bacteria and can become infected.
  A.   True
  B.   False

154. The mainstem bronchus that leaves the trachea at almost a straight angle is the right mainstem bronchus.

    A.   True

    B.   False

155. BUN, or blood urea nitrogen, and creatinine are both measured in blood as part of assessment of kidney function.

    A.   True

    B.   False

156. The urethra in men is much shorter than it is in women, and this is one reason why there is a gender difference in the incidence of lower urinary tract infections.

    A.   True

    B.   False

Matching

The Cell

Write the letter of the term in the space provided next to the description or definition to which it applies.

Term

A. cytoplasm		**F.**	granulocyte
B. cytoskeleton		**G.**	leukocyte
C. cytosol		**H.**	lymphocyte
D. cytotoxin		**I.**	monocyte
E. erythrocyte		**J.**	phagocyte

Description

157. Cell with the ability to ingest other cells and substances such as cell debris and bacteria

158. Clear liquid portion of the cytoplasm in a cell

159. Red blood cell

160. Structure of protein filaments that supports the internal structure of a cell

161. Substance that is toxic to cells

162. Thick fluid that fills a cell

163. Type of leukocyte that attacks foreign substances

164. White blood cell

165. White blood cell with a single nucleus

166. White blood cell with multiple nuclei

Skeletal organization

Write the letter of the appropriate anatomical structure in the space provided below. List the structures from most proximal to most distal.

Structure

    A. carpals

    B. clavicle

C. humerus
D. metacarpals
E. olecranon
F. phalanges
G. radius
H. scapula

Order

_____ **167.** Most proximal.

_____ **168.**

_____ **169.**

_____ **170.**

_____ **171.**

_____ **172.**

_____ **173.**

_____ **174.** Most distal

Cardiovascular Terms

Write the letter of the paramedic role in the space provided next to the functions to which it applies.

Term

A. action potential
B. ~~automaticity~~
C. ~~conductivity~~
D. diastole
E. resting potential
F. ~~excitability~~
G. systole

Description

_C___ **175.** ability of the cells to propagate the electrical impulse from one cell to another.

_f___ **176.** ability of the cells to respond to an electrical stimulus

_a___ **177.** the stimulation of myocardial cells that subsequently spreads across the myocardium.

_d___ **178.** period of time when the myocardium is contracting

_b___ **179.** pacemaker cells' capability of self-depolarization

_g___ **180.** period of time when the myocardium is relaxed and cardiac filling occurs

Chapter 13

General Principles of Pathophysiology

Part 1: How Normal Body Processes Are Altered by Disease and Injury

Review of Chapter Objectives

Introduction to Advanced Prehospital Care
Because Chapter 13 is lengthy, it has been divided into parts to aid your study. Read the assigned textbook pages, then progress through the objectives and self-evaluation materials as you would with other chapters. When you feel secure in your grasp of the content, proceed to the next part.

After reading this part of the chapter, you should be able to:

1. **Discuss cellular adaptation, injury, and death.**   **pp. 633-639**

   Cellular adaptation involves the ability of the body cell to change and adapt based upon normal and abnormal stresses. Cellular adaptation includes atrophy, hypertrophy, hyperplasia, metaplasia, and dysplasia.

   • Atrophy is the process of decreasing cell size due to a decrease in cell workload.
   • Hypertrophy is an increase in cell size resulting from an increase in workload.
   • Hyperplasia is an increase in the number of cells in response to an increase in workload.
   • Metaplasia is a replacement of one type of cell with another type of cell not normal for that tissue.
   • Dysplasia is an abnormal change in cell size, shape, and appearance due to an external stressor.

   Cellular injury is most commonly due to hypoxia, chemicals, infectious agents, inflammatory reactions, physical agents, nutritional factors, or genetic factors.

   • Hypoxic injury results when a cell is deprived of oxygen due to a respiratory or cardiovascular problem. Ultimately, the cell cannot efficiently produce its energy source, ATP, and acids and fluids accumulate.
   • Chemical injury results when agents such as ethanol, lead, carbon monoxide, drugs, or insecticides enter the body and injure the cell.

• Infectious injury causes cell damage when disease-causing agents (pathogens) enter the body. These agents damage and destroy cells, create toxins, or instigate an allergic reaction.
• Immunologic/inflammatory injury results as the body attempts to ward off invading foreign substances. Although the response is intended to attack the foreign substance, it also damages body cells.
• Physical injury results from exposure to temperature extremes, electrical current, pressure, radiation, noise, and mechanical stresses.
• Injuries due to nutritional imbalance include atherosclerosis, exacerbation of diabetes, insufficient intake of proteins, carbohydrates, lipids, vitamins, and minerals, or malnutrition and starvation.
• Genetic injury results from defective DNA that creates a predisposition toward (like diabetes) or directly causes (like sickle cell disease) a disease.

Cellular death occurs through one of two processes. They are apoptosis and necrosis.

• Apoptosis is a natural elimination of damaged, destroyed, or non-functioning cells. This response involves scattered individual cells and allows tissue to repair itself.
• Necrosis is the result of a pathological process and generally involves a grouping or region of cells. In necrosis, cells swell and rupture and take on a different appearance. The process disrupts the normal physiological activity of the tissue.

2. Describe factors that precipitate disease in the human body.   pp. 639-645

The body goes to great lengths to maintain a constant internal and cellular environment (homeostasis). Major factors of this environment include hydration, the movement of substances into and out of the cell, and acid/base balance.

• **Hydration.** Water composes about 60 percent of the total body weight and plays a very important role in the body's internal environment. Some 75 percent of the body's water is contained within the cells (intracellular fluid), while 7.5 percent is contained within the vascular system (intravascular fluid). The remaining water is found between cells (interstitial fluid) and in other spaces within the body. An abnormal decrease in body hydration (dehydration) may be caused by increased gastrointestinal losses, sweating, internal (third space) losses, plasma losses, or other types of losses. An abnormal increase in body water is called overhydration.

• **Electrolytes.** Electrolytes are molecules that dissociate into negatively and positively charged particles (called ions) when dissolved in water. The normal distribution of body water is dependent on the distribution of electrolytes among the body spaces (intravascular, interstitial, and intracellular).

• **Osmosis and diffusion.** Diffusion is the movement of molecules from an area of higher concentration to one of lower concentration. Osmosis is the movement of a solvent (like water) through a membrane to equalize the concentration of electrolytes on each side of the membrane. The body also moves electrolytes through cell membranes (against the osmotic gradient) by active transport and facilitated diffusion. These processes are responsible for maintaining a fluid electrolyte balance among the intravascular, interstitial, and intracellular spaces.

• **Acid/base balance.** The concentration of free hydrogen ions in a fluid reflects its acidity and is noted as a logarithmic value called pH. A pH of 1 is extremely acidic, while a pH of 14 is without hydrogen ions and extremely basic (or alkalotic). The body maintains a slightly alkalotic environment by regulating the quantity of free hydrogen ions. Normal body pH ranges from 7.35 to 7.45. The body maintains its pH through a bicarbonate buffer system, the respiratory system, and the kidneys.

3. Analyze disease risk.   pp. 646-652

Disease risk arises from several sources including genetic, environmental, life-style, age, and gender factors. Genetic factors are transferred from parents to offspring through genes and may cause frank disease or predispose an individual to disease. Environmental factors include violence, toxins, climate, socioeconomic conditions, exposure to bacteria, and other factors. Life-style factors include diet, exercise, smoking, and drug use. Age results in a progressive diminution of body functions and the increasing presence of progressive diseases. Gender risk is associated with hormonal protection or predisposition to disease. Often disease risk is associated with a combination of genetic, environmental, life-style, age, and gender factors.

4. Describe environmental risk factors and combined effects and interactions among risk factors.   pp. 646-652

Environmental risk factors include violence that may induce trauma, toxins that may cause chemical trauma, poisoning, or cancers, and adverse climates that may cause UV skin and eye damage as well as hyper- and hypothermia, frostbite, and freezing injuries. Poor water supplies, poor nutrition, inadequate housing, and poor medical care may also increase the risk for disease. Frequently, environmental and other disease risk factors combine to induce disease. Type II diabetes, for example, is associated with a familial history but is also associated with a high-fat and high-carbohydrate diet, lack of exercise, and obesity. Heart disease is associated with a familial history, diet, gender, and age factors.

5. Discuss familial diseases and associated risk factors.   pp. 646-652

Diseases such as allergies, asthma, rheumatic fever, some cancers, diabetes, cardiovascular disease, cystic fibrosis, sickle cell disease, and some neuromuscular diseases are caused directly by defective genes or related to a genetic predisposition to the disease. Often these predispositions are then triggered by environmental or life-style factors that lead to the disease. For example, a familial history of heart disease is exacerbated with smoking, obesity, poor diet, and a sedentary life style.

6. Discuss hypoperfusion. pp. 652-657

Hypoperfusion is inadequate blood flow to and past the body cells. This means that blood flow is insufficient to provide oxygen and necessary nutrients and to remove carbon dioxide and other metabolic wastes. If permitted to continue, hypoperfusion progresses and leads to failure of compensatory mechanisms, decompensation, irreversible shock, and death. Hypoperfusion (or shock) may be caused by trauma, fluid loss, myocardial infarction, infection, allergic reaction, spinal cord or brain injury, and other causes.

7. Define cardiogenic, hypovolemic, neurogenic, anaphylactic, and septic shock.   pp. 657-661

Cardiogenic shock is due to the inability of the heart to pump enough blood to meet the body's needs. It is commonly caused by severe left ventricular failure secondary to a myocardial infarction or congestive heart failure. Cardiac output decreases and workload increases, while coronary artery flow decreases and myocardial oxygen demand increases. These factors begin a vicious cycle that often ends in complete heart failure.

Hypovolemic shock is due to the loss of blood volume through internal or external hemorrhage, dehydration, plasma losses from burns, excessive sweating, or third space losses. As the vascular volume decreases, the body compensates by releasing catecholamines, increasing heart rate and inducing vasoconstriction. This produces the classical signs and symptoms of shock—a rapid weak pulse, cool, clammy, ashen skin, dyspnea, anxiety, combativeness—and, ultimately, hypotension.

Neurogenic shock results from injury to the brain or spinal cord that interrupts the body's control over the vascular system. The vessels lose tone and dilate, increasing the size of the vascular container and producing a relative hypovolemia. The body's normal response is muted because the adrenal glands do not secrete catecholamines and the central nervous system cannot induce vasoconstriction. The injury may also affect the heart and respiratory system.

Anaphylactic shock is an exaggerated and severe allergic reaction to a foreign substance that enters the body. It usually occurs rapidly and may be triggered by many substances. The most severe of anaphylactic reactions are triggered when substances are injected directly into the bloodstream, as with bee and wasp stings and injected medications.

Septic shock is caused by an infection that progresses and enters the bloodstream. The toxins produced by the overwhelming infection increase capillary permeability and overcome the compensatory mechanisms, and shock results.

8. Describe multiple organ dysfunction syndrome.   pp. 662-664

Multiple organ dysfunction syndrome (MODS) is a progressive impairment of two or more body organs, usually after an initial insult and apparently successful resuscitation. It is caused by an uncontrolled inflammatory response and occurs most commonly after septic shock. The syndrome is caused by an exaggerated immune response in which hormones are released, causing vasodilation, increased capillary permeability, and increased metabolic demands. The syndrome usually begins within 24 hours of the initial insult and progresses over several weeks.

CONTENT SELF-EVALUATION

_____   **1.** Atrophy, hypertrophy, hyperplasia, metaplasia, and dysplasia are examples of:
        A.   pathogens   **D.**   physiological responses.
        B.   cellular adaptation.   **E.**   pathophysiological responses.
        C.   cellular injury.

_____   **2.** An increase in cell size due to an increase in workload is an example of the process known as:
        A.   atrophy.   **D.**   metaplasia.
        B.   hypertrophy.   **E.**   dysplasia.
        C.   hyperplasia.

_____   **3.** An abnormal change in cell size or shape due to some external stressor is an example of the process known as:
        A.   atrophy.   **D.**   metaplasia.
        B.   hypertrophy.   **E.**   dysplasia.
        C.   hyperplasia.

_____   **4.** A decrease in cell size resulting from decreased workload is an example of the process known as:
        A.   atrophy.   **D.**   metaplasia.
        B.   hypertrophy.   **E.**   dysplasia.
        C.   hyperplasia.

_____   **5.** An increase in the number of cells resulting from an increased workload is an example of the process known as:
        A.   atrophy.   **D.**   metaplasia.
        B.   hypertrophy.   **E.**   dysplasia.
        C.   hyperplasia.

_____   **6.** The most common cause of cellular injury is:
        A.   hypoxia.   **D.**   ischemia.
        B.   anoxia.   **E.**   infarction.
        C.   hypoperfusion.

_____   **7.** A blockage or reduction in the delivery of oxygenated blood to body cells is:
        A.   hypoxia.   **D.**   ischemia.
        B.   anoxia.   **E.**   infarction.
        C.   hypoperfusion.

_____   **8.** Ischemia can result from:

A. increasing number of red blood cells.
B. an increase of hemoglobin in the blood.
C. ineffectiveness of oxygen binding sites.
D. an increase in the size of red blood cells.
E. a lack of red blood cells.

9. Cellular infarction occurs when:
   A. cellular injury progresses from reversible to irreversible.
   B. oxygen is resupplied to damaged tissue.
   C. cells move from aerobic to anaerobic metabolism.
   D. cells move from anaerobic to aerobic metabolism.
   E. a blockage reduces the delivery of oxygen to the cells.

10. Which of the following types of cellular injuries is caused by pathogens?
    A. hypoxic   D. immunologic
    B. chemical   E. infectious
    C. inflammatory

11. A pathogen's virulence is described as its ability to:
    A. invade cells.   D. produce hypersensitivity reactions.
    B. destroy cells.   E. all of the above
    C. produce toxins.

12. A change in cellular structure due to an alteration in the permeability of the cell's membrane is:
    A. fatty alteration.   D. cellular swelling.
    B. anabolism.   E. apoptosis.
    C. catabolism.

13. Cellular destruction caused by an internal release of enzymes is:
    A. apoptosis.   D. gangrene.
    B. fatty change.   E. hemoptysis.
    C. necrosis.

14. Which of the following is NOT a type of necrosis?
    A. fatty   D. coagulative
    B. liquefactive   E. caseous
    C. bilateral

15. The blood component that contains proteins, electrolytes, and clotting factors is:
    A. plasma.   D. leukocytes.
    B. platelets.   E. none of the above
    C. erythrocytes.

16. Which of the blood components below is/are responsible for a portion of the clotting process?

    A. lipids   D. leukocytes
    B. platelets   E. hemoglobin
    C. erythrocytes

17. The percentage of blood accounted for by red blood cells is termed the:
    A. component count.   D. oncotic pressure.
    B. hematocrit.   E. leukocyte level.
    C. hemoglobin level.

18. The most desirable fluid for blood loss replacement is:
    A. whole blood.   D. lactated Ringers.
    B. packed red cells.   E. plasma.
    C. normal saline.

19. Which of the following is NOT a colloid solution?

- A. plasmanate
- B. hetastarch
- C. dextran
- D. lactated Ringers
- E. salt-poor albumin

20. A solution with a lower solute concentration than the cells is known as:

- A. a colloid solution.
- B. a hypertonic solution.
- C. a hypotonic solution.
- D. an isotonic solution.
- E. a normotonic solution.

21. A solution with a higher solute concentration than the cells is known as:

- A. a colloid solution.
- B. a hypertonic solution.
- C. a hypotonic solution.
- D. an isotonic solution.
- E. a normotonic solution.

22. Which of the following solutions will cause a net movement of water into erythrocytes?

- A. a colloid solution
- B. a hypertonic solution
- C. a hypotonic solution
- D. an isotonic solution
- E. a normotonic solution

23. A common cause of metabolic alkalosis is the administration of:

- A. sedatives.
- B. analgesics.
- C. bronchodilators.
- D. diuretics.
- E. antibiotics.

24. Which of the following is a factor that can influence disease risk?

- A. family history
- B. environment
- C. gender
- D. life style
- E. all of the above

25. Somatic cells contain:

- A. 12 chromosomes.
- B. 23 chromosomes.
- C. 24 chromosomes.
- D. 46 chromosomes.
- E. 48 pairs of chromosomes.

26. Sex cells contain:

- A. 12 chromosomes.
- B. 23 chromosomes.
- C. 24 chromosomes.
- D. 46 chromosomes.
- E. 48 pairs of chromosomes.

27. The death rate from disease is reported as its:

- A. prevalence.
- B. morbidity.
- C. mortality.
- D. incidence.
- E. none of the above

28. Which of the following disorders is not associated with genetic history?

- A. cardiomyopathy
- B. prolongation of the QT interval
- C. hemophilia
- D. coronary artery disease
- E. mitral-valve prolapse

29. Hypertension is a risk factor for which of the following?

- A. stroke
- B. kidney disease
- C. cancer
- D. cardiovascular disease
- E. all except C

30. What percentage of lung cancers in women are associated with smoking?

- A. 40 percent
- B. 60 percent
- C. 70 percent
- D. 80 percent
- E. 90 percent

31. Obesity is defined as having a body weight that is over ideal body weight by:

A. 20 percent.	**D.** 35 percent.
B. 25 percent.	**E.** 40 percent.
C. 30 percent.	

32. For which of the following diseases is obesity NOT a risk factor?

A. hypertension	**D.** vascular disease
B. heart disease	**E.** diabetes
C. breast cancer	

33. Shock, resulting in an inadequate supply of oxygen and nutrients to the body tissues is also known as:

A. shunt.	**D.** hyptension.
B. hypertension.	**E.** hypoperfusion
C. hyperperfusion.	

34. Hypoperfusion may occur with all of the following EXCEPT:

A. low heart rate.	**D.** reduced blood volume.
B. dilated vascular container.	**E.** excessive afterload.
C. excessive vascular constriction.	

35. The second stage of cellular metabolism that breaks glucose down into energy that can be used by the body requires the presence of:

A. sodium bicarbonate.	**D.** pyruvic acid.
B. glucagon.	**E.** sodium chloride.
C. oxygen.	

36. The Krebs' cycle produces a chemical energy form used by the body that is called:

A. adenosine triphosphate.	**D.** citric acid.
B. lactic acid.	**E.** sodium bicarbonate.
C. pyruvic acid.	

37. The process by which glycogen is converted into glucose in the cells is:

A. glycolysis.	**D.** gluconeogenesis.
B. glycogenesis.	**E.** lipolysis.
C. glycogenolysis.	

38. The body's process of compensation for hypoperfusion is initiated by:

A. glucose.	**D.** pyruvic acid.
B. oxygen.	**E.** cortisol.
C. norepinephrine.	

39. During the body's response to hypoperfusion , the catecholamines epinephrine and norepinephrine are responsible for:

A. decreasing heart rate.
B. decreasing cardiac contractile strength.
C. arteriolar dilation.
D. increasing blood pressure.
E. decreasing blood volume.

40. During shock, the spleen may expel blood back into the circulatory system up to a volume of:

A. 200 ml.	**D.** 500 ml.
B. 300 ml.	**E.** 600 ml.
C. 400 ml.	

41. During hypoperfusion, the renin-angiotensin compensatory system:

A. increases red blood cell production.
B. causes the spleen to release blood.
C. produces a potent vasoconstrictor.

D.   induces beneficial fluid shifts.

E.   reduces the production of lactic acid.

_____ 42. The stage of shock in which medical intervention is no longer effective is:

    A.   compensated shock.   D.   irreversible shock.

    B.   decompensated shock.   E.   septic shock.

    C.   progressive shock.

_____ 43. During decompensated shock, which of the following is likely to occur?

    A.   fluid shift from the interstitial spaces

    B.   systemic alkalosis

    C.   cardiac excitation

    D.   dropping blood pressure

    E.   all of the above

_____ 44. What type of shock is due to plasma loss from burns?

    A.   cardiogenic   D.   septic

    B.   hypovolemic   E.   anaphylactic

    C.   neurogenic

_____ 45. What type of shock is due to a severe allergic reaction?

    A.   cardiogenic   D.   septic

    B.   hypovolemic   E.   anaphylactic

    C.   neurogenic

_____ 46. Which type of shock results from infection that enters the bloodstream and is carried throughout the body?

    A.   cardiogenic   D.   septic

    B.   hypovolemic   E.   anaphylactic

    C.   neurogenic

_____ 47. A relaxing of the blood vessel walls is the cause of which type of shock?

    A.   cardiogenic   D.   septic

    B.   hypovolemic   E.   anaphylactic

    C.   neurogenic

_____ 48. A loss of water caused by greatly increased urination and dehydration due to high levels of glucose that cannot be reabsorbed into the blood from the kidney tubules is known as:

    A.   septicemia.   D.   renal failure.

    B.   MODS.   E.   dysplasia.

    C.   osmotic diuresis.

_____ 49. The first evidence of MODS usually presents within:

    A.   12 hours.   D.   7 to 10 days.

    B.   24 hours.   E.   14 to 21 days.

    C.   72 hours.

_____ 50. Death from MODS usually occurs after:

    A.   24 hours.   D.   14 days.

    B.   48 hours.   E.   21 days.

    C.   72 hours.

True/False

_____ 51. Hypertrophy most commonly affects cells of the heart, brain, and sex organs.

    A.   True

    B.   False

_____ 52. The process by which damaged or destroyed cells of one type are replaced by cells of another type is called metaplasia.

A. True
B. False

53. Hypoxia is most often caused by a deficit in the cardiovascular or neurological system.
A. True
B. False

54. The most desirable fluid for blood loss replacement is normal saline.
A. True
B. False

55. When in a solution, colloids, unlike crystalloids, can diffuse through a membrane such as a capillary wall.
A. True
B. False

56. Metabolic alkalosis is often caused by diuresis, vomiting, or ingestion of too much sodium bicarbonate.
A. True
B. False

57. Metabolic acidosis is increased acidity caused by abnormal retention of carbon dioxide resulting from impaired ventilation.
A. True
B. False

58. In addition to treating the underlying cause, the care of metabolic acidosis includes ensuring adequate ventilation.
A. True
B. False

59. Most disease processes are simply caused by either an environmental or genetic factor, rarely both.
A. True
B. False

60. People with genetic predispositions to certain diseases can frequently take actions that modify the risk factors associated with acquiring the disease.
A. True
B. False

61. Rheumatic fever is an infectious condition that may have a hereditary factor.
A. True
B. False

62. The greatest risk factor for breast and colorectal cancers is age.
A. True
B. False

63. Hypoperfusion can develop even when cardiac output is adequate.
A. True
B. False

64. The Krebs cycle, which yields a high amount of energy occurs during anaerobic metabolism.
A. True
B. False

65. MODS – multiple organ dysfunction syndrome – can result from any sever disease or injury that triggers a massive systemic inflammatory response..
A. True
B. False

Matching

Match the type of shock with the characteristic of its presentation.

Type of shock

      A.   cardiogenic
      B.   hypovolemic
      C.   neurogenic
      D.   septic
      E.   anaphylactic

Pathology or presentation

_____   **66.** pulmonary edema

_____   **67.** warm, red skin

_____   **68.** itching and skin flushing

_____   **69.** history of recent illness

_____   **70.** hives

_____   **71.** possible high fever

_____   **72.** classic signs of shock

_____   **73.** laryngeal edema

_____   **74.** dry skin

_____   **75.** history of diarrhea

Chapter 13

General Principles of Pathophysiology

Part 2: The Body's Defences against Disease and Injury

Review of Chapter Objectives

Introduction to Advanced Prehospital Care

After reading this part of the chapter, you should be able to:

1. Define the characteristics of the immune response.   **pp. 668-670**

Foreign and invading cells or substances often have unique proteins on their surfaces called antigens. The immune system detects these antigens as being unlike those of the body's cells and initiates a response. This response uses antibodies to selectively control or destroy the foreign substance. As a result of the first contact with the foreign agent, the body develops a "memory" that produces a more rapid and effective response should the same antigen be recognized again. This response is called immunity.

Immunity can be acquired or natural. Natural immunity is not generated by the immune response but is a genetically inhospitable environment for a particular organism—for example, human resistance to canine distemper. Active acquired immunity is that immunity gained from a response to an invading antigen and is long lasting. Passive immunity is acquired from an outside source such as an immunization or from maternal blood during gestation and is temporary.

The primary immune response occurs with the first exposure to an antigen and lags from five to seven days after exposure. The secondary response occurs as the immune system is sensitized to the antigen by the first response. If it is again exposed to the antigen, it presents a more aggressive and faster response.

Humoral immunity is immunity resident in the blood and lymphatic fluid, primarily from B lymphocytes that produce antibodies. Cell-mediated immunity is immunity provided by T lymphocytes that recognize and directly attack the foreign antigen.

2. Discuss induction of the immune system. pp. 669-670

The immune system must be triggered or induced. This may occur due to the actions of antigens and immunogens, histocompatibility, and blood groupings.

Antigens that induce an immune response are called immunogens. Generally an antigen must be sufficiently foreign and sufficient in size, complexity, and number to generate an immune response.

Histocompatibility locus antigens are antigens that the body recognizes as either foreign or self. Those that are recognized as self (or non-foreign) do not generate an immune response, while those that are recognized as foreign (non-self) stimulate an immune response. It is extremely important to find compatible tissue for organ donation or tissue rejection may result.

Blood group antigens are associated with a different grouping of antigens than those associated with the histocompatibility response. The major blood group antigens consist of the Rh factor (present in about 85% of the population) and the A and B antigens associated with the ABO blood typing system.

3. Describe the inflammation response and its systemic manifestations. pp. 670-676

The inflammatory response is a swift, short-acting, non-specific internal response to cellular injury from trauma or disease. It involves several plasma protein systems and provides four major functions. They are destroying and removing the unwanted substances, walling off the infected or inflamed area, stimulating the immune response, and promoting the healing process.

There are three major manifestations of the acute inflammatory response. They are fever, an increase in circulating white blood cells, and an increase in circulating plasma proteins. Fever is a result of fever-causing chemicals (endogenous pyrogens) released during phagocytosis and is caused by toxins released by bacteria or as a response to an antigen-antibody complex. The elevation in body temperature may make the environment less hospitable to the invading pathogen. Both the number of circulating white blood cells and plasma proteins increase as the body tries to defeat the infection.

The chronic inflammatory response is a response that lasts longer than two weeks. During chronic inflammation, the body tries to isolate the agent by forming a barrier around it. Sometimes this cavity is filled with a fluid mixture of cellular debris, dead white blood cells, and tissue fluid called pus.

4. Discuss the role of mast cells, the plasma protein system, and cellular components plus resolution and repair as part of the inflammation response. pp. 672-676

Mast Cells. Specialized cells called mast cells that resemble bags of granules are the chief activators of the inflammatory response. When injured, they initiate the inflammatory response by releasing their granules (degranulation) or by constructing substances that play important roles in the inflammatory response (synthesis).

Degranulation occurs as the mast cell is injured and releases vasoactive amines and chemotactic factors. The principle vasoactive amine is histamine, a potent agent that increases blood flow through the affected area and increases capillary permeability to permit fluid and white blood cells to migrate into the interstitial space. Chemotactic factors are agents that attract white blood cells to the site of inflammation.

Synthesis is the construction of leukotrienes and prostaglandins to enhance the inflammatory response. Leukotrienes have actions similar to histamine and chemotactic factors; however, they promote a slower and longer lasting response. Prostaglandins cause increased perfusion and capillary permeability but limit the effects of histamine and reduce the release of enzymes from some white blood
    cells.

Plasma Protein Systems. In addition to the antigen-antibody system, there are three plasma protein systems that complement the inflammatory response system. They are the complement system, the coagulation system, and the kinin system.

The complement system is a complicated cascade system that is activated by antigen-antibody complexes, by products released by the invading bacteria, or by components of other plasma protein systems. The later portions of the cascade produce proteins that may coat the invading agent (opsonization), ingest the agent (phagocytosis), rupture the bacteria's cell membrane (lysis), cause the invading agents to clump together (agglutination), or neutralize the virus through actions similar to the degranulation of the mast cell. Complement proteins may also clog the tissues surrounding the infection and isolate it.

The coagulation or clotting system produces fibrin at the end of a clotting cascade. Fibrin is a sticky protein fiber that traps red blood cells to form a clot, prevents microorganism movement, increases vascular permeability, and produces some chemotactic substances.

The kinin system produces bradykinin, a protein that causes vasodilation, extravascular smooth muscle contraction, increased vascular permeability, and some chemotaxis.

Cellular components of the inflammatory response include the vascular response, increased capillary permeability, and exudation of white blood cells. The vascular response causes blood to flow more strongly into the injured area and helps push both plasma and white blood cells into the inflamed area. The increased capillary permeability is due to a constriction in the capillary wall cells that opens the spaces in between the cells and permits the large white blood cells to squeeze through (diapedesis). The white blood cells are phagocytes that engulf and digest invading cells and debris.

Resolution is the complete restoration of the structure and function of injured tissue. If the injury was more than minor and complete restoration is not possible, then repair will take place. **Repair** replaces original tissue with scar tissue.

5. Discuss hypersensitivity. pp. 676-678

Usually, hypersensitivity triggers an inflammation response that injures healthy tissue. There are four types of hypersensitivity that cause this destructive reaction. They are IgE-mediated reactions (type I), tissue-specific reactions (type II), immune complex-mediated reactions (type III), and cell-mediated reactions (type IV).

Type I reactions involve the immunoglobulin (antibody) IgE. These antibodies are created in great numbers with the first exposure to an antigen and are released with subsequent exposures, leading to a release of histamine and triggering of the inflammatory response. This results in skin flushing, itching, urticaria and edema, dyspnea, laryngeal edema, laryngospasm, bronchospasm, vasodilation and increased permeability, tachycardia, hypertension, nausea, vomiting, cramping and diarrhea, dizziness, headache, convulsions, and tearing. This type of reaction (anaphylactic) may be life threatening.

Type II reactions are directed to specific types of tissue. The tissue is destroyed by either the complement cascade, which causes destruction of the target cell's membrane, by clearance of the target cell by macrophage action, by the antigen binding cytotoxic cells to the target cell, and finally by the antigen disabling receptor sites on the target cell.

Type III reactions are either localized or systemic reactions as the complement cascade system attracts neutrophils. They are unable to destroy the invading pathogen and release agents that destroy neighboring healthy cells.

Type IV reactions are activated directly by T cells and do not involve antibodies. The T cells activate other immune cells and attack antigen-bearing cells directly with toxins they produce.

6. Describe deficiencies in immunity and inflammation. pp. 678-680

Congenital or primary immunity deficiencies occur when the development of lymphocytes is impaired during fetal development. Differing immune deficiencies may develop depending upon whether T cells, B cells, or both are affected. In some cases just a small portion of the immune system is deficient and the body is unable to respond to one or a few antigens.

Acquired deficiencies occur after birth and do not result from genetic factors. Nutritional, iatrogenic (caused by medical care), trauma, and stress factors may also result in a decrease in the body's resistance to illness. A specific type of immune deficiency is acquired immune deficiency syndrome (AIDS). AIDS develops from an infection caused by human immunodeficiency virus (HIV). It carries its genetic information on RNA that converts into DNA when it invades a cell and then becomes part of the infected cell's genetic material. The virus may remain dormant for years until it becomes active and kills the host cell and infects other cells. It results in a pervasive invasion of the body's immune defenses.

7. Describe homeostasis as a dynamic steady state. p. 682

Homeostasis is often defined as a constant environment within the body and one that the body tries to maintain. In reality, this state is always changing due to turnover of body cells, to the aging process, to continuing body processes like synthesis and breakdown of all body substances, and to the effects of stressors. The body tries, however, to maintain a relatively constant environment.

8. Describe neuroendocrine regulation. pp. 682-685

When a psychologic stressor affects an individual, the sympathetic nervous system is stimulated and there is a release of catecholamines, cortisol, and other hormones.

Catecholamines (norepinephrine and epinephrine) are released when sympathetic nerve impulses (from the thoracic and lumbar portions of the spinal cord) stimulate the adrenal medulla. These catecholamines act on four different receptors: Alpha 1, alpha 2, beta 1, and beta 2. Alpha 1 receptors cause peripheral vasoconstriction and mild bronchoconstriction and increase metabolism. Alpha 2 receptors mediate the actions of alpha 1 agents. Beta 1 receptors increase the heart rate, contractile strength, automaticity, and conductivity. Stimulation of beta 2 receptors causes vasodilation and bronchodilation.

Sympathetic stimulation also causes the adrenal cortex to produce a steroid hormone, cortisol. Cortisol stimulates the creation of glucose (gluconeogenesis) and limits glucose up-take by cells, increasing blood glucose levels. It also promotes the breakdown of proteins and lipids and acts as an immunosuppressant. While its effects do not support the inflammation and immune responses, cortisol ensures there are adequate energy sources and may help direct blood flow to critical organs during stress.

9. Discuss the interrelationships between stress, coping, and illness. pp. 686-687

The ability to cope with stress appears to have an impact on how effectively the body deals with disease. Positive coping mechanisms support the resolution of disease, while ineffective coping mechanisms exacerbate symptoms and the illness.

CONTENT SELF-EVALUATION

_____ **1.** Which of the following are single-cell organisms consisting of cytoplasm surrounded by a rigid cell membrane?

A.	viruses		**D.**	parasites
B.	bacteria		**E.**	prions
C.	fungi			

2. Which of the following are released by bacterial cells during their growth?
  A. antibiotics
  B. gram-negative material
  C. exotoxins
  D. endotoxins
  E. none of the above

3. The body's anatomical barrier against infection (the skin and linings of the respiratory and digestive systems) is considered:
  A. an external, specific barrier.
  B. an external, nonspecific barrier.
  C. an internal, specific barrier.
  D. an internal, nonspecific barrier.
  E. none of the above

4. The body's immune response against infection is considered:
  A. an external, specific response.
  B. an external, nonspecific response.
  C. an internal, specific response.
  D. an internal, nonspecific response.
  E. none of the above

5. The proteins located on the surface of many substances that enter the body and are used during the immune response to identify foreign organisms are:
  A. antigens.
  B. antibodies.
  C. B cells.
  D. T cells.
  E. lymphocytes.

6. Which types of immunity refers to the body's initial response to exposure to an antigen?
  A. primary
  B. acquired
  C. natural
  D. secondary
  E. humoral

7. The type of immunity, resident in the blood that produces antibodies and remembers a specific antigen is:
  A. cell-mediated.
  B. humoral
  C. natural.
  D. primary.
  E. extrinsic.

8. Which of the following is NOT an essential characteristic of an antigen required to trigger an immune response?
  A. sufficient foreignness
  B. sufficient size
  C. sufficient complexity
  D. sufficient quantity
  E. sufficient lability

9. What percentage of the North American population has the Rh factor present in their blood?
  A. 15 percent
  B. 25 percent
  C. 45 percent
  D. 75 percent
  E. 85 percent

10. Under the ABO classification system, the universal blood donor is identified as having blood type:
  A. A.
  B. B.
  C. O.
  D. AB.
  E. B and O.

11. Individuals with which of the following blood types would have the anti-A antibody?
  A. A
  B. B
  C. O
  D. AB
  E. B and C

12. Which of the following is NOT true of inflammatory response?
  A. It is of relatively short duration.
  B. It begins after 5 to 7 days.
  C. It involves many types of cells.

D. It involves several protein systems.

E. It is considered part of the body's immune system.

13. Which of the following is NOT a function of the inflammatory response?
    - **A.** to destroy and remove unwanted substances
    - **B.** to wall off the infected and inflamed area
    - **C.** to stimulate the immune response
    - **D.** to promote healing
    - **E.** to agglutinate viruses

14. Degranulation by the mast cells occurs when the cell is stimulated by all of the following EXCEPT:
    - **A.** physical injury.
    - **B.** toxins.
    - **C.** allergic reactions.
    - **D.** histamines.
    - **E.** venoms.

15. The attraction of white blood cells to the site of infection is called:
    - **A.** synthesis.
    - **B.** chemotaxis.
    - **C.** allergy.
    - **D.** the complement system.
    - **E.** agglutination.

16. The action of histamine during the inflammatory response is to:
    - **A.** increase capillary permeability.
    - **B.** increase blood flow to the injured area.
    - **C.** attack the invading cells.
    - **D.** attract white blood cells.
    - **E.** both A and B

17. The best outcome from the wound healing process is:
    - **A.** debridement.
    - **B.** repair.
    - **C.** resolution.
    - **D.** scarring.
    - **E.** granulation.

18. Which of the following describes a disturbance in the body's normal tolerance for self antigens?
    - **A.** allergy
    - **B.** anaphylaxis
    - **C.** autoimmunity
    - **D.** isoimmunity
    - **E.** granulation

19. Which of the following is a hypersensitivity response associated with antigens from another person?
    - **A.** allergy
    - **B.** anaphylaxis
    - **C.** autoimmunity
    - **D.** isoimmunity
    - **E.** monoimmunity

20. The common allergic and anaphylactic responses are caused by which immunoglobulin (antibody)?
    - **A.** IgM
    - **B.** IgG
    - **C.** IgA
    - **D.** IgE
    - **E.** IgD

21. Most cases of infection by the human immunodeficiency virus (HIV) in the United States result from:
    - **A.** injection.
    - **B.** droplet inhalation.
    - **C.** skin contamination.
    - **D.** body fluids during sexual intercourse.
    - **E.** both A and D

22. A state of physical or psychological arousal to stimuli is:

A.	disease.	D.	general adaptation syndrome.
B.	homeostasis.	E.	turnover.
C.	stress.		

23. The initial stage of the general adaptation syndrome in response to stress is:

A.	exhaustion.	D.	alarm.
B.	resistance.	E.	turnover.
C.	withdrawal.		

24. The second stage of the general adaptation syndrome in response to stress is:

A.	exhaustion.	D.	alarm.
B.	resistance.	E.	turnover.
C.	withdrawal.		

25. The final stage of the general adaptation syndrome in response to stress is:

A.	exhaustion.	D.	alarm.
B.	resistance.	E.	turnover.
C.	withdrawal.		

26. During the initial stage of stress, which of the following is NOT likely to occur?
   A. tachycardia
   B. levels of circulating hormones returning to normal
   C. hypertension
   D. digestion slowing
   E. blood flow to skeletal muscles increasing

27. The interactions that contribute to the alteration of the immune system as an outcome of a stress response are called:

A.	GAS alliance.	D.	stress-stressor combination.
B.	homeostatic return.	E.	pyschoneuroimmunological
	regulation.		
C.	turnover response.		

28. The continual synthesis and breakdown of body substances that results in homeostasis is:

A.	autocombustion.	D.	oxidation.
B.	turnover.	E.	plasmodynamics.
C.	recycling.		

29. Catecholamines include which of the following hormones?

A.	endorphins	D.	norepinephrine
B.	epinephrine	E.	both B and D
C.	cortisol		

30. Stimulation of the alpha 1 receptors will cause:
   A. increased heart rate.
   B. inhibition of the effects of norepinephrine.
   C. vasoconstriction.
   D. bronchodilation.
   E. all of the above

31. Stimulation of the beta 2 receptors will cause:
   A. increased heart rate.
   B. inhibition of the effects of norepinephrine.
   C. vasoconstriction.
   D. bronchodilation.
   E. increase contractility.

True/False

32. Most infections are caused by bacteria.

A. True
B. False

_____ **33.** The immune response to infection is more rapid than the inflammatory response and is not specific to the invading organism.
A. True
B. False

_____ **34.** Both the inflammatory response and immune response are internal lines of defense.
A. True
B. False

_____ **35.** The two main functions of mast cells are granulation and synthesis.
A. True
B. False

_____ **36.** Occasionally, when macrophages are unable to destroy foreign invaders, a granuloma will form to isolate the infection.
A. True
B. False

_____ **37.** Repair is the outcome of healing that result in complete healing of a wound and return of tissues to their normal structure and function.
A. True
B. False

_____ **38.** Isoimmunity is an immune response to antigens from another member of the same species.
A. True
B. False

_____ **39.** Iatrogenic deficiencies are a congenital condition in which there is a lack or partial lack of thymus development.
A. True
B. False

_____ **40.** The hormone released in the greatest quantity by the adrenal medulla is norepinephrine.
A. True
B. False

_____ **41.** Effective stress coping mechanisms have an apparent impact on how people deal with disease but do not effect the seriousness of the associated illness.
A. True
B. False

Matching

Write the letter of the appropriate term in the space provided next to the definition to which it applies.

Term

A. chemotactic factors
B. degranulation
C. fibroblasts
D. histamine
E. prostaglandins

Description

_____ **42.** the emptying of granules from the interior of a mast cell inot the extracellular environment

_____ **43.** a substance release during the degranulation of mast cells that causes increased blood flow to the injury site and increased permeability of vessel walls

_____ **44.** substances synthiesized by mast cells during inflammatory response that cause vasoconstriction, vascular permeability, and chemotaxis.

_____ **45.** cells that secrete collagen

Chapter 14

General Principles of Pharmacology

Part 1: Basic Pharmacology

Review of Chapter Objectives

Because Chapter 14 is lengthy, it has been divided into parts to aid your study. Read the assigned textbook pages, then progress through the objectives and self-evaluation materials as you would with other chapters. When you feel secure in your grasp of the content, proceed to the next part.

After reading this part of the chapter, you should be able to:

1. Describe important historical trends in pharmacology.   p. 690

The use of herbs and minerals has been documented in the treatment of illness and injury since as early as 2000 b.c. Before that, the ancient Egyptians, Arabs, and Greeks probably passed formulations down through the generations by word of mouth. During the 17th and 18th centuries, tinctures of opium, coca, and digitalis were available, and the concept of inoculation with biologic extracts was developed by the late 19th century. By the end of that century, atropine, chloroform, codeine, ether, and morphine were in use. This past century has seen an explosion in the number and types of pharmaceuticals in use. As we begin the 21st century, recombinant DNA technology has produced human insulin and tissue plasma activator (tPA).

2. Differentiate among the chemical, generic (nonproprietary), official (USP), and trade (proprietary) names of a drug.   pp. 690-691

The chemical name of a drug represents its chemical composition and molecular structure. An example is 7-chloro-1,3-dihydro-1-methyl-5-phenyl-2H-1,4-benzodiazepine-2-one.

The generic name of a drug is suggested by the original manufacturer. An example, for which the chemical name is given above, is diazepam. The brand, trade, or proprietary name of a drug is the name given the drug by a specific manufacturer. This name is a proper name and should be capitalized and may be followed by a trademark insignia. An example is Valium®, a brand name for diazepam.

3. List the four main sources of drug products.   p. 691

There are four main sources of drugs. They are plants, animals, minerals, and synthetic substances (laboratory).

4. List the authoritative sources for drug information.   pp. 691-692

Drug inserts usually accompany prescription drugs and list information as required by Health Canada.

The *Compendium of Pharmaceuticals and Specialites (CPS)* is a compilation of materials supplied by the Canadian Pharmacists Association. It also contains indexing and some drug photos. *The Physician's Desk Reference* is a common American publication It is an authoritative listing of virtually every drug used in the United States.

5. List legislative acts controlling drug use and abuse in Canada.   pp. 692-694

Health Canada's Therapeutic Products Directorate regulates pharmaceutical drugs and medical devices. The Food and Drugs Act and Regulations require manufactures to present scientific evidence of a product's safety, efficacy, and quality before Health Canada will grant market authorization. The federal government strictly regulates controlled substances because of thei high potential for abuse.

6. Differentiate among the schedules of controlled drugs and list examples of substances in each schedule.   p. 693

The narcotics schedule contains stringently restricted drugs. The letter N must appear on all labels and professional advertisements. Examples include cocaine, morphine, codeine, methadone, hydromorphone, meperidine, phencyclidine, cannabis.

Schedule F contains prescription drugs such as benzodiazepines. The symbol PR must appear on the label.

Schedule G lists controlled drugs. Prescriptions are controlled because of the abuse potential with these duugs. Examples include nalbupine, butorphanol, amphetamines, Phenobarbital, amobarbital, and secobarbital.

Schedule H are restricted street drugs that typically have no recognized medicinal properties. Examples include Peyote, LSD, and Mescaline.

Nonprescription Drug Schedule (Group 3) drugs are available only in a pharmacy and are used only on the recommendation of a physician. These include low-dose codeine preparations, insulin, nitroglycerine, and muscle relaxants.

7. Discuss standardization of drugs.   p. 694

Drugs may contain the same active ingredient yet be far different in the way they are delivered to the body. To recognize this, an assay of the drug determines the amount and purity of the drug in the preparation. A bioassay determines the amount of drug that is available in a biological model and thereby establishes its bioequivalence, or relative therapeutic effectiveness compared with drugs with chemically equivalent compositions.

8. Discuss the paramedic's responsibilities and scope of management pertinent to the administration of medications.   pp. 694-696

There are six basic "rights" of drug administration that indicate the paramedic's essential responsibilities and practices. They are the right medication, the right dose, the right time, the right route, the right patient, and the right documentation.

The right medication. Ensure the medication is what is intended for the patient. Review your standing orders or, if an order is received from medical direction, repeat the order back to the physician so you are both clear on the medication, dose, route, and timing of the administration. Also examine the drug packaging to ensure it is the medication you wish to administer.

The right dose. Carefully calculate the dose (usually weight dependent) for the patient before you draw up the medication and again just before you administer it. Prehospital medications are usually packaged to accommodate a single administration. If the drug package you select has much more or less than you intend to use, recheck the packaging to ensure it is the right drug and right concentration and recheck your calculations to ensure the right dosage.

The right time. Usually prehospital medications are given rather rapidly and not on a schedule. Check the packaging and your protocols for administration rate and ensure you follow the sequencing, time intervals, and drip rates for emergency drugs.

The right route. While most emergency drugs are administered by the IV route, be aware of the alternate routes of drug administration, the drugs administered via those routes, and the circumstances requiring the use of those routes. With each medication administration, ensure you are using the right route.

The right patient. It is imperative to ensure that the patient is properly matched to medication. A patient/drug mismatch is an infrequent problem in prehospital care, but as EMS moves to the out-of-hospital environment, paramedics may be treating some patients on a routine basis. Always ensure that the medication order is for the patient you are attending.

The right documentation. Thoroughly document all aspects of patient care, including what drugs were administered in what dosage.

9. Discuss special consideration in drug treatment with regard to pregnant, pediatric, and geriatric patients.   pp. 696-697

Pregnancy alters the mother's physiology and also adds a second party, the developing fetus, to the concerns regarding medication administration. The increased maternal heart rate, cardiac output, and blood volume can affect the onset and actions of many medications. Drugs may also alter fetal development and result in fetal injury, deformity, or death. During the third trimester, some drugs may pass through the placenta and affect the fetus directly.

Several anatomic and physiological differences between pediatric patients and adults result in differences in the ways drugs are absorbed and metabolized. Differences in gastric pH and emptying time and lower digestive enzyme levels in children change the way enteral medications are absorbed. A child's thinner skin causes topical agents to be absorbed more quickly. Lower plasma protein levels in children affect the availability of agents that usually bind to them. Higher water content in the neonate also affects drug absorption and distribution, as does the slower, then faster metabolism of the neonate and child, respectively. Organ maturity also affects drug metabolism and elimination. For children, drug administration is often guided by weight and in some cases guided by height (the Broselow tape).

With advancing age, the body's metabolism, gastric motility, decreased plasma proteins, reduced body fat and muscle mass, and depressed liver function all affect the absorption, metabolism, and elimination of drugs. Older patients are also likely to be on multiple medications for multiple diseases, thereby increasing the likelihood of adverse medication interactions.

10. Review the specific anatomy and physiology pertinent to pharmacology.   pp. 698-710

Drugs modify or exploit the existing functions of cells; they do not confer any new properties. They also often have several sites of action throughout the body and must be thought of for their systemic actions. Drugs may cause their effects by binding to cell receptor sites, changing the physical properties of a cell, chemically combining with other chemicals, or altering a normal metabolic pathway.

The most common mechanism of action for drugs administered in the prehospital setting involves drugs that bind to receptor sites. These receptor sites are most commonly associated with the nervous system because this system is responsible for overall body control. Drugs frequently affect the receptors for pain and those of the autonomic nervous system, including the sympathetic and parasympathetic nervous systems. Autonomic effects include changes in the rate and strength of cardiac contraction, in the degree of peripheral vascular contraction (resistance), and in bronchoconstriction or dilation to name just a few.

Other drugs act by changing the physical properties of the body, for example, by altering the osmolarity of the blood or by chemically combining with other substances to change the internal environment (as sodium bicarbonate combines with acids to make the blood more alkaline). Finally, some drugs alter a metabolic pathway to obtain their intended effect. Some anticancer drugs act in this way.

11. List and describe general properties of drugs.   p. 704

• **Affinity** is the force of attraction between the drug and the receptor site.
• **Efficacy** is the drug's ability to cause its expected effect.
• An **agonist** is a drug that causes the expected effect when bound to the receptor site.
• An **antagonist** is a drug that does not cause the expected effect when bound to the receptor site.
• An **agonist-antagonist** is a drug that binds to a receptor site, causing some expected effects and blocking others.
• A **competitive antagonist** is a drug that causes some effects as it binds to a receptor site but blocks the binding of another drug.
• A **noncompetitive antagonist** is a drug that binds to and deforms a receptor site so other drugs cannot bind there.

12. List and describe liquid and solid drug forms.   Pp. 705 - 707

Drugs come in many different forms. Solid drug forms include the following:
• **Pills** are drugs that are shaped spherically for easily swallowing.
• **Powders** are drugs simply in a powder form.
• **Tablets** are powders compressed into a disk-like form
• **Suppositories** are drugs mixed with a wax-like base that melts at body temperature. They are usually inserted into the rectum or vagina.
• **Capsules** are gelatin containers filled with the drug powder or tiny pills. When the container dissolves, the drug is released into the gastrointestinal tract.
Liquid forms include the following:
• **Solutions** are drugs dissolved in a solvent, usually water- or oil-based.
• **Tinctures** are medications extracted using alcohol with some alcohol usually remaining.
• **Suspensions** are mixtures of a solvent and drug in which the solid portion will precipitate out.
• **Emulsions** are suspensions with an oily substance in the solvent that remains as globules even when mixed.
• **Spirits** are solutions of volatile drugs in alcohol.
• **Elixirs** are drugs mixed with alcohol and water, often with flavorings to improve taste.
• **Syrups** are solutions of sugar, water, and drugs.

13. List and differentiate routes of drug administration.   pp. 702-704

Enteral routes deliver medications by absorption through the gastrointestinal tract. There are several routes of enteral administration. Oral routes are the most common for drug administration and are well suited for self-administration of medication. Naso- or orogastric tube administration uses either type of tube to direct medications into the stomach. Sublingual administration permits the drug to be absorbed by the capillaries under the tongue. Buccal (between the cheek and gum) absorption is similar to sublingual drug administration. Rectal administration is a route used for unconscious, vomiting, seizing, or uncooperative patients.

Routes outside the gastrointestinal tract are referred to as parenteral and typically use needles to inject medications into the circulatory system or tissues. With intravenous drug administration, a drug is injected directly into the veins, leading to rapid distribution of the medication. Endotracheal medication administration uses the endotracheal tube to place the medication into the lung field, where it is quickly absorbed by the bloodstream. Intraosseous administration directs medication into the medullary space of a long bone in the pediatric patient. Umbilical drug administration uses the umbilical artery or vein as an alternate IV site in the neonate. With intramuscular administration, the medication is injected into the muscle tissue, where it is rapidly absorbed by the bloodstream. Subcutaneous administration is just slightly slower than intramuscular administration. Transdermal administration is slightly slower than subcutaneous, and topical administration has the slowest absorption rate of all routes. With administration by inhalation/nebulization, a drug is introduced into the lung field, where it is absorbed. Nasal medications are introduced into the mucous membranes of the nose and are rapidly absorbed. With instillation, a drug is placed (topically) into a wound or the eye. Intradermal medications are delivered between dermal layers.

14. Differentiate between enteral and parenteral routes of drug administration.   pp. 703-704

Enteral routes of administration are those that direct drugs into the gastrointestinal system and include oral (PO), orogastric or nasogastric tube (OG/ON), sublingual (SL), buccal, and rectal. Parenteral routes are routes of administration outside the gastrointestinal tract and include intravenous (IV), endotracheal (ET), intraosseous (IO), umbilical, intramuscular (IM), subcutaneous (SQ), inhalation/nebulization, topical, transdermal, nasal, instillation, and intradermal.

15. Describe mechanisms of drug action.   pp. 705-707

How a drug interacts with the body to cause its effects is referred to as pharmacodynamics. Drugs induce their effects by binding to a receptor site, changing the physical properties of the body, chemically combining with other substances, or altering a normal metabolic pathway.

16. List and differentiate the phases of drug activity, including the pharmaceutical, pharmacokinetic, and pharmacodynamic phases.   pp. 698-710

The pharmaceutical phase of drug activity addresses the drug's intrinsic characteristics such as how the drug dissolves or disintegrates once injected or ingested. Pharmacokinetics refers to the processes by which a drug is absorbed, distributed, biotransformed, and eliminated by the body. Pharmacodynamics is the mechanism (or mechanisms) by which a drug interacts with the body to accomplish its action.

17. Describe the processes called pharmacokinetics and pharmocodynamics, including theories of drug action, drug-response relationship, factors altering drug responses, predictable drug responses, iatrogenic drug responses, and unpredictable adverse drug responses. pp. 698-710

There are two important elements of pharmacology: how drugs are transported into or out of the body (pharmacokinetics) and how drugs interact with the body to cause their effects (pharmacodynamics).

Pharmacokinetics examines the absorption, distribution, biotransformation, and elimination of drugs.

For a drug to perform its action, it must first reach its site of action, a process referred to as **absorption.** While some drugs affect target tissue directly (like antacids in the stomach), most must first find their way to the bloodstream. Drugs administered directly into a venous or arterial vessel are quickly transported to the heart, mixed with the blood, and distributed throughout the body. A drug injected into the muscle tissue and, to a somewhat lesser degree, into the subcutaneous tissue, is transported quickly to the bloodstream because of the more than adequate circulation in these tissues. However, shock and hypothermia may slow the process, while fever and hyperthermia may speed it. Oral medications must survive the gastric acidity and be somewhat lipid soluble to be transported across the intestinal membrane. The differing acid content of the digestive tract also impacts the dissociation of the drug into ions that are more difficult to move into the circulation. And finally, the drug's concentration affects its uptake by the bloodstream and, ultimately, its distribution. The end result of the absorption process is the concentration of the drug in the bloodstream and its availability for activation of the target tissue, called its bioavailability.

Once a drug enters the bloodstream, it must be carried throughout the body and to its site of action. This term for this process is **distribution.** Many factors affect the release and uptake of a drug by the body's cells. Some drugs bind to the plasma proteins of the blood and are released over a prolonged period of time. An increase in the blood's pH may increase the rate of release of the drug, or competition from other drugs for binding sites may cause more of a drug to become available. Distribution of some drugs is dependent upon their ability to cross the blood-brain or placental barriers. Other drugs are easily deposited in fatty tissue, bones, and teeth.

Once in the body, drugs are broken down into metabolites in a process called **biotransformation.** This process makes the drug more or less active and can make the drug more water soluble and easier to eliminate. Some drugs are totally metabolized, some are partially metabolized, while still others are not metabolized at all. The liver is responsible for most biotransformation, while the lungs, kidneys, and GI tract do some limited biotransformation.

Elimination is the excretion of the drug in urine, expired air, or in feces. Renal excretion is the major mechanism for eliminating drugs from the body. Drugs are eliminated as the blood pressure pushes and filters blood through kidney structures. This effect is enhanced by special cells that "pump" (active transport) some metabolites into the tubules. Kidney reabsorption also plays a part in drug excretion. Protein-soluble molecules and electrolytes are easily absorbed, but the uptake may be affected by the blood's pH.

A drug's effects on the body are referred to as **pharmacodynamics.** Drugs may cause their effects by binding on a receptor site, by changing physical properties, by chemically combining with other substances, or by altering a normal metabolic pathway.

Most drugs effect their actions by binding to receptor sites, especially those of the autonomic nervous system. The drug either inhibits or stimulates the cells or tissue. The force of attraction of a drug is referred to as its **affinity.** Affinity becomes important when different drugs compete for a site. The drug's **efficacy** is its ability to cause the expected response. Binding to a receptor site causes a change within the cell and induces the drug's effect. However, some drugs may establish a chain-reaction effect whereby other drugs are released and cause the desired effect. The number of receptor sites may change as the drug becomes available and uses them, thereby reducing the drug's continuing effect. Chemicals that bind to the receptor and cause the expected response are termed **agonists. Antagonists** bind to the site and do not cause the expected response. Some drugs have both properties. Often drugs compete for receptor site in a process called **competitive antagonism,** while a situation in which a drug attaches to a receptor, effectively locking out other drugs, is termed **noncompetitive antagonism.** Permanent binding to a receptor site is **irreversible antagonism.**

Drugs may also act by modifying the physical properties of a part of the body. For example, the drug mannitol changes the blood's osmolarity and increases urine output.

Some drugs chemically combine with other substances to cause their desired effect. For example, antacids interact with the hydrochloric acid in the stomach to reduce the pH.

Other drugs act by altering normal biologic processes and the metabolic pathways. Such drugs are used to treat cancers and viral infections.

The **drug-response relationship** is the relationship between a drug's pharmaceutical, pharmacokinetic, and pharmacodynamic properties. It most commonly relates to the blood plasma level of the drug. Other important factors include the speed of onset, duration of action, minimum effective concentration, and biologic half-life. Another very important factor in the drug-response relationship is the **therapeutic index,** or the ratio between the drug's lethal and effective doses.

Factors altering drug response include the patient's age, body mass, sex, pathologic state, genetic factors, and psychological factors as well as environmental considerations and the time of administration. These factors may increase or decrease the drug's ability to generate its desired affect.

Responses to drug administration may include unintended responses, or **side effects.** These are care-provider induced (iatrogenic) and include allergic reactions, idiosyncratic (unique to an individual) reactions, tolerance, cross tolerance, tachyphylaxis, cumulative effects, dependency, drug interactions, drug antagonisms, summation, synergistic reactions (a result greater than the expected additive result of two drugs administered together), potentiation, and interference. Some of these effects may be predictable and desired and some may be unexpected.

18. Differentiate among drug interactions.　　p. 709-710

Drugs have the potential to interact, cause, and alter the effects of other drugs taken by a patient. One drug may alter the effects of another by altering the rate of intestinal absorption, by competing for the same plasma protein binding site, by altering the other's metabolism and hence bioavailability, by causing an antagonistic or synergistic action at a receptor site, by altering the excretion rate of another drug through the kidneys, or by altering the electrolyte balance necessary for the other drug's actions.

19. Discuss considerations for storing and securing medications.　　p. 704

Temperature, humidity, ultraviolet radiation (sunlight), and time affect the potency of many drugs. It is important that they be stored under proper conditions and that they are rotated so they are utilized (or discarded) before their shelf life expires.

20. List the components of a drug profile by classification.　　p. 692

Names: The generic, trade, and sometimes the chemical names.

Classification: The broad group to which the drug belongs.

Mechanism of action: The way the drug causes it desired effects (its pharmacodynamics).

Indications: The conditions appropriate for the drug's administration.

Pharmacokinetics: How the drug is absorbed, distributed, and eliminated, including its onset and duration of action.

Side effects/adverse reactions: The drug's untoward or undesired effects.

Routes of administration: How the drug is given.

Contraindications: Conditions that make it inappropriate to administer a drug (including conditions in which administration is likely to cause a harmful outcome).

Dosage: The amount of drug that should be given.

How supplied: The typical concentrations and preparations of the drug.

Special considerations: How the drug may affect pregnant, pediatric, and geriatric patients.

CONTENT SELF-EVALUATION

_____ 1. The study of drugs and their interactions with the body is:
- **A.** pharmaceutics.
- **B.** pharmacokinetics.
- **C.** pharmacodynamics.
- **D.** pharmacology.
- **E.** pharmacopedia.

_____ 2. Which of the following types of drug names is 7 chloro-1,3-dihydro-1-methyl-5-phenyl-2H-1,4 benzodiazepine-2-one?
- **A.** chemical name
- **B.** generic name
- **C.** official name
- **D.** brand name
- **E.** common name

_____ 3. Which of the following types of drug names is diazepam?
- **A.** chemical name
- **B.** generic name
- **C.** official name
- **D.** brand name
- **E.** common name

_____ 4. Digitalis is an example of a drug derived from:
- **A.** a plant.
- **B.** an animal.
- **C.** a mineral.
- **D.** synthetic production.
- **E.** a lipid base.

_____ 5. Bovine insulin is an example of a drug derived from:
- **A.** a plant.
- **B.** an animal.
- **C.** a mineral.
- **D.** synthetic production.
- **E.** a lipid base.

_____ 6. The drug reference that presents manufacturer-provided drug information and some photos of drugs is the:
- **A.** _EMS Guide to Drugs._
- **B.** _CMA Drug Evaluations._
- **C.** _Compendium of Pharmaceuticals & Specialties._
- **D.** _Monthly Prescribing Reference._
- **E.** all of the above

_____ 7. The broad group to which a drug belongs is its:
- **A.** indication.
- **B.** pharmacokinetics.
- **C.** classification.
- **D.** mechanism of action.
- **E.** none of the above

_____ 8. Conditions in which it is inappropriate to give a drug are referred to as its:
- **A.** mechanisms of action.
- **B.** indications.
- **C.** contraindications.
- **D.** side effects.
- **E.** special considerations.

_____ 9. Which of the following drugs is classified as a Schedule G controlled substance?
- **A.** heroin
- **B.** morphine
- **C.** codeine
- **D.** diazepam
- **E.** B and C

_____ 10. The assay of a drug in a preparation determines its:
- **A.** potency.
- **B.** amount and purity.
- **C.** effectiveness.
- **D.** availability in a biological model.
- **E.** effectiveness compared to other like drugs.

11. The bioequivalence of a drug in a preparation refers to its:

    A.   potency.

    B.   amount and purity.

    C.   effectiveness.

    D.   availability in a biological model.

    E.   effectiveness compared to other like drugs.

12. Which of the following is NOT one of the six rights of medication administration?

    A.   right dose   **D.**   right time

    B.   right patient   **E.**   right mechanism

    C.   right documentation

13. Hallucinogens such as peyote are examples of drugs found in the:

    A.   Narcotics Schedule.

    B.   Schedule F: prescriptions drugs.

    C.   Schedule G: controlled drugs.

    D.   Schedule H: restricted drugs.

    E.   Nonprescription drug schedule.

14. Low-dose codeine preparations are examples of drugs found in the:

    A.   Narcotics Schedule.

    B.   Schedule F: prescriptions drugs.

    C.   Schedule G: controlled drugs.

    D.   Schedule H: restricted drugs.

    E.   Nonprescription drug schedule.

15. Which of the following is NOT true regarding the newborn patient?

    A.   The neonate has less gastric acid than an adult.

    B.   The neonate has diminished blood plasma levels.

    C.   The neonate has immature renal and hepatic systems.

    D.   The neonate has less body water than an adult.

    E.   The neonate has lower enzyme levels than an adult.

16. Drugs in which of the following FDA categories have demonstrated definite risks to the fetus?

    A.   R   **D.**   C

    B.   A   **E.**   D

    C.   B

17. Which of the following is NOT true regarding the geriatric patient?

    A.   The geriatric patient has decreased gastrointestinal motility.

    B.   The geriatric patient has decreased body fat.

    C.   The geriatric patient has decreased muscle mass.

    D.   The geriatric patient is more likely to be disease free.

    E.   The geriatric patient has decreased liver function.

18. The study of how drugs are transported into and out of the body is known as:

    A.   Pharmacokinetics.   **D.**   Pharmacodynamics.

    B.   Pharmacology.   **E.**   Pathopharmacology.

    C.   Polypharmacy.

19. Which of the following is NOT one of the four basic processes of pharmacokinetics?

    A.   absorption   **D.**   biotransformation

    B.   distribution   **E.**   elimination

    C.   receptor binding

20. Which of the following represents an energy-consuming movement of ions against the concentration gradient?

    A.   diffusion   **D.**   filtration

    B.   active transport   **E.**   facilitated transport

    C.   osmosis

21. Which of the following represents movement of molecules across a membrane from an area of higher pressure to an area of lower pressure?
- **A.** diffusion
- **B.** active transport
- **C.** osmosis
- **D.** filtration
- **E.** facilitated transport

22. The measure of the amount of a drug that is still active after it reaches the target organ is its:
- **A.** bioavailability.
- **B.** biotransformativity.
- **C.** metabolism.
- **D.** pro-drug effect.
- **E.** active distribution.

23. Which of the following is NOT a significant medium for elimination of drugs from the body?
- **A.** urine
- **B.** respiratory air
- **C.** feces
- **D.** sweat
- **E.** all are significant

24. Which of the following is NOT an enteral route of drug administration?
- **A.** oral
- **B.** umbilical
- **C.** buccal
- **D.** sublingual
- **E.** rectal

25. Which of the following is the preferred route for medication administration in most emergencies?
- **A.** intramuscular
- **B.** inhalation
- **C.** endotracheal
- **D.** intravenous
- **E.** subcutaneous

26. Drugs that are spherically shaped to be easy to swallow are:
- **A.** pills.
- **B.** suppositories.
- **C.** tablets.
- **D.** capsules.
- **E.** suspensions.

27. Drugs that are powders compressed into disks are:
- **A.** pills.
- **B.** suppositories.
- **C.** tablets.
- **D.** capsules.
- **E.** suspensions.

28. Preparations in which the solid does not dissolve in the solvent are:
- **A.** solutions.
- **B.** tinctures.
- **C.** suspensions.
- **D.** spirits.
- **E.** elixirs.

29. Preparations made with alcohol and water solvent, often with flavorings, are:
- **A.** solutions.
- **B.** tinctures.
- **C.** suspensions.
- **D.** spirits.
- **E.** elixirs.

30. Pharmacodynamics are best described as:
- **A.** interactions between drugs.
- **B.** the processes by which drugs are eliminated from the body.
- **C.** the effects of a drug on the body.
- **D.** the processes by which drugs bind to receptor sites.
- **E.** the process by which a drug is administered.

31. The location where a drug combines with a protein, resulting in a biochemical effect, is a:
- **A.** second messenger.
- **B.** antagonist.
- **C.** receptor.
- **D.** agonist.
- **E.** protein block.

32. A drug's ability to cause its expected response is referred to as its:
    A. affinity.
    B. efficacy.
    C. agonism.
    D. antagonism.
    E. equilibrium.

33. A chemical that binds to a receptor site but does not cause the expected effect is a(n):
    A. partial-antagonist.
    B. competitive antagonist.
    C. agonist.
    D. antagonist.
    E. noncompetitive antagonist.

34. A chemical that binds to a receptor site, causes the expected effect, and prevents other drugs from activating the receptor site is a(n):
    A. partial antagonist.
    B. competitive antagonist.
    C. agonist.
    D. antagonist.
    E. noncompetitive antagonist.

35. The drug morphine sulfate is an example of a(n):
    A. agonist-antagonist.
    B. competitive antagonist.
    C. agonist.
    D. antagonist.
    E. noncompetitive antagonist.

36. The drug nalbuphine (Nubain) is an example of a(n):
    A. agonist-antagonist.
    B. competitive antagonist.
    C. agonist.
    D. antagonist.
    E. noncompetitive antagonist.

37. A drug reaction that is unique to an individual is referred to as:
    A. idiosyncrasy.
    B. tachyphylaxis.
    C. antagonism.
    D. synergism.
    E. potentiation.

38. A drug reaction that is greater than expected from the administration of two drugs that have the same effect at the same time is referred to as:
    A. idiosyncrasy.
    B. tachyphylaxis.
    C. antagonism.
    D. synergism.
    E. potentiation.

39. The time span between when a drug drops below its minimum effective concentration and its complete elimination from the body is its:
    A. onset of action.
    B. duration of action.
    C. therapeutic index.
    D. biologic half-life.
    E. termination of action.

40. The ratio between a drug's lethal dose and its effective dose is its:
    A. onset of action.
    B. duration of action.
    C. therapeutic index.
    D. biologic half-life.
    E. termination of action.

True/False

41. Generic names, also known as trade names, are selected by the manufacturer.
    A. True
    B. False

42. The majority of drugs used in the prehospital setting are controlled substances such as morphine sulfate, or are prescription drugs.
    A. True
    B. False

43. Nitroglycerine is an example of a Schedule G: controlled drug.

A. True
B. False

44. Dosages of many emergency drugs are based upon patient weight, so unit dose packaging may not contain the right amount for every patient.
A. True
B. False

45. Intravenous administration of epinephrine is more effective than subcutaneous administration for patients in anaphylaxis.
A. True
B. False

46. Children are, for the most part, just small adults, so drug dosages just need to be reduced proportionally by weight.
A. True
B. False

47. Teratongenic drugs are medications used to treat the fetus during pregnancy.
A. True
B. False

48. A newborn's low metabolic rate and incompletely developed hepatic system put him or her at higher risk for toxic drug interactions.
A. True
B. False

49. Due to changes in gastrointestinal motility, geriatric patients absorb oral medications more quickly than younger adults.
A. True
B. False

50. Drugs do not confer anynew properties on cells or tissues; they only modify or exploit existing functions.
A. True
B. False

51. A mechanism that uses energy to move a substance at the cellular level is known as active transport..
A. True
B. False

52. In diffusion, solvent molecules move from an area of low solute concentration to an area of higher solute concentration.
A. True
B. False

53. Bioavailability is the proportion of a drug availabie in the body to cause either desired or undesired effects.
A. True
B. False

54. PO, SL, and PR are examples of enteral medication routes..
A. True
B. False

55. Efficacy is the force of attraction between a drug and a receptor.
A. True
B. False

Matching

Pharmacokinetics

Write the letter of the term in the space provided next to the definition or description to which it applies.

Term

A. active transport	**F.** free drug availability
B. bioavailability	**G.** facilitated diffusion
C. bioequivalence	**H.** osmosis
D. diffusion	**I.** oxidation
E. filtration	**J.** ionization

Definition

_____ **56.** movement of solute from an area of higher concentration to an area of lower concentration.

_____ **57.** proportion of a drug available in the body to cause either desired or undesired effects

_____ **58.** requires the use of energy to move a substance

_____ **59.** movement of molecules across a membrane from an area of higher pressure to an area of lower pressure.

_____ **60.** movement of solvent from an area of lower solute concentration to an area of higher solute concentration.

_____ **61.** amount of a drug that is still active after it reaches its target tissue.

_____ **62.** relative therapeutic effectiveness of chemically equivalent drugs

_____ **63.** process in which carrier proteins transport large molecules a cross the cell membrane

_____ **64.** to become electrically charged or polar

_____ **65.** the loss of hydrogen atoms or the acceptance of an oxygen atom.

Pharmacodynamics

Write the letter of the term in the space provided next to the definition or description to which it applies.

Term

A. agonist
B. antagonist
C. competitive antagonism
D. irreversible antagonism
E. Noncompetitive antagonism

Definition

_____ **66.** the binding of an antagonist causes a deformity of the biding site that prevents an agonist from fitting and binding

_____ **67.** drug that binds to a receptor but does not cause it to initiate the expected response

_____ **68.** drug that binds to a receptor and causes it to initiate the expected response

_____ **69.** a competitive antagonist permanently binds with a receptor site

_____ **70.** one drug binds to a receptor and causes the expected effect while also blocking another drug from triggering the same receptor.

Chapter 14

General Principles of Pharmacology

Part 2: Drug Classifications

Review of Chapter Objectives

After reading this part of the chapter, you should be able to:

1. Describe how drugs are classified.   **pp. 710-711**

The Food and Drug Administration classifies a new drug using one-digit and one-letter designations. The numerical classification describes its origin: a new molecular drug, a new salt of a marketed drug, a new formulation or dosage, a new combination not previously marketed, a generic duplication of an existing drug, a new indication for an already marketed drug, and a drug on the market prior to the existence of the FDA. The letter classification identifies the treatment or therapeutic potential of a drug: an important therapeutic gain, a similarity to an existing drug or drugs, whether the drug is indicated in the treatment of AIDS and HIV disease, whether the drug has been developed to treat a severely debilitating or life-threatening disease, or whether the drug is an orphan drug (a drug developed for a relatively uncommon disease).

2. Review the specific anatomy and physiology pertinent to pharmacology with additional attention to autonomic pharmacology.   **pp. 711-760**

Drugs affect many systems of the body including the central nervous system, the autonomic nervous system, the cardiovascular system, the respiratory system, the gastrointestinal system, and the endocrine system. Drugs are also used to treat infectious disease and inflammation.

Central Nervous System Pharmacology
The central nervous system consists of the brain and spinal column and all neurons that both originate and terminate within these structures. Since this system is responsible for conscious thought and affects many bodily functions, it is the target for many drugs used in medical care. These agents include analgesics, anesthetics, antianxiety and sedative-hypnotic drugs, antiseizure and antiepileptic drugs, CNS stimulants, and psychotherapeutic drugs.

    Analgesics are used to reduce the sensation of pain. These drugs include the opioid and nonopioid analgesics, adjunctive medications (to enhance the effects of the analgesics), and opioid agonists-antagonists. Agents that block the actions of analgesics, opioid antagonists and in some cases analgesic antagonists, are used in cases of overdose or to reverse or negate the undesired effects of analgesics.

Anesthetics are used to decrease the sensation of both touch and pain. Anesthetics may be given locally or systemically and in lower doses may produce a decreased sensation of pain while the patient may remain conscious. At higher doses, anesthetics generally induce unconsciousness.

Antianxiety and sedative-hypnotic drugs are used to reduce anxiety, induce amnesia, assist sleeping, and may be used as a part of a balanced approach to anesthesia. These drugs include the benzodiazepines, barbiturates, and alcohol. They decrease (depress) the central nervous system's response to stimuli.

Antiseizure and antiepileptic agents are used to prevent seizure activity and are often associated with undesirable side effects. Antiseizure agents generally act on the sodium and calcium channels in the neural membrane and include phenytoin, carbamazepine, valproic acid, and ethosuximide.

CNS stimulants are used to treat fatigue, drowsiness, narcolepsy, obesity, and attention deficit disorders. They cause their actions by either increasing the release and effectiveness of excitatory neurotransmitters or decreasing the release or effectiveness of inhibitory neurotransmitters. These agents include amphetamines, methylamphetamines, and methylxanthines.

Psychotherapeutic medications treat mental dysfunction, including schizophrenia, depression, and bipolar disorder. Schizophrenia is treated with neuroleptic (affecting the nerves) and antipsychotic drugs (phenothiazines and butyrophenones), which block numerous peripheral neuroreceptor sites. Antidepressants increase the availability, release, or effectiveness of norepinephrine and serotonin and are used to treat depression. These medications include the tricyclic antidepressants (TCAs), the selective serotonin reuptake inhibitors (SSRIs), and monoamine oxidase inhibitors (MAOIs). Bipolar disorder (manic depression) is manifested by dramatic mood swings and is treated with lithium.

Parkinson's disease is another central nervous system disorder caused by the destruction of dopamine-releasing neurons in the portion of the brain controlling fine motor movements. This disease is treated by stimulating the dopamine release (Sinemet) or with anticholinergic agents (benztropine).

Autonomic Nervous System Pharmacology

The autonomic nervous system is located within the peripheral nervous system and consists of the sympathetic (fight-or-flight) and parasympathetic (feed-and-breed) systems. These systems are antagonistic and provided control over body functions. The autonomic nervous system controls virtually every organ and body structure not under conscious control and is responsible for maintaining the internal human environment. The nerves of the two systems do not actually touch other nerves or target organs. Messages are carried through the small space between them (synapse) via chemical messengers (neurotransmitters). Acetylcholine is the neurotransmitter at the target organs of the parasympathetic nervous system, while norepinephrine is the neurotransmitter at the target organs for the sympathetic nervous system.

Stimulation of the parasympathetic nervous system causes pupillary constriction, digestive gland secretion, decreased cardiac rate and strength of contraction, bronchoconstriction, and increased digestive activity. Cholinergic (effecting the acetylcholine receptors) drugs stimulate the parasympathetic nervous system and produce salivation, lacrimation, urination, defecation, gastric motility, and emesis (signs suggested by the acronym SLUDGE). They cause their actions directly by acting on the receptor sites (bethanechol and pilocarpine) or indirectly by inhibiting the degradation of acetylcholine (neostigmine and physostigmine). Anticholenergic (parasympatholytic) drugs oppose the actions of acetylcholine and the parasympathetic nervous system. Atropine is the prototype anticholinergic drug, while scopolamine (transdermal) is used to treat motion sickness and ipratropium bromide (Atrovent) is inhaled to treat bronchoconstriction caused by asthma. Ganglionic blocking agents compete for the acetylcholine receptors at the ganglia and can effectively turn off the parasympathetic nervous system. Neuromuscular blocking agents produce a state of paralysis without inducing unconsciousness. Ganglionic stimulating agents (nicotine) stimulate the ganglia of both the parasympathetic and sympathetic nervous systems yet have no therapeutic purpose.

Stimulation of the sympathetic nervous system causes an increased heart rate and strength of contraction, bronchodilation, increased blood flow to the muscles, decreased blood flow to the skin and abdominal organs, decreased digestive activity, release of glucose stores from the liver, increased energy production, decreased digestive activity, and the release of epinephrine and norepinephrine. Sympathetic receptors include four adrenergic receptors (alpha 1, alpha 2, beta 1, and beta 2) and dopaminergic receptors. Alpha 1 stimulation causes peripheral vasoconstriction, mild bronchoconstriction, and increased metabolism. Alpha 2 stimulation prevents the over-release of norepinephrine at the synapse. Beta 1 stimulation exclusively affects the heart and causes increased heart rate, cardiac contractile force, automaticity, and conduction. Beta 2 stimulation causes bronchodilation and selective vasodilation. Dopaminergic stimulation causes increased circulation to the kidneys, heart, and brain. Sympathomimetic (adrenergic) drugs stimulate the effects of the sympathetic nervous system, while sympatholytic drugs block the actions of the sympathetic nervous system. Alpha 1 drugs increase peripheral vascular resistance, preload, and blood pressure. Alpha 1 agonists are used to control blood pressure or to control injury due to the infiltration of an alpha 1 drug. Beta 1 drugs stimulate the heart and are primarily used in cardiac arrest or cardiogenic shock. Beta 1 antagonists are used to control blood pressure, suppress tachycardia, and reduce cardiac workload in angina. Beta 2 agonists are used to treat asthma.

Cardiovascular System Pharmacology

The cardiovascular system consists of the heart, blood vessels, and the blood. The heart is a four-chambered muscular organ that pumps most of the blood around the body. It is controlled by an intrinsic electrical system that coordinates cardiac muscular response and pumping action. The myocardium is unique in that it has the ability to generate an electrical impulse (automaticity) and conduct an impulse to surrounding tissue (conductivity). The heart muscle contracts and relaxes (depolarizes and repolarizes) as sodium, calcium, and potassium ions flow into and out of the cell.

Antidysrhythmic drugs are used to prevent or treat abnormal variations in the cardiac electrical cycle. Sodium channel blockers slow the influx of sodium back into the cell and, in effect, slow conduction through the atria and ventricles. Class IA sodium channel blockers (quinidine, procainamide, and disopyramide) slow repolarization, while class IB drugs (lidocaine, phenytoin, tocainide, mexiletine) speed repolarization and reduce automaticity in the ventricles. Class IC drugs (flecainide, propafenone) decrease conduction velocity through the atria, ventricles, bundle of His, and the Purkinje network and delay ventricular repolarization. Beta blockers (propranolol, acebutolol, esmolol) are antagonistic to the beta 1 actions of the sympathetic nervous system. Since the beta receptors are attached to the calcium channels of the heart, these agents act in a manner very similar to the calcium channel blockers. Potassium channel blockers (bretylium, amiodarone) block the efflux of calcium; these agents prolong repolarization and the effective refractory period (the period before the myocardium can contract again). Calcium channel blockers (verapamil, diltiazem) decrease conductivity through the AV node and slow conduction of atrial flutter or fibrillation to the ventricles. Other antidysrhythmics include adenosine (a fast and short-acting potassium and calcium blocker), digoxin (decreases SA node firing rate and conduction velocity through the AV node), and magnesium (effective in treating a polymorphic ventricular tachycardia—*torsade de pointes*).

Antihypertensive drugs manipulate peripheral vascular resistance, heart rate, or stroke volume to reduce blood pressure. Diuretics reduce the amount of circulating blood (and hence the cardiac preload and stroke volume) by increasing the urine output of the kidneys. They include loop diuretics (furosemide), thiazides (HydroDIURIL), potassium-sparing diuretics (spironolactone), and the osmotic diuretics (mannitol). Beta adrenergic antagonists (metoprolol) act by reducing the heart's rate and contractility as well as by reducing the release of hormones (renin) from the kidneys that ultimately cause vasoconstriction (through the renin-angiotensin-aldosterone system). Centrally acting adrenergic inhibitors (clonidine) stimulate alpha 2 receptors and inhibit the release of norepinephrine. Alpha 1 antagonists (prazosin, terazosin) competitively block the alpha 1 receptors, mediating sympathetic increases in peripheral vascular resistance. Finally, some drugs (labetalol, carvedilol) have combined alpha and beta antagonistic effects. Angiotensin converting enzyme (ACE) inhibitors (captopril, enalapril, lisinopril, enalaprilat) block the production of angiotensin II, a very potent vasoconstrictor, through the renin-angiotensin-aldosterone system. Angiotensin II receptor antagonists act on the renin-angiotensin-aldosterone system by blocking the actions of angiotensin II at its receptor site. Calcium channel blockers (nifedipine) are also effective at controlling hypertension by selectively acting on the smooth muscles of the arterioles and reducing peripheral vascular resistance without reducing cardiac preload. Direct vasodilators (hydralazine, minoxidil, sodium nitroprusside) selectively dilate arterioles and decrease peripheral vascular resistance. Hypertension may also be controlled by agents that block the autonomic nervous system (trimethaphan) or with cardiac glycosides (digoxin, digitoxin) that affect the ion pumps of the myocardium and increase cardiac contraction strength but reduce heart rate.

Angina is treated with calcium channel blockers (verapamil, diltiazem, nifedipine) because they reduce cardiac workload and slow the heart rate. Organic nitrates (nitroglycerin, isosorbide, amyl nitrite) relax vascular smooth muscle, decreasing cardiac preload and workload, and, in Prinzmetal's angina, may increase coronary blood flow.

Three agents are used to prevent and break up blood clots that obstruct either the heart chambers or the blood vessels. Antiplatelet drugs (aspirin, dipyridamole, abciximab, ticlopidine) decrease the formation of platelet plugs during the clotting process. Anticoagulants (heparin, warfarin) interrupt the clotting cascade. Thrombolytics (streptokinase, alteplase, reteplase, anistreplase) dissolve the fibrin mesh of clots and thereby help break apart clots after they form.

Antihyperlipidemic agents (lovastatin, simvastatin, cholestyramine) are used to reduce the level of low-density lipoproteins, a causative factor for coronary artery disease.

Respiratory System Pharmacology

The respiratory system is basically a pathway through which air travels in from the exterior to the air-exchange sacs, the alveoli, and then out again. Indications for pharmacologic intervention include asthma, rhinitis, and cough.

Asthma is a pathologic condition caused by an allergy to pet dander, dust, or mold that causes respiratory restriction or obstruction. The allergic response releases histamine, leukotrienes, and prostaglandins, producing immediate bronchoconstriction and then inflammation. Treatment includes beta$_2$ agonists (albuterol) to reduce bronchoconstriction and epinephrine for severe reactions not responding to beta$_2$ agonists. Anticholinergic agents (ipratropium) act along different pathways to the beta$_2$ agonists and may provide an additive effect in limiting bronchoconstriction. Glucocorticoids (beclomethasone, methylprednisolone, cromolyn) have anti-inflammatory properties that reduce the amount of mucus and the edema in the airway and alveolar walls. Lastly, leukotriene antagonists (zileuton) block the formation of, or the receptors for (zafirlukast), leukotriene. Leukotrienes are mediators released from mast cells that contribute powerfully to both bronchoconstriction and inflammation.

Rhinitis is the inflammation of the mucosa of the nasal cavity and may cause nasal congestion, itching, sneezing, and rhinorrhea (runny nose). Nasal decongestants (phenylephrine, pseudoephedrine, phenylpropanolamine) are alpha$_1$ agonists that reduce vasodilation and are given in mist or oral form. Antihistamines (alkylamines, ethanolamines, clemastine, phenothiazines, loratadine, cetirizine, fexofenadine) are used for more serious allergic reactions and block the action of histamine and thereby relieve bronchoconstriction, capillary permeability, and vasodilation. Cough suppressants (antitussive agents, both opioid and nonopioid) dull the cough reflex and are designed to treat unproductive coughing due to an irritated oropharynx. Expectorants are intended to increase the productivity of the cough while mucolytics make the mucus more watery and possibly more effective.

Gastrointestinal System Pharmacology

Drugs used to treat the gastrointestinal system are primarily for gastric ulcers, constipation, diarrhea, emesis, and to aid digestion. Peptic ulcer disease occurs as the balance between the protective coating of the stomach and its acidity is no longer maintained. The acid may then eat away at the intestinal lining and tissues underneath. The injury may result in internal hemorrhage. Peptic ulcer disease is treated with antibiotics (bismuth, metronidazole, amoxicillin, tetracycline) to treat the underlying cause and drugs (cimetidine, ranitidine, famotidine, nizatidine, omeprazole, lansoprazole, antacids, pirenzepine) that block or decrease the secretion of acid. Constipation is treated with bulk-forming (methlycellulose, psyllium), surfactant (docusate sodium), stimulant (phenolphthalein, bisacodyl) or osmotic (magnesium hydroxide) laxatives. Diarrhea is often caused by an underlying disease and is usually self-correcting. In severe cases, It is treated with antibiotics. Input from the inner ear, nose, and eyes or a response to anxiety or fear triggers the vomiting reflex (emesis), which can be useful for certain poisonings and overdoses (Ipecac). Antiemetics that reduce the vomiting reflex include serotonin antagonists (ondansetron), dopamine antagonists (phenothiazines, butyrophenones, metoclopramide), anticholenergics, and cannabinoids (dronabinol, nabilone). Finally, drugs used to aid ingestion are enzymes (pancreatin, pancrelipase) similar to endogenous enzymes found in the intestinal tract.

Endocrine System Pharmacology

The endocrine system provides the body with hormones essential to maintaining homeostasis and controlling overall body activity. It consists of the following glands: pituitary, pineal, thyroid, thymus, parathyroid, adrenal, pancreas, ovaries, and testes. These organs produce hormones that then circulate throughout the body and affect target organs. Drugs can affect the anterior and posterior pituitary, parathyroid and thyroid, adrenal, pancreas, and reproductive glands or simulate the hormones they produce.

The pituitary gland is made up of the anterior and posterior lobes and resides deep within the skull. The anterior pituitary gland releases hormones related to growth. Dwarfism results from a deficiency in growth hormone and is treated with somatrem and somatropin. Gigantism and acromegaly usually result from a tumor and are treated by surgical removal of the tumor or with the drug octreotide, which inhibits the release of the growth hormone. The posterior pituitary produces oxytocin and antidiuretic hormone (ADH). Oxytocin induces uterine contractions and precipitates delivery, while antidiuretic hormone increases water reabsorption in the kidneys and thereby regulates electrolyte balance, blood volume, and blood pressure. Diabetes insipidus is caused by inadequate circulating ADH and is treated with vasopressin, desmopressin, and lypressin.

The parathyroid gland regulates the levels of calcium and vitamin D. Chronic low calcium and vitamin D levels are treated with supplements, while high levels (usually due to tumors) are treated with surgical removal of all or part of the parathyroid gland.

The thyroid gland hormones play vital roles in growth, maturation, and metabolism. Child onset hyperthyroidism results in dwarfism and mental retardation, while adult onset hyperthyroidism manifests with a decreased metabolism, weight gain, fatigue, and bradycardia. Hypothyroidism is treated with levothyroxine, a synthetic analog of thyroxine, the major thyroid hormone. Goiters occur as a result of inadequate iodine in the diet and are treated with iodine supplements. Thyroid tumors often cause hyperthyroidism and are treated with surgery, radiation therapy, or the drug propylthiouracil or a combination of therapies.

The adrenal cortex secretes glucocorticoids that increase the glucose in the bloodstream, mineralocorticoids that regulate the salt/water balance, and androgens that regulate sexual development and maturity. Cushing's disease results in increased glucocorticoid secretion and hyperglycemia, obesity, hypertension, and electrolyte imbalances. It is usually treated surgically, with pharmacological intervention aimed at the symptoms; drugs used for this include antihypertensive agents (spironolactone), ACE inhibitors (captopril), and drugs that inhibit corticoid synthesis. Addison's disease is characterized by hyposecretion of corticoids and presents with hypoglycemia, emaciation, hypotension, hyperkalemia, and hyponatremia. It is treated with cortisone, hydrocortisone, and fludrocortisone.

The pancreas produces two hormones important to glucose metabolism. They are insulin and glucagon. Insulin is essential for the transport of glucose, potassium, and amino acids into the cells. It stimulates cell growth and division and converts glucose into glycogen in the liver and skeletal muscles. Glucagon increases blood glucose levels by promoting the synthesis of glucose from glycerol and amino acids and from breaking down glycogen into glucose. Diabetes is an inappropriate carbohydrate metabolism due to an inadequate release of insulin (type I, juvenile onset) or a decreased responsiveness to insulin (type II, adult onset). Oral hypoglycemic agents stimulate insulin release from the pancreas and are administered to the type II diabetic. They are from four classes: sulfonylureas (tolbutamide, chlorpropamide, glipizide, glyburide), biguanides (metformin), alpha-glucosidase inhibitors (acarbose, miglitol), and thiazolidinediones (troglitazone). Pork, beef, or human insulin is injected subcutaneously daily for the type I diabetic. Hyperglycemic agents (glucagon and diazoxide) act to increase blood glucose levels while 50 percent dextrose in water ($D_{50}W$) is an intravenous sugar solution intended to supply carbohydrates to the hypoglycemic patient.

The genitalia release hormones that regulate human sexuality and reproduction. In the female, the ovaries, ovarian follicles, and, during pregnancy, the placenta release these hormones. Drug therapy can supplement these hormones, provide contraception, stimulate or relax the pregnant uterus, or assist in fertility. Estrogen is administered post-menopause to reduce the risk of osteoporosis and coronary artery disease. It is also administered in delayed puberty. Progestins counteract the untoward effects of estrogen and are used to treat amenorrhea, endometriosis, and dysfunctional uterine hemorrhage. Estrogen and progestin (or progestin alone) are commonly used as contraceptives. Their side effects include a predisposition to thromboembolisms, hypertension, and uterine bleeding. Oxytocic agents (oxytocin) induce uterine contractions to induce or speed up labor, while tocolytics (terbutaline, ritodrine) relax the smooth muscle of the uterus and delay labor. Female infertility is treated with agents (clomiphene, urofollitropin, menotropin) that promote maturation of ovarian follicles. In the male, testosterone replacement therapy (testosterone enanthate, methlytestosterone, fluoxymesterone) is provided for deficiency or delayed puberty. An enlarged prostate is cared for with surgery or drug (finasteride) therapy. A recent drug, sildenafil, is used for erectile dysfunction and acts by relaxing vascular smooth muscle. However, in combination with nitrates, it may lead to decreased cardiac preload and profound hypotension.

Pharmacology of Infectious Disease

Infectious diseases are typically caused by bacteria, viruses, or fungi and are treated by antimicrobial drugs including antibiotics and antifungal, antiviral, and antiparasitic agents. Symptoms of microbial infection are treated with nonsteroidal anti-inflammatory drugs (NSAIDs), and some diseases are treated prophylactically with serums and vaccines.

Antibiotics either kill the offending bacteria or decrease their ability to grow and reproduce. Penicillin, cephalosporin, and vancomycin act by inhibiting cell wall synthesis and causing the walls to rupture. Macrolide, aminoglycoside, and tetracycline antibiotics prevent cells from replicating.

Antifungal agents inhibit fungal growth (ketoconazole), while antiviral drugs act through various mechanisms (indinavir, acyclovir, zidovudine). Antiparasitic agents are used to treat malaria (chloroquine, mefloquine, quinine), amebiasis (paromomycin, metronidazole), and helminthiasis (mebendazole, niclosamide).

Other antimicrobials are used to treat diseases such as tuberculosis (isoniazid, refampin) and leprosy (dapsone, clofazimine).

Nonsteroidal anti-inflammatory drugs (ketorolac, piroxicam, naproxen) limit the fever (antipyretics) and pain (analgesics) associated with headache, arthritis, dysmenorrhea, and orthopedic injuries

3. List and describe common prehospital medications, including indications, contraindications, side effects, routes of administration, and dosages.   **pp. 711-760**

At the back of this workbook you will find a series of pages with drug cards. Each card contains the name/class, description, indications, contraindications, precautions, routes of administration, and dosages for a drug commonly used in prehospital emergency care. Detach the cards and begin to use them as flash cards. This will help you learn essential information about the drugs you will use during your career as a paramedic.

4. Given several patient scenarios, identify medications likely to be prescribed and those that are likely to be a part of the prehospital treatment regimen.   **pp. 711-760**

Prescribed Medications
As you arrive at the side of and begin to assess and treat a patient, an important aspect of assessment will be to determine what medications the patient is taking (both prescribed and over-the-counter). Since many drugs are given for specific pathologies, the drugs prescribed may give you clues as to the patient's underlying problem. The general pathology classification and the drugs used to care for that pathology are listed below. As you progress through your training, and especially as you enter the medical emergencies portion of your training, the classification of pathologies and the drugs prescribed for such will become more specific and extensive.

Central Nervous System

Analgesics	Opoid agonists	opium,morphine
	Nonopioids	aspirin, NSAIDs, ibuprofen, acetaminophen
	Benzodiazepines	diazepam, lorazepam, midazolam
	Antihistamines	promethazine, caffeine
	Opioid agonist-antagonists	pentazocine, nalbuphine, butorphanol
Antianxiety	Benzodiazepines	diazepam, lorazepam, midazolam
	Barbiturates	phenobarbital
Antiseizure	Benzodiazepines	diazepam, lorazepam, midazolam
	Barbiturates	phenobarbital
	Hydantoins	phenytoin, fosphenytoin
	Succinimides	ethosuimide
	Miscellaneous	valproic acid
CNS stimulants	Amphetamines	amphetamine sulfate, methamphetamine, extroamphetamine
	Methyphenidates	methyphenidate
	Methylxanthines	caffeine, aminophylline, theophylline
Antipsychotics	Phenothiazines	chlorpromazine
	Butyrophenones	haloperidol
	Miscellaneous	clozapine, risperidone
Antidepressant	TCAs	imipramine, amitriptyline, desipramine, ortriptyline
	SSRIs	fluoxetine, sertraline, paroxetine
	MAOIs	phenelzine
Bipolar disorder		lithium (bipolar disorder)
Parkinson's disease		levodopa, Sinemet, amantadine, bromocriptine

| | MAOIs | selegiline |
| | Anticholenergics | benztropine, diphenhydramine |

Autonomic Nervous System

Parasympathetic
nervous system

| | Cholinergics | bethanechol, pilocarpine, neostigmine, physostigmine, echothiophate |
| | Anticholinergics | atropine, scopolamine, ipratropium bromide, dicyclomine, benztropine |

Sympathetic
nervous system

	Adrenergics	norepinephrine, epinephrine, dopamine, dolbutamine, isoproterenol, ephedrine phenylephedrine, terbutaline
	Antiadrenergics	phenoxybenzamine, prazosin, phentolamine
	Beta-blockers	propranolol, metoprolol, atenolol
	Skeletal muscle relaxants	baclofen, cyclobenzaprine, carisoprodol dantrolene

Sense Organs

Eyes

	Glaucoma	timolol, betaxolol, pilocarpine
	Diagnostic procedures	atropisol, scopolamine, phenylephrine
	Anesthetic	tetracaine

Ears

| | Antibiotics | chloramphenicol, gentamicin sulfate |
| | Wax removal | carbamide peroxide and glycerin |

Cardiovascular System

Antidysrhythmics

	Sodium channel blockers	quinidine, procainamide, disopyramide, lidocaine, phenytoin, mexiletine, flecainide, propafenone, moricine
	Beta-blockers	propranolol, esmolol
	Potassium channel blockers	bretylium, amiodarone
	Calcium channel blockers	verapamil, diltiazem
	Miscellaneous	adenosine, digoxin, magnesium

Diuretics

	Loop	furosemide
	Thiazides	hydrochlorothiazide
	Potassium sparing	spironolactone

Antihypertensives

	Adrenergic inhibitors	clonidine, methyldopa, reserpine, guanethidine, guanadrel, prazosin, terazosin, labetalol, carvedilol, nifedipine
	ACE inhibitors	captoril, enalapril, lisinopril
	Angiotension II antagonist	losartan
	Calcium channel blockers	nifedipine
	Vasodilators	hydralazine, minoxidil, sodium nitroprusside, trimethaphan, digoxin, digitoxin
	Antianginals	verapamil, diltiazem, nifedipine, nitroglycerin

Hemostatic agents

	Antiplatelets	aspirin, dipyridamole, abciximab, ticlopidine
	Anticoagulants	heparin, warfarin
	Thrombolitics	streptokinase, alteplase, reteplase, anistreplase
	Antihyperlipidemics	lovastatin, simvastatin, cholestyramine

Respiratory System

Antiasthmatics	Beta 2 agents	salbutomol, terbutaline
	Sympathomimetics	epinephrine, ephedrine, isoproterenol
	Methylxanthines	methylxanthine, theophylline, aminophylline
	Anticholinergics	ipratropium
	Glucocorticoids	methylprednisolone, cromolyn
	Leukotriene antagonists	zileuton, zafirlukast
Rhinitis and cough	Nasal decongestants	phenylephedrine, pseudoephedrine, phenylpropanolamine
	Antihistamines	
	Alkylamines	chlorpheniramine
	Ethanolamines	diphenhydramine, clemastine
	Phenothiazines	promethiazine, dimenhydrinate, loratadine, cetirizine, fexofenadine
	Cough suppressants	
	antitussive	codeine, hydrocodone, dextromethorphan, diphenhydramine, benzonatate

Gastrointestinal System

Peptic ulcer disease	H_2 receptor agonists	cimetidine, ranitidine, famotidine, nizatidine
	Proton pump inhibitors	omeprazole, lansoprazole
	Antacids	aluminum, magnesium, calcium, or sodium compound
	Anticholinergics	pirenzepine
Laxatives	Bulk-forming	methylcellulose, psyllium
	Surfactant	docusate sodium
	Stimulant	phenolphthalein, bisacodyl
	Osmotic	magnesium hydroxide
Antidiarrheal	Antibiotics	
Antiemetics	Serotonin antagonists	ondansetron
	Dopamine antagonists	
	Phenothiazines	prochlorperazine, promethazine
	Butyrophenones	haloperidol, droperidol
	Miscellaneous	metoclopramide
	Cannabinoids	dronabinol, nabilone
To aid digestion		pancreatin, pancrelipase

Endocrine System

Pituitary gland	Anterior pituitary	somatrem, somatropin, octreotide
	Posterior pituitary	vasopressin, desmopressin, lypressin
Parathyroid glands		calcium and vitamin D supplements
Thyroid gland		levothyroxine
Adrenal cortex	Cushing's disease	spironolactone, captopril
	Addison's disease	cortisone, hydrocortisone, fludrocortisone

Pancreas	Insulin	
	Oral hypoglycemics	
	sulfonylureas	tolbutamide, chlorpropamide, glipizide, glyburide
	Biguanides	metformin
	Alpha-glucosidase inhibitors	acarbose, miglitol
	Thiazolidinediones	troglitazone
	Hyperglycemic agents	glucagon, diazoxide

Reproductive System

Female	Estrogen/Progestins	
	Oral contraceptives	
	Oxytocics	oxytocin, ergonovine
	Tocolytics	terbutaline, ritodrine
	Infertility agents	clomiphene, urofollitropin, menotropin

Male	Testosterone	enanthate, methyltestosterone, fluoxymesterone
	Enlarged prostate	finasteride

Sexual performance		levodopa, sildenafil

Cancer Drugs

	Antimetabolites	fluorouracil
	Alkylating agents	cyclophosphamide, mechlorethamine
	Mitotic inhibitors	vinblastine, vincristine

Infectious Disease

	Antibiotics	penicillin, cephalosporin, vancomycin
	Antifungals	ketoconazole
	Antivirals	acyclovir, zidovudine, indinavir
	Antiparasitics	
	Malaria	chloroquine, mefloquine, quinine
	Amebiasis	paromomycin, metronidazole
	Helminthiasis	mebendazole, niclosamide
	Antimicrobial	
	Tuberculosis	isoniazid, rifampin
	Leprosy	dapsone, clofazimine
	Nonsteroidal anti-inflammatories	acetaminophen, ibuprofen, ketorolac, piroxicam, naproxen

Immune System

	Immunosuppressants	azathioprine
	Immunomodulators	zidovudine, rotonavir, saquinavir

Note that this is not a complete list of common prescription drugs. As you continue your studies and career as a paramedic, many prescription drugs will become familiar to you. It is also recommended that you obtain a small pocket book that lists common prescription drugs and the conditions for which they are normally prescribed.

Prehospital Medications

Indications for the drugs commonly used in prehospital emergency medical care are contained on the drug cards in at the end of this Workbook. Review them with special attention to the conditions in which each drug is used.

5. Given various patient medications, assess the pathophysiology of a patient's condition by identifying classifications of drugs.   pp. 710-760

Within the discussion of the previous objective and throughout the text of this part of Chapter 6, drugs prescribed frequently for each common medical condition are noted. Finding one or more of these drugs with a patient might suggest pre-existing medical conditions and, possibly, the underlying reason the patient called for your assistance. Whenever you find prescription drugs with a patient, you should determine what they were prescribed for and if the patient has been compliant with his or her drug administration. There are numerous pocket EMS drug guides that identify the most common prescription drugs by their various names and give the common reasons they are prescribed. If you are ever unsure of the nature and use of a patient's medication, contact your medical direction physician.

CONTENT SELF-EVALUATION

1. Drugs can be classified by:
   - A.   the body system they affect.
   - B.   the mechanism of their action.
   - C.   their indications.
   - D.   their source.
   - E.   all of the above

2. The drug that demonstrates the common properties of a class of drugs is called a:
   - A.   root drug.
   - B.   prototype drug.
   - C.   characteristic drug.
   - D.   primary drug.
   - E.   none of the above

3. Which of the following is NOT a division of the nervous system?
   - A.   central nervous system
   - B.   peripheral nervous system
   - C.   autonomic nervous system
   - D.   sympathetic nervous system
   - E.   antagonistic nervous system

4. Which nervous system controls motor functions?
   - A.   somatic
   - B.   autonomic
   - C.   sympathetic
   - D.   parasympathetic
   - E.   antagonistic

5. Which nervous system is responsible for the "feed-or-breed" response?
   - A.   somatic
   - B.   autonomic
   - C.   sympathetic
   - D.   parasympathetic
   - E.   antagonistic

6. A drug that relieves pain only is termed a(n):
   - A.   anesthetic.
   - B.   endorphin.
   - C.   analgesic.
   - D.   opioid.
   - E.   antimanic.

7. The prototype opioid drug is:
   - A.   heroin.
   - B.   morphine.
   - C.   aspirin.
   - D.   ibuprofen.
   - E.   acetaminophen.

8. Naloxone (Narcan) is the principle:
   - A.   non-opioid analgesic.
   - B.   opioid agonist.
   - C.   opioid antagonist.
   - D.   prehospital anesthetic.
   - E.   opioid agonist-antagonist.

9. Anesthetics, as a group, tend to cause which of the following?
   - A.   reconfigured sensation
   - B.   respiratory stimulation
   - C.   central nervous system depression
   - D.   cardiovascular stimulation
   - E.   endorphin stimulation

10. The absence of all sensation is:

    A. anesthesia.
    B. anesthetic.
    C. analgesia.
    D. neuroleptanesthesia.
    E. coma.

11. Which of the following is the only anesthetic gas given in the prehospital setting?

    A. ether
    B. halothane
    C. enflurane
    D. nitrous oxide
    E. sodium pentothal

12. Sedative is a term that describes a drug that:

    A. decreases anxiety.
    B. deters sleep.
    C. reduces sensation.
    D. decreases pain sensation.
    E. is an opioid antagonist.

13. The antagonist for the benzodiazepines is:

    A. naloxone.
    B. flumazenil.
    C. thiopental.
    D. diazepam.
    E. midazolam.

14. Amphetamines cause which of the following?

    A. release of epinephrine
    B. release of dopamine
    C. decreased wakefulness
    D. increased appetite
    E. weight gain

15. Caffeine is classified as a(n):

    A. methylxanthine.
    B. methylphenidate.
    C. amphetamine.
    D. opioid.
    E. endorphin.

16. The drug class used to care for patients with mental dysfunctions is:

    A. neuroleptic.
    B. psychotherapeutic.
    C. extrapyramidal.
    D. schizophrenic.
    E. antimanic.

17. Which of the following acts to inhibit the influx of sodium into cells, thus decreasing the cell's ability to depolarize and propagate a seizure?

    A. Dilantin
    B. valporic acid
    C. Ativan
    D. benzodiapepines
    E. barbiturates

18. As a result of the extrapyramidal effects of antipsychotic drugs, these drugs are termed:

    A. Parkinsonian agents.
    B. extrapyramidogenics.
    C. neuroleptics.
    D. dopamine agonists.
    E. neurotransmitters.

19. The drug of choice for treating the extrapyramidal symptoms associated with antipsychotic drugs is:

    A. diazepam.
    B. furosemide.
    C. chlorpromazine.
    D. diphenhydramine.
    E. epinephrine.

20. Which of the following is NOT a sign or symptom of depression?

    A. weight loss
    B. weight gain
    C. sleep disturbances
    D. excessive energy
    E. inability to concentrate

21. Expected side effects of tricyclic antidepressants include all of the following EXCEPT:

    A. blurred vision.
    B. dry mouth.
    C. urinary retention.
    D. bradycardia.
    E. orthostatic hypotension.

22. A significant effect of tricyclic antidepressants (TCAs) rtaken in overdose is:

   A. seizure.
   B. MI or dysrhythmias.
   C. respiratory arrest.
   D. hyperthermia.
   E. pulmonary edema.

23. The drug of choice for the management of bipolar disorder is:

   A. valium.
   B. lithium.
   C. imipramine.
   D. phenelzine.
   E. morphine sulfate.

24. Parkinson's disease may present with which characteristic signs and symptoms?

   A. elation
   B. unsteady gait
   C. postural rigidity
   D. tachykinesia
   E. aggressiveness

25. Parkinson's disease begins:

   A. in middle age with subtle signs.
   B. in middle age with rapid onset.
   C. in late middle age and rapidly progresses to incapacitation.
   D. in later years with subtle signs.
   E. in later years and rapidly progresses to incapacitation.

26. The goal of pharmacological therapy in Parkinson's disease is to::

   A. increase acetylcholine production.
   B. restore the balance between dopamine and acetylcholine.
   C. decrease dopamine production.
   D. decrease stimulation of dopamine receptors.
   E. increasing stimulation of acetylcholine receptors.

27. Which nervous system works in opposition to the parasympathetic nervous system?

   A. central
   B. sympathetic
   C. autonomic
   D. somatic
   E. antagonistic

28. The agents that transport impulses through the synapse between neurons and between nerve cells and the target organs are called:

   A. neuroeffectors.
   B. neurotransmitters.
   C. intrasynaptic agents.
   D. neuroleptic ions.
   E. transport cells.

29. The cholinergic neurotransmitter is:

   A. acetylcholine.
   B. epinephrine.
   C. norepinephrine.
   D. muscarinic antagonist.
   E. muscarinic agonist.

30. Which neurotransmitter serves both the sympathetic and parasympathetic nervous systems?

   A. acetylcholine
   B. epinephrine
   C. norepinephrine
   D. dopamine
   E. none of the above

31. A drug that stimulates the parasympathetic nervous system is called a(n):

   A. sympatholytic.
   B. sympathomimetic.
   C. parasympatholytic.
   D. parasympathomimetic.
   E. antiemetic.

32. A cholinergic drug is also which of the following:

   A. a sympatholytic.
   B. a sympathomimetic.
   C. a parasympatholytic.
   D. a parasympathomimetic.
   E. an antiemetic.

33. The acronym that describes the effects of cholinergic stimulation is:

A.	SARIN.	**D.**	ALPHA.
B.	2-PAM.	**E.**	BETA.
C.	SLUDGE.		

34. The effects of cholinergic stimulation include all of the following except:

A.	salivation.	**D.**	urination.
B.	bradycardia.	**E.**	emesis.
C.	defecation.		

35. The prototype anticholenergic drug is:

A.	epinephrine.	**D.**	atropine.
B.	norepinephrine.	**E.**	dopamine.
C.	acetylcholine.		

36. Anticholinergic agenst:
- **A.** oppose the parasympathetic nervous system.
- **B.** oppose the sympathetic nervous system.
- **C.** stimulate the sympathetic nervous system.
- **D.** stimulate the parasympathetic nervous system.
- **E.** have no effect on the parasympathetic nervous system.

37. Which of the following is NOT an action caused by nicotine?

A.	tachycardia	**D.**	hypotension
B.	increased salivation	**E.**	increased gastric secretion
C.	vasoconstriction		

38. Bronchodilators are termed:

A.	beta selective.	**D.**	beta agonists.
B.	alpha antagonists.	**E.**	beta antagonists.
C.	alpha agonists		

39. What effect does alpha stimulation have on the heart?

A.	increases heart rate	**D.**	increases oxygen consumption
B.	increases automaticity	**E.**	none of the above
C.	increases contractile strength		

40. Which type of drug decreases cardiac contractility and heart rate?

A.	beta 2 agonists	**D.**	alpha 1 antagonists
B.	beta 1 antagonists	**E.**	alpha 1 agonists
C.	beta 1 agonists		

41. The prototype beta-blocker is:

A.	isoproterenol.	**D.**	propranolol.
B.	dopamine.	**E.**	none of the above.
C.	atropine.		

42. Which of the following is NOT a naturally occurring catecholamine?

A.	dopamine	**D.**	isoproterenol
B.	epinephrine	**E.**	A and C
C.	norepinephrine		

43. Which type of drug causes bronchodilation?

A.	beta 2 agonists	**D.**	alpha 1 antagonists
B.	beta 1 antagonists	**E.**	alpha 1 agonists
C.	beta 1 agonists		

44. Construction of arterioles and veins is a response to stimulation of what types of adrenergic receptors?

A.	alpha 1	**D.**	beta 2
B.	alpha 2	**E.**	dopaminergic
C.	beta 1		

45. Adenosine produces which of the following?
- **A.** facial pallor
- **B.** chest pain
- **C.** bronchodilation
- **D.** marked tachycardias
- **E.** all of the above

46. Cardiac output is equal to:
- **A.** heart rate times systolic blood pressure.
- **B.** heart rate times diastolic blood pressure.
- **C.** heart rate times stroke volume.
- **D.** heart rate times pulse pressure.
- **E.** none of the above

47. Which of the following is an osmotic diuretic?
- **A.** hydrochlorothiazide
- **B.** furosemide
- **C.** potassium chloride
- **D.** mannitol
- **E.** spironolactone

48. The renin-angiotensin-aldosterone system performs what function?
- **A.** increasing hepatic function
- **B.** decreasing blood volume
- **C.** increasing vasoconstriction
- **D.** causing severe bronchoconstriction
- **E.** all of the above

49. Which of the following drug types is used in the treatment of hypertension?
- **A.** antihyperlipidemics
- **B.** glucocorticoids
- **C.** calcium channel blockers
- **D.** cardiac glycosides
- **E.** all of the above

50. Which of the following are actions caused by the administration of digoxin?
- **A.** decreases intracellular sodium levels
- **B.** decreases intracellular calcium
- **C.** increases the strength of cardiac muscle contraction
- **D.** increases ventricular engorgement during left heart failure
- **E.** all of the above

51. The primary action of nitroglycerin in angina is to:
- **A.** reduce preload.
- **B.** reduce peripheral vascular resistance.
- **C.** dilate the coronary arteries.
- **D.** reduce the anginal pain.
- **E.** increase blood pressure.

52. Thrombi are the primary pathologies for which of the following?
- **A.** stroke
- **B.** myocardial infarction
- **C.** pulmonary embolism
- **D.** hypertension
- **E.** all of the above except D

53. Which of the following prevents thrombi by interrupting the clotting cascade?
- **A.** antiplatelets
- **B.** anticoagulants
- **C.** thrombolytics
- **D.** hemostatic agents
- **E.** all of the above

54. All of the following are used to treat or prevent thrombi EXCEPT:
- **A.** antiplatelets.
- **B.** antihyperlipidemic agents.
- **C.** thrombolitics.
- **D.** oral anticoagulants.
- **E.** parenteral anticoagulants.

55. Warfarin is contraindicated in pregnant mothers because it is likely to cause:
- **A.** uterine bleeding.
- **B.** birth defects.
- **C.** maternal hypertension.
- **D.** vitamin K toxicity.
- **E.** placenta previa.

56. Of the hemostatic agents, which can dissolve clots once they have formed?
- **A.** aspirin
- **B.** heparin
- **C.** warfarin
- **D.** streptokinase
- **E.** thrombarin

57. Which of the following is of greatest help in reducing cholesterol levels in the blood?
- **A.** low density lipoproteins (LDL)
- **B.** very low density lipoproteins (VLDL)
- **C.** high density lipoproteins (HDL)
- **D.** intermediate density lipoproteins (IDL)
- **E.** neutral density lipoproteins (NDL)

58. Which of the events below occurs first in an asthma attack?
- **A.** inflammatory response
- **B.** mast cell rupture
- **C.** release of histamine and leukotrienes
- **D.** immediate bronchospasm
- **E.** allergen binding to antibody on the mast cell

59. Which of the following groups is NOT used to treat asthma?
- **A.** leukotriene antagonists
- **B.** glucocorticoids
- **C.** ganglionic blocking agents
- **D.** methylxanthines
- **E.** anticholinergics

60. Which of the following is the first line therapy for asthma?
- **A.** selective beta 2 agonists
- **B.** nonselective sympathomimetics
- **C.** anticholinergics
- **D.** glucocorticoids
- **E.** leukotriene antagonists

61. Nasal decongestants act by which of the following actions?
- **A.** restricting histamine release
- **B.** blocking histamine action
- **C.** constricting nasal capillaries
- **D.** thinning nasal mucus
- **E.** all of the above

62. Which of the following is an inhaled short-acting beta 2 specific agonist?
- **A.** epinephrine
- **B.** Ventolin
- **C.** Belovent
- **D.** prednisone
- **E.** ephedrine

63. Stimulation of histamine receptors in the vasculature causes:
- **A.** vasodilation
- **B.** vasoconstriction
- **C.** trachycardia
- **D.** decreased capillary permeability
- **E.** bronchoconstriction

64. A drug that suppresses the urge to cough is a(n):
- **A.** expectorant.
- **B.** mucolytic.
- **C.** antitussive.
- **D.** surfactant.
- **E.** cannabinoid.

65. Most peptic ulcer disease is caused by:
- **A.** over-secretion of gastric acid.
- **B.** stress.
- **C.** alcohol consumption.
- **D.** decreased gastric circulation.
- **E.** a bacterium.

66. Which of the following is a type of laxative?
- **A.** bulk-forming
- **B.** osmotic
- **C.** surfactant
- **D.** stimulant
- **E.** all of the above

67. The drug chloramphenicol is used to treat what condition involving the ears?

A.	bacterial infections	**D.**	inflammation/irritation
B.	viral infections	**E.**	all of the above
C.	impacted wax		

68. Which of the following drugs have ototoxic properties?
- **A.** aspirin
- **B.** other nonsteroidal anti-inflammatory drugs
- **C.** some antibiotics
- **D.** furosemide
- **E.** all of the above

69. The gland of the endocrine system that is regarded as the master gland is the:

A.	pituitary.	**D.**	pancreas.
B.	thyroid.	**E.**	adrenal.
C.	parathyroid.		

70. The hormones produced by the thyroid play vital roles in growth, maturation, and:

A.	acromegaly.	**D.**	gastric secretion regulation.
B.	electrolyte balance.	**E.**	all of the above
C.	metabolism.		

71. Goiters are typically caused by an insufficiency in:

A.	potassium.	**D.**	vitamin K.
B.	calcium.	**E.**	hemoglobin.
C.	iodine.		

72. The adrenal cortex is responsible for the production of hormones for all the following purposes EXCEPT:

A.	to regulate salt balance.	**D.**	to regulate water balance.
B.	to regulate immunity.	**E.**	to regulate sexual maturity.
C.	to regulate glucose production.		

73. The type of diabetes that typically manifests during childhood is:

A.	gestational.	**D.**	type III.
B.	type I.	**E.**	type IV.
C.	type II.		

74. The pancreas secrets two hormones important to the regulation of glucose. They are insulin and:

A.	glucagon.	**D.**	cortisol.
B.	glycogen.	**E.**	orinase.
C.	dextrose.		

75. Which of the following forms of insulin is not likely to cause an allergic reaction?

A.	lente	**D.**	recombinant
B.	pork	**E.**	bovine
C.	beef		

76. The principle indication for estrogen replacement therapy in women is:

A.	postmenopause replacement.	**D.**	in delayed puberty.
B.	contraception.	**E.**	all of the above
C.	to delay childbirth.		

77. Serious hypotension may occur in a patient who takes sildenafil when also taking:

A.	glucagon.	**D.**	antibiotics.
B.	nitrates.	**E.**	thyroxine.
C.	$D_{50}W$.		

78. Antibiotics act by:
- **A.** killing the bacteria outright.
- **B.** creating antigens to de-activate the bacteria.

  C. engulfing the bacteria.
  D. decreasing the bacteria's growth rate.
  E. both A and D

79. The best age for vaccination against disease is:
  A. under 6 months.   **D.** over 5 years of age.
  B. under 2 years.   **E.** over 8 years of age.
  C. from 2 to 5 years.

80. The number associated with each B vitamin relates to:
  A. its order of discovery.   **D.** its point of absorption.
  B. its molecular size.   **E.** none of the above
  C. its importance to the body.

True/False

81. When using neuromuscular blocking agents, it is common to use antianxiety, amnesic, and analgesic agents as well.
  A. True
  B. False

82. It appears that dopamine, norepinephrine, and serotonin play a role in psychotic pathologies.
  A. True
  B. False

83. Tricyclic antidepressants (TCAs) raise the seizure threshold and are effective antiseizure medications.
  A. True
  B. False

84. Parkinson's disease is caused by a reduced number of presynaptic terminals that release dopamine.
  A. True
  B. False

85. Dopamine is given directly to the Parkinson's disease patient to help balance the dopamine/acetylcholine balance.
  A. True
  B. False

86. Neuromuscular blockade produces paralysis and amnesia to the event.
  A. True
  B. False

87. Alpha 1 antagonist drugs are used almost exclusively to control hypertension.
  A. True
  B. False

88. Beta-blockers and calcium channel blockers have similar effects on the heart.
  A. True
  B. False

89. Histamine is a major agent in the severe anaphylactic reaction.
  A. True
  B. False

90. Antihistamine drugs are not indicated for asthma patients because they thicken bronchial secretions.
  A. True
  B. False

Matching

Write the letter of the term in the space provided next to the definition or description to which it applies.

Term

      A. analgesic
      B. analgesia
      C. anesthesia
      D. anesthetic
      E. neuroleptanesthesia
      F. sedation

Definition

_____   **91.** The absence of the sensation of pain

_____   **92.** state of decreased anxiety and inhibitions

_____   **93.** the absence of all sensations

_____   **94.** medication that induces a loss of sensation to touch or pain

_____   **95.** anesthesia that combines decreased sensation of pain with amnesia while the patient remains conscious

Common Medications

Write the letter of the medication in the space provided next to the condition or effect associated with it.

Medication

      A. Bretylium
      B. digoxin
      C. lidocaine
      D. lithium
      E. salbutamol
      F. streptokinase

Effect or Associated Condition

_____   **96.** the absence of the sensation of pain

_____   **97.** state of decreased anxiety and inhibitions

_____   **98.** the absence of all sensations

_____   **99.** medication that induces a loss of sensation to touch or pain

_____   **100.** anesthesia that combines decreased sensation of pain with amnesia while the patient remains conscious

Adrenergic Receptors Effects

Write the letter of the adrenergic receptor in the space provided next to the effects to which it applies.

Adrenergic Receptor

      A. alpha 1
      B. alpha 2

C. beta 1
D. beta 2
E. dopaminergic

Effect

_____   **101.** increased heart rate

_____   **102.** constriction of veins

_____   **103.** bronchodilation

_____   **104.** constriction of arterioles

_____   **105.** increased conductivity

Chapter 15

Medication Administration

Part 1: Principles and Routes of Medication Administration

Review of Chapter Objectives

Because Chapter 15 is lengthy, it has been divided into parts to aid your study. Read the assigned textbook pages, then progress through the objectives and self-evaluation materials as you would with other chapters. When you feel secure in your grasp of the content, proceed to the next part.

After reading this part of the chapter, you should be able to:

1. **Review the specific anatomy and physiology pertinent to medication administration. pp. 766-796**

Chapter 6 reviewed human anatomy as it pertains to the absorption, distribution, metabolization, and elimination of the drugs we use to treat disease and trauma. This chapter identifies the anatomy and physiology related to medication administration.

The percutaneous routes of drug administration include transdermal and mucous membrane administration. Transdermal administration permits drug absorption through the skin via topical application in which the medication is slowly and steadily absorbed. Mucous membrane administration methods include sublingual, buccal, ocular, nasal, and aural administration, in which a drug is given under the tongue, between the cheek and gum, in the eye, into the nose, or into the ear respectively. Sublingual and buccal routes result in systemic absorption, while the remaining routes result in more local effects.

Pulmonary administration introduces a drug by nebulizer or metered dose inhaler or through an endotracheal tube. All three methods direct the drug to the lung tissue for action; however, endotracheal administration is an emergency route for systemic administration.

Enteral administration delivers a drug to the gastrointestinal tract, where it is absorbed. This is a relatively safe and simple route for drug administration and is the most common route for over-the-counter and prescription drug administration. The disadvantage of this route is that many factors can affect absorption including stress, diet, and metabolic rate. Liver function metabolizes some drugs, and a dysfunctional liver may alter the medication's metabolization or distribution. The enteral methods of administration include oral, gastric tube, and rectal administration. (Rectal administration is not subject to hepatic [liver] alteration.)

With parenteral administration, a drug is injected into the dermis (intradermal), the subcutaneous layer (subcutaneous), muscle (intramuscular), or veins (intravenous). The intradermal route provides little or no systemic absorption and is used for diagnostic testing and for the administration of local anesthetic. Subcutaneous injection promotes slow, sustained systemic absorption of a drug, while intramuscular injection permits systemic drug absorption at a moderate rate. Because intravenous drug administration injects the drug directly into the bloodstream, where it is directed to the heart, mixed with the returning venous blood, and then distributed systemically, it is the fastest parenteral administration route.

Anatomically, subcutaneous injections may be made into the skin regions over the deltoid muscle, the thighs, and, in some cases, the upper abdomen. Intramuscular injections may be given into the deltoid muscle, 2 inches below the acromial process; into the gluteal muscle, in the upper outer quadrant of the buttocks; into the anterolateral aspect of the thigh muscle (vastus lateralis); and into the central and lateral segment of the mid-thigh (rectus femoris).

2. Describe the indications, equipment needed, technique used, precautions, and general principles for the following.

All administration of medication requires the use of body substance isolation measures and medically clean techniques. The six rights of medication administration must be observed (see objective 5). With drug administration, you must watch carefully for the desired and adverse effects of the drug administration.

a. inhalation routes of medication administration. pp. 770-773

Pulmonary medications are administered via nebulizer, metered dose inhaler, and endotracheal tube. Drugs indicated for inhalation include those that cause bronchodilation, mucolytics, antibiotics, and topical steroids for respiratory emergencies, congestion, infection, and inflammation respectively.

A nebulizer aerosolizes a small volume of liquid (or dissolved) medication using oxygen, which is then inhaled into the lungs and absorbed quickly. The device is assembled (mouth piece, medication reservoir, oxygen port, relief valve, and oxygen tubing and source), and 3 to 5 ml of solution (or a medication dissolved in 3 to 5 ml of sterile water) is placed in the medication reservoir. Oxygen is set to run at 5 to 8 liters per minute (without a humidifier), and the mouthpiece is placed in the patient's mouth. The patient should hold the nebulizer and inhale slowly and deeply with each breath, then hold the breath for 1 to 2 seconds before exhaling. The patient should continue doing this until the medication is gone (about 3 to 5 minutes). For nebulized medications to be effective, the patient must have an adequate tidal volume and respiratory rate, although nebulizers can be connected to an endotracheal tube during positive pressure ventilation.

Metered dose inhalers are frequently used in patients with COPD and asthma to deliver agents to induce bronchodilation. The device consists of a pressurized medication canister, plastic shell and mouthpiece, and possibly a spacer. The patient self-administers the drug by assembling the inhaler, shaking it for 2 to 5 seconds, inverting it, placing the mouthpiece in the mouth, and sealing the lips against the mouthpiece. Then, during the beginning of a deep inhalation, the patient presses the canister downward to release a dose of medication. A second dose may be necessary. Nebulizers are preferable to metered dose inhalers in acute respiratory emergencies because they administer the drug over more time and are less dependent on a single deep inspiration.

Endotracheal administration of a drug involves expressing the drug down the endotracheal tube (in a volume of 10 ml and from 2 to 2.5 times the normal intravenous dose). Narcan, atropine, lidocaine, and epinephrine can be administered this way in an emergency when IV access is not otherwise available. Once the drug is injected down the endotracheal tube, the ventilator provides several deep ventilations to deliver the drug to the pulmonary tissue.

b. parenteral routes of medication administration. pp. 780-796

Parenteral administration includes the routes utilizing needles to administer drugs into the tissues or vascular system—intradermal, subcutaneous, intramuscular, intravenous, and intraosseous routes. Begin the parenteral administration process by cleansing the patient's skin at the injection site with an antiseptic such as alcohol or a betadine solution. The medication for injection is in solution and drawn up in a syringe, then injected with a needle (bevel up). For subcutaneous and intramuscular injection, consider injecting a 0.1-ml air bubble after the medication to limit leakage, and then massage the region to enhance absorption. Most emergency medications are injected via the intravenous route because of its rapid distribution throughout the body.

Intradermal drug administration calls for insertion of a 25- to 27-gauge needle at a 10- to 15-degree angle just into a segment of skin that is pulled taut. Slow injection of up to 1 ml of solution will create a small wheal of medication. Then remove the needle. Intradermal injection results in a very slow absorption rate greatly affected by local perfusion rates and is used for diagnostic testing and the administration of local anesthetics.

For subcutaneous administration, place a 24- to 26-gauge needle into a 2.5 cm "pinch" of the patient's skin at a 45-degree angle and inject no more than 1 ml of medication. The skin must be free of scarring, superficial nerves, blood vessels and tendons, tattoos, and bruising. Pulling the plunger back ensures that the needle is not in a blood vessel (aspiration of blood indicates a blood vessel entry). Subcutaneous injection may be given at many locations around the body, including the tissue under the tongue.

For intramuscular injections, use a 21- to 23-gauge needle inserted at a 90-degree angle into the deltoid (up to 2 ml), dorsal gluteal (up to 5 ml), vastus lateralis (up to 5 ml), or rectus femoris (up to 5 ml) muscle. Again, pulling back on the plunger ensures that the needle is not in a blood vessel. Intramuscular injection provides a predictable systemic absorption and is used for several prehospital drugs including glucagon and morphine. Careful placement of parenteral needles is important because of potential damage to nerves and arteries. Needles for intradermal, subcutaneous, and intramuscular injection are 3/8 to 1 inch in length.

c.   **percutaneous routes of medication administration.pp. 766-770**

Transdermal drug administration is indicated for drugs that are readily absorbed through the skin, when slow, steady absorption is required, or for topical administration for local effects (anti-inflammatories, bacteriostatics, and softening agents). Transdermal medications include lotions, creams, foams, wet dressings, adhesive-backed applications, and suppositories. The medication is applied to a clean, dry portion of skin according to the manufacturer's instructions. The medication is left for the required time and watched for the desired and adverse effects, and a dressing is placed over the application if necessary. Care must be taken not to get the drug on your skin and to watch for overdosing due to thin skin, increasing absorption rates, or for underdosing due to thick skin, scar tissue, or peripheral vascular disease, slowing absorption.

The mucous membrane route for drug administration permits drug absorption through the capillaries of the sublingual, buccal, ocular, nasal, or aural mucous membranes. With the sublingual route, a spray is applied or a tablet placed beneath the tongue, where the patient must let it dissolve and be absorbed. Nitroglycerin is a drug commonly administered via the sublingual route. With buccal administration a pill or other preparation is placed between the cheek and gum to permit absorption. Hormonal and enzyme preparations are commonly administered via the buccal route. Ocular administration involves one or both eyes. The patient lies supine or tips his head back and looks at the ceiling. The eyelid is pulled down and the droplet of a liquid medication (using an medicine dropper) or an ointment is placed into the conjunctival sac. Do not touch the eye or administer drugs directly on the eye unless specifically instructed to do so. Medications administered via this route include agents to treat eye pain, infection, or increased intraocular pressure or to lubricate the eyelid. Nasal administration involves the topical absorption of drops or sprays through the nasal mucosa for nasal congestion, hemorrhage, or infection. The patient is directed to blow his nose and tilt his head back. A medicine dropper or squeezable nebulizer expresses the drug into the nare(s), then the nare(s) is (are) held shut and/or the head is tilted forward to enhance the distribution of the medication. Aural administration is used to treat local infection or ear pain. Droplets or medicated gauze are placed into the affected ear while the patient lies supine with his head turned. The adult's pinna is pulled up and back, while the child's is pulled down and back to expose the auditory canal. Do not pack the canal tightly.

d.   **enteral routes of medication administration, including gastric tube administration and rectal administration.   pp. 773-780**

Enteral drug administration includes oral, gastric tube, and rectal administration routes and results in drug absorption through the gastrointestinal tract. Medications administered this way (excepting the rectal route) are processed through the liver, affecting their metabolism and elimination.

Oral medications are introduced as capsules, tablets, pills, time release capsules, elixirs, emulsions, lozenges, suspensions, or syrups introduced into the oral cavity and swallowed with 4 to 8 ounces of water. This is the most common method of over-the-counter and prescription drug administration because of its ease of administration.

Gastric tube administration introduces a drug down the naso- or orogastric tube and into the stomach. It is used when the patient has difficulty swallowing and in instances of overdose, trauma, upper gastrointestinal bleeding, or the need for nutritional support. Drugs in solid forms may be crushed (so as to move easily down the tube), mixed with water, and administered through the gastric tube, although such action will destroy the time release action of coated drugs. When administering a drug via the gastric tube route, ensure proper placement by injecting air and auscultating over the epigastric area and by aspirating gastric contents through the tube. Flush the tube with 50 to 100 ml of saline, then prepare a volume of about 30 ml of medication (diluted to volume with normal saline) and administer the solution through the gastric tube. Follow administration with 50 to 100 ml of normal saline and clamp off the tube for about 30 minutes.

Rectal administration involves topical administration of a medication to the rectal mucosa and provides rapid predictable absorption. Use a syringe and 14-gauge needleless catheter (or small endotracheal tube) to introduce the medication into the rectum, then hold the buttocks closed to promote retention and absorption. A suppository is a soft, pliable form of drug that melts at body temperature and is inserted into the rectum for absorption. An enema is a liquid bolus of medication introduced through the rectum.

3. Describe the indications, contraindications, side effects, dosages, and routes of administration for medications commonly administered by paramedics.   pp. 766-796

There are many drugs used in the prehospital setting to care for the common medical and trauma emergencies. The Emergency Drug Cards at the back of this workbook list many of these drugs, including the drug name/class, indications, contraindications, precautions, dosages, and routes of administration. Detach these cards and review them frequently to become familiar with the medications you will use during your prehospital patient care.

4. Discuss legal aspects affecting medication administration. pp. 763-764, 766

The administration of the wrong medication or withholding the right medication or providing it in the wrong dose or by the wrong route can have catastrophic consequences. Hence, medication administration is an area of paramedic practice where the paramedic is exposed to legal liability. You must ensure that you receive informed and expressed consent from the patient (when possible), provide medications in strict compliance with system protocols and the direction of on-line medical control, and follow proper administration techniques. Once a medication is administered, it is essential that you document the indication for the drug, any online authorization for the administration, the name of the person who delivered the drug, the drug name, dose, route and rate of delivery, and the resulting patient response, whether positive or negative. These actions will go a long way to limiting your liability in drug administration.

5. Discuss the "six rights" of drug administration and correlate them with the principles of medication administration. p. 763

There are basically six rights of drug administration. They are the right patient, the right drug, the right dose, the right time, the right route, and the right documentation.
The right patient. Ensure that the patient is the right person and properly matched to the medication. This is an infrequent problem in prehospital care, but as EMS moves to the out-of-hospital environment, we may be treating some patients on a routine basis. Ensure the medication order is for the patient you are attending.
The right drug. Ensure the drug is what is intended for the patient. Review your standing orders or, if the order is received from medical direction, repeat ("echo") the order back to the physician so you are both clear on the drug, dose, route, and timing of the order. Also examine the drug packaging to ensure that it contains the medication you wish to administer and that the medication is still sterile, has not expired, and is not contaminated or discolored.

The right dose. Carefully calculate the exact dose (usually weight dependent) for the patient before you draw up the medication and again just before you administer it. If the drug package you select has significantly more or less of the drug than you intend to use, recheck the packaging to ensure it is the right drug and right concentration, and recheck your calculations to ensure the right dosage. Never overdose or underdose your patient.

The right time. Usually prehospital medications are given rather rapidly and not on a schedule. Check the packaging and your protocols for administration rates and ensure that you follow the sequencing, time intervals between, and drip rates for emergency drugs.

The right route. Specific drugs require specific routes of administration. While most emergency drugs are administered by the IV route, be aware of alternate drug administration routes, the drugs that can be administered by those routes, and the circumstances requiring the use of those routes. With each medication administration, ensure you are using the right route.

The right documentation. Documentation of drug administration is of paramount importance. You must carefully record the patient's condition (the circumstances that require the drug's administration), the drug name, dose, and route of administration, and who administered the drug and at what time. It is also essential that you record the patient's response to the drug, whether good or bad.

6. Differentiate among the percutaneous routes of medication administration. pp. 766-770

The **transdermal** route of medication administration promotes slow, steady absorption of the drug across the dermis. Nitroglycerin is frequently administered for its systemic effects via this route, while lidocaine, anti-inflammatories, and bacteriostatic solutions are administered for their local effects.

Sublingual drugs are absorbed through the mucous membranes beneath the tongue, where the medication is rapidly absorbed by the extensive vasculature there. Tablets or sprays are often used, and nitroglycerin is frequently administered this way in the emergency setting.

Buccal medications (usually tablets) are placed between the cheek and gums for absorption. Enzymes and hormonal preparations are also administered this way.

Ocular drug administration involves topical administration of a medication (usually drops or ointment) into one or both eyes. This route is typically used for treating eye pain or local infections, decreasing intraocular pressure, or lubrication of the eyelid.

Nasal medications are usually drops or sprays given through the nares to treat nasal congestion, hemorrhage, or infection.

Aural medications are delivered into the auditory canal using a medicine dropper (solution) or medicated gauze. These drugs are used to treat localized infection and ear pain.

7. Discuss medical asepsis and the differences between clean and sterile techniques. pp. 764-765

Medical asepsis describes a medical environment free of pathogens. The most aseptic environment is a sterile one, one free of all living organisms. However, in prehospital care we frequently cannot attain such a state. We utilize equipment and supplies that are sterile when packaged and then use medically clean techniques to reduce the risk of spreading infection. These techniques include the use of disinfectants to kill microorganisms on equipment and in the ambulance and of antiseptics to reduce the bacterial load on the patient's skin when we utilize procedures like venipuncture.

8. Describe uses of antiseptics and disinfectants. pp. 764-765

Antiseptics are agents are designed for topical use to destroy or inhibit pathogenic microorganisms already on living tissue. They are used to cleanse the skin before parenteral drug administration to prevent infection secondary to the needle stick.

Disinfectants are powerful agents that are toxic to living tissue. They are not designed for topical administration but for the direct cleaning of durable patient care equipment.

9. Describe the use of body substance isolation (BSI) procedures when administering a medication.   p. 764

Any time there is the possibility of contact with body substances or patient wounds, you must use body substance isolation measures. Gloves, at a minimum, provide barrier protection to the care giver from possibly infectious material at the scene and to the patient from the care giver. Goggles and a mask also provide protection, as does hand washing after contact with a patient or possibly infected material.

10. Describe disposal of contaminated items and sharps.   p. 765

Sharps and contaminated materials pose a risk for the spread of infection. Do not recap needles unless absolutely necessary and, in such instance, do so using only one hand. Used needles represent a real risk for introducing pathogens from the patient's blood into someone stuck with the needle. Dispose of all needles in a puncture-proof biohazard container. Ensure all medical waste is placed in a biohazardous waste bag and is not left at the scene. Follow your service's biohazard exposure plan should you receive a needle stick.

11. Synthesize a pharmacologic management plan including medication administration. pp. 763-796

As you care for patients with serious medical and trauma emergencies, you will often need to administer medications to them via the sublingual, oral, pulmonary, subcutaneous, intramuscular, intravenous, and interosseous routes. The procedures described in this chapter must become an integral part of your patient management skills.

The following objective, while not listed in the chapter, will help in your understanding of the chapter content.

12. Describe the equipment and procedures for preparing and drawing up a medication in anticipation of parenteral administration.   pp. 787-796

A syringe is a plastic, hollow, calibrated barrel into which fits a plunger that is used to draw up and administer very accurate volumes of a solution or liquid. Syringes range in size from 1 ml to 100 ml. A hypodermic needle is a hollow metal tube, one end of which is beveled and very sharp while the other end is equipped with an adapter to fit a syringe. Needles are measured in diameter or gauge from 14 (largest) to 27 (smallest) and vary in length from 1 to 4 cm.

Medications come packaged for administration in glass ampules, single and multidose vials, nonconstituted vials, prefilled syringes, and premixed IV solutions. Ampules are sealed glass containers that must be broken to obtain the drug. A sterile gauze pad is wrapped around the ampule neck and the top is broken off. The needle from a syringe is placed within the ampule to draw out the necessary volume of solution. Single and multidose vials are glass containers with self-sealing rubber tops, usually protected with a metal cap. The cap is removed and the stopper cleansed with alcohol. A syringe is filled with a volume of air, equivalent to the desired volume of drug. The needle is inserted into the vial, the air is expressed inside, and the drug is withdrawn. The needle is then withdrawn from the vial, and the drug is ready for administration. Nonconstituted drug vials come either in the form of pairs of vials (the drug and solvent) that require you to introduce the solvent into the powdered drug vial or in specially designed vials (Mix-o-Vials) that permit mixing after you pop the seal between the drug and solvent. Once the drug is constituted, you withdraw it as from a standard vial. Preloaded syringes are vials containing the drug that screw into a syringe barrel and permit direct administration of the drug by pushing the vial barrel into the syringe. Intravenous premixed solutions for IV infusion come in bottles or plastic bags (plastic bags are use for prehospital administration). They contain a solution of drug and solvent for direct administration via an intravenous line with administration volume (and hence dose) controlled by setting the rate of administration.

CONTENT SELF-EVALUATION

_____ 1. Which of the following is NOT one of the six rights of drug administration?
- A. the right dosage
- B. the right indication
- C. the right time
- D. the right documentation
- E. the right patient

_____ 2. The process you use to ensure you hear and correctly understand the medical direction physician's order to administer a medication is:
- A. protocol compliance.
- B. order confirmation with your partner.
- C. redundant physician orders.
- D. echoing the order back to the physician.
- E. asking the physician to repeat the order.

_____ 3. Which of the following must you know about the drugs you are authorized to administer?
- A. their usual dosages
- B. their contraindications
- C. their common side effects
- D. their routes of administration
- E. all of the above

_____ 4. When you administer drugs, which of the following body substance isolation measures should you always employ?
- A. gloves
- B. a mask
- C. goggles
- D. a gown
- E. A and D

_____ 5. The condition in which a medical environment is free of all pathogens is described as:
- A. asepsis.
- B. uncontaminated.
- C. medically clean.
- D. disinfection.
- E. none of the above

_____ 6. The environment that paramedics should strive to maintain while delivering prehospital emergency care is:
- A. aseptic.
- B. sterile.
- C. medically clean.
- D. disinfected.
- E. none of the above

_____ 7. To cleanse the site of a parenteral injection, you would use a(n):
- A. aseptic.
- B. disinfectant.
- C. detergent.
- D. antiseptic.
- E. dilutant.

_____ 8. You should recap needles:
- A. as a last resort.
- B. in a moving ambulance only.
- C. only when the ambulance is at a full stop.
- D. only when they have not been used on a patient.
- E. when directed by a physician.

_____ 9. Documentation regarding the administration of a drug should include all of the following EXCEPT the:
- A. time of administration.
- B. route of administration.
- C. class of drug administered.
- D. positive patient responses.
- E. negative patient responses.

_____ 10. Transdermal medications are provided in which of the following forms?
- A. ointments
- B. wet dressings
- C. foams
- D. lotions
- E. all of the above

11. Which of the following factors can decrease the absorption rate with transdermal medication administration?

    A.   thin skin   **D.**   peripheral vascular disease

    B.   overdose   **E.**   all of the above

    C.   penetrating solvents

12. The term buccal refers to:

    A.   the area between the tongue and the cheek.

    B.   the area under the tongue.

    C.   the roof of the mouth.

    D.   the large fleshy area on the lateral aspect of the shoulder.

    E.   the flank.

13. Which of the following is a common emergency drug administered sublingually?

    A.   sodium bicarbonate   **D.**   aspirin

    B.   epinephrine   **E.**   magnesium

    C.   nitroglycerin

14. Buccal medications are generally given as:

    A.   injections   **D.**   pills

    B.   pastes   **E.**   liquids

    C.   tablets

15. Ocular medications are given for which conditions?

    A.   eye pain   **D.**   lubricating the eyelid

    B.   eye infection   **E.**   all of the above

    C.   increased intraocular pressure

16. Ocular medications are most commonly administered:

    A.   over the pupil.   **D.**   into the conjunctival sac.

    B.   over the iris.   **E.**   all of the above

    C.   over the sclera.

17. The small volume nebulizer often used in prehospital emergency medical service administers what volume of medication?

    A.   1 to 2 ml   **D.**   10 to 15 ml

    B.   3 to 5 ml   **E.**   15 to 20 ml

    C.   5 to 10 ml

18. The metered dose inhaler is activated to release its medication:

    A.   just before the patient seals his lips to the mouthpiece.

    B.   as the patient exhales.

    C.   as the patient inhales.

    D.   during both inhalation and exhalation.

    E.   between inhalation and exhalation.

19. Endotracheal medication administration calls for drugs to be diluted to what volume?

    A.   1 ml   **D.**   5 ml

    B.   2 ml   **E.**   10 ml

    C.   3 ml

20. Which of the following drugs is NOT administered via the endotracheal route?

    A.   meperidine   **D.**   lidocaine

    B.   naloxone   **E.**   epinephrine

    C.   atropine

21. Enteral medications are absorbed through the:

    A.   liver.   **D.**   portal system.

    B.   gastrointestinal tract.   **E.**   accessory organs.

    C.   mucous membranes.

22. When using a medicine cup to measure an oral dose of medication, you should use what aspect of fluid level to determine the fluid volume?
    A.   the highest point of the meniscus
    B.   the lowest point of the meniscus
    C.   between the high and low point of the meniscus
    D.   one calibration below the lowest point of the meniscus
    E.   none of above

23. The normal teaspoon holds about what volume of fluid?
    A.   2 ml   **D.**   10 ml
    B.   3 ml   **E.**   12 ml
    C.   5 ml

24. The advantage of rectal administration over the other enteral drug routes is that:
    A.   the rectal route is easier to administer drugs through.
    B.   there is no hepatic alteration of the drug.
    C.   the rectal route can absorb more medication.
    D.   rectal irritation is rare.
    E.   all of the above

25. To inject a drug rectally you may use:
    A.   a large catheter with needle removed.
    B.   a special enema container with a rectal tip.
    C.   a small endotracheal tube attached to a syringe.
    D.   all of the above
    E.   none of the above

26. What is the total dose of a drug contained in an ampoule with 5 ml of a drug in a 0.3 mg/ml concentration?
    A.   0.3 mg   **D.**   15 mg
    B.   1.5 mg   **E.**   none of the above
    C.   5 mg

27. Which of the following drug containers may contain multiple doses of a drug?
    A.   vial   **D.**   preloaded syringe
    B.   ampoule   **E.**   medicated solutions
    C.   Mix-o-vial

28. Which of the following forms of packaging extends the viability and storage time of drugs that have a short shelf life or are unstable in liquid form?
    A.   vial   **D.**   preloaded syringe
    B.   ampoule   **E.**   medicated solutions
    C.   Mix-o-vial

29. When giving multiple medications in a syringe for a single delivery, you should:
    A.   anticipate total volume and select an appropriate syringe.
    B.   be aware of potential drug incompatibilities.
    C.   draw each medication in order according to local protocols.
    D.   all of the above.
    E.   you should not give multiple medications in a single syringe

30. The advantage of preloaded syringes is that they:
    A.   are quicker to employ in an emergency situation.
    B.   do not require additional preparation before use.
    C.   contain standard dosages, thus decreasing waste.
    D.   contain standard dosages, thus decreasing the chance of dosage error.
    E.   all of the above.

31. Which of the following must be cleansed with an alcohol swab before the drug is withdrawn?

	A.	vial	D.	preloaded syringe
	B.	ampule	E.	A and C
	C.	Mix-o-Vial		

_____ 32. The drug route that calls for insertion of the needle at 10 to 15 degrees is:

	A.	intradermal.	D.	intraosseous.
	B.	subcutaneous.	E.	none of the above
	C.	intramuscular.		

_____ 33. Which of the following is most likely to be an acceptable site for subcutaneous injection?

	A.	forearms	D.	buttocks
	B.	calves	E.	all of the above are acceptable
	C.	thighs		

_____ 34. Through which of the following routes should you inject no more than 1 ml of a drug?

	A.	intradermal	D.	A and B
	B.	subcutaneous	E.	all of the above
	C.	intramuscular		

_____ 35. At which of the following intramuscular injection sites should you administer a maximum of 2 ml of a drug?

	A.	deltoid	D.	rectus femoris
	B.	gluteal	E.	both B and C
	C.	vastus lateralis		

_____ 36. When you pull back on the syringe plunger during subcutaneous or intramuscular injection and blood appears, you should:

- A. inject the drug.
- B. inject the drug followed by a small bubble of air.
- C. insert the needle 1 cm further.
- D. attempt the injection at another site.
- E. consider the appearance of blood insignificant.

_____ 37. The drug route that calls for use of a 21- to 23-gauge needle is:

	A.	intradermal.	D.	intraosseous.
	B.	subcutaneous.	E.	none of the above
	C.	intramuscular.		

_____ 38. The drug route that calls for use of a needle 1 to 2.5 cm long is:

	A.	intradermal.	D.	all of the above
	B.	subcutaneous.	E.	none of the above
	C.	intramuscular.		

_____ 39. The recommended angle of insertion for the needle when administering an intramuscular injection is:

	A.	10 degrees.	D.	90 degrees.
	B.	15 degrees.	E.	between 10 and 15 degrees.
	C.	45 degrees.		

_____ 40. The two most important routes of parenteral drug administration are:

	A.	intravenous and intradermal.	D.	intravenous and oral.
	B.	intravenous and intraosseous.	E.	intraosseous and oral.
	C.	intravenous and inhaled.		

True/False

_____ 41. You must receive authorization from your online medical director before administering any medication.

A. True
B. False

_____ 42. Hand washing, glove changing, and discarding equipment in opened packages are examples of maintaining a medically clean environment.
  A. True
  B. False

_____ 43. Percutaneous medications use the transdermal, sublingual, and buccal routes of administration.
  A. True
  B. False

_____ 44. The metered dose inhaler and spacer are complex delivery systems that may be difficult for the elderly or young children to use.
  A. True
  B. False

_____ 45. When administering medications via the ET route, you should use 2 – 2 ½ times the conventional IV dose diluted in 10 mL of Normal Saline.
  A. True
  B. False

_____ 46. Absorption of drugs given via enteral routes is unreliable and can be affected by physical activity or emotions.
  A. True
  B. False

_____ 47. The gauge and diameter of hypodermic needle are directly related: the higher the gauge, the larger the diameter.
  A. True
  B. False

_____ 48. Subcutaneous tissue has large numbers of blood vessels which allows for rapid absorption and onset of injected medications.
  A. True
  B. False

_____ 49. The preferred sites for subcutaneous injection are the thighs or upper arm.
  A. True
  B. False

_____ 50. After injecting an intramuscular drug, massaging the site is contraindicated because it will slow absorption.
  A. True
  B. False

Matching

Write the letter of the appropriate term in the space provided next to the description to which it applies.

Term

  A. asepsis   **D.** medically clean
  B. antiseptic   **E.** personal protective equipment
  C. body substance isolation   **F.** sterile

Description

_____ 51. careful handling of equipment to prevent contamination.

_____ **52.** cleansing agent that is not toxic to living tissue.

_____ **53.** measures that decrease the risk of exposure to blood and body fluids.

_____ **54.** free of all forms of life.

_____ **55.** an environment that is free of pathogens.

Drug Administration Routes

Write the letter of the appropriate route of drug administration in the space provided next to the description to which it applies.

Term

A. aural		**I.**	intravenous
B. buccal		**J.**	occular
C. enteral		**K.**	parenteral
D. injection		**L.**	percutaneous
E. intradermal		**M.**	subcutaneous
G. intramuscular		**N.**	sublingual
H. intraosseous		**O.**	transdermal

Description

_____ **56.** within a vein..

_____ **57.** within the layer of loose connective tissue between the skin and muscle.

_____ **58.** medications absorbed through the gastrointestinal tract.

_____ **59.** beneath the tongue.

_____ **60.** through the mucous membranes of the ear and ear canal.

_____ **61.** between the cheek and gums.

_____ **62.** within the bone.

_____ **63.** absorbed through the skin.

_____ **64.** through the mucous membranes of the eye.

_____ **65.** medications administered outside the gastrointestinal tract.

Chapter 15

Medication Administration

Part 2: Intravenous Access, Blood Sampling, and Intraosseous Infusion

Review of Chapter Objectives

After reading this part of the chapter, you should be able to:

1. **Review the specific anatomy and physiology pertinent to medication administration.**
   pp. 796-835

Various veins are found close to the surface of the skin and are relatively easy to locate because of their prominence, color, and/or feel. Common vessels used for peripheral venipuncture include those of the back of the hand, those of the arms, the vein of the antecubital fossa, and those of the feet and legs. An additional large vein available for catheter insertion is the external jugular vein on the lateral neck. The more distal veins should be used, when possible, as using a vein generally limits the use of veins distal to the site. Large veins must be used for blood administration, in the administration of some drugs, and in cases where large volumes of drugs must be administered. Central veins are not usually used in the prehospital setting because of the time needed to initiate the access, the difficulty in determining proper placement, and the incidence of complications.

Intraosseous infusion directs the flow of fluid or a drug into the medullary space of a long bone, where it is available to the venous circulation. The tibia is the most frequent location of cannulation, with the proximal anterior and medial tibia just below the tibial tuberosity used for pediatric patients and the distal tibia just above the medial malleolus and just medial to the tibial crest for adults. A special needle is inserted through the compact bone and into the medullary space.

2. **Describe the indications, equipment needed, technique used, precautions, and general principles for the following:**

   a. **peripheral venous or external jugular cannulation.** **pp. 797-824**
   Peripheral venous access is the preferable route for medication administration in the emergency prehospital setting. Most emergency drugs are administered this way because it provides a direct route into the venous system, then to the heart, where the drug and blood are further mixed, and then to the body as distributed by the arterial system. Vascular access can be obtained using a steel needle with a beveled sharp edge. Most commonly, an over-the-needle catheter is advanced into the vein, with the needle then withdrawn, leaving the catheter to permit introduction of drugs or fluid or withdrawal of

blood for diagnostic testing. The veins of the hands, arms, antecubital fossa, feet, and legs and the external jugular veins are common sites for intravenous cannulation.

The equipment used for intravenous therapy includes a venous constricting band to help engorge the veins; the needle for venipuncture; an antiseptic to cleanse the site; administration tubing to direct and control fluid administration from an IV bag or a syringe to draw up, then administer medication; tape or commercial devices to secure the intravenous catheter; and bacteriostatic ointment to protect the site from infection. An ideal location for venipuncture is free of injury and with relatively prominent veins. The care giver should take appropriate body substance isolation measures before beginning the procedure. Then the venous constricting band is secured just proximal to the selected site and a vein is chosen. The area is cleansed with an alcohol or betadine swab, using concentric circles moving outward from the selected site. An over-the-needle catheter is selected, with 14- to 18-gauge for blood, thick medications such as glucose, or fluid volume administration or a 20- to 22-gauge catheter for pediatric or geriatric patients or patients who do not need a larger catheter. The catheter is directed, bevel up, through the skin at an angle of 10 to 30 degrees until a "pop" is felt or blood appears in the flash chamber. Once in the vein, the catheter is advanced an additional 0.5 cm and then the catheter is threaded into the vein. The needle is withdrawn, the constricting band is released, and the administration set or saline or heparin lock is attached. A small amount of fluid is run to ensure that the catheter is patent. Watch for edema around the site, which is suggestive of infiltration. Intravenous cannulation and infusion may result in local pain, infiltration, pyrogenic reactions, allergic reactions, catheter shear and embolism, inadvertent arterial puncture, circulatory overload, thrombophlebitis, thrombus formation, air embolism, and necrosis.

Fluid is infused through a venipuncture site to hydrate the patient or to keep the drug route open and quickly available. Most prehospital infusions use isotonic (same osmotic pressure as the plasma) solutions such as normal saline, 5 percent dextrose in water, or lactated Ringer's solution. These solutions flow through the administration set, where their rate of administration is regulated by adjusting the drip rate in a chamber. Most commonly 10 (macro) or 60 (micro) drops traveling through a drip chamber equal 1 milliliter. The administration set contains one or more injection ports to accommodate the administration of drugs or additional fluid administration. A special type of administration set is the measured volume administration set, which contains a calibrated chamber that will permit the discrete administration of a volume of fluid.

The external jugular vein is an alternate venous access site located on the lateral anterior neck. It is a large, easily found vein that permits venous access when other veins are collapsed due to hypovolemia or other vascular problems. It is close to the central circulation, so it provides almost immediate absorption of any drugs administered through it. The jugular vein can be engorged by placing digital pressure along the vein just above the clavical. External jugular cannulation is painful and risks damage to the airway or arterial structures in the neck.

b.   intraosseous needle placement and infusion.   pp. 828-835

Intraosseous needle placement is indicated for the critical pediatric patient under 5 when you cannot establish other IV access sites or for the adult patient when you also cannot perform peripheral venous access because of disease or extreme hypovolemia. A special needle is introduced through the compact bone of the tibia and into the medullary space. There fluids or drugs are readily available for absorption and distribution by the venous system.

In the child, the needle is placed at 90 degrees to the tibial plateau, just medial and about two finger widths below the tibial tuberosity (the anterior bump just below the patella). Don gloves and cleanse the site with an antiseptic swab. With a firm twisting motion, introduce the needle into the bone for a few centimeters until you feel a "pop" or reduced resistance. Remove the trocar, attach a syringe, and draw back on the syringe to aspirate bone marrow and blood. Rotate the plastic disk to engage the skin and secure the needle. Connect the IV fluid administration set and secure the needle with bulky dressings and tape. Adult or geriatric IO administration uses the flat tibial plate just two finger widths above the medial malleolus. IO infusion may result in bone fracture, infiltration, growth-plate damage, pulmonary embolism, and the problems associated with venous cannulation. This site is not very effective for extensive fluid resuscitation in the adult.

c.   obtaining a blood sample.   pp. 824-828

Blood composition, the presence of toxins, and blood gas levels are important values to determine for learning what is wrong with a patient. Since emergency care may alter these figures, it is sometimes important to draw blood in the prehospital setting. Blood is withdrawn from a vein through either a needle or catheter and is either directly placed in special containers (blood tubes) or into a syringe for distribution into the blood tubes. A large vein must be used, because the withdrawal of blood may collapse smaller veins. A needled vacutainer is introduced into an engorged vein and blood tubes are introduced, one at a time. The vacuum withdraws blood from the vein and into the tubes, which are then manually agitated to mix the blood with an anticoagulant (all but the red top tube). If a vacutainer is not available, 20 ml of blood may be drawn up in a syringe and distributed among the containers. It is important to fill the containers in order of red, blue, green, purple, and gray (as available), because they contain various anticoagulants and another order may cross-contaminate the blood.

CONTENT SELF-EVALUATION

_____   1.   Which of the following is an indication for intravenous administration?
           A.   fluid replacement   **D.**   need of blood for analysis
           B.   blood replacement   **E.**   all of the above
           C.   drug administration

_____   2.   Which of the following is a likely site for intravenous cannulation?
           A.   the hands   **D.**   the neck
           B.   the arms   **E.**   all of the above
           C.   the legs

_____   3.   Which of the following is NOT a central venous vessel?
           A.   the internal jugular
           B.   the subclavian
           C.   the femoral
           D.   the antecubital
           E.   all of the above are central venous vessels

_____   4.   The solution that contains large proteins is a(n):
           A.   colliod.   **D.**   hypotonic.
           B.   crystalloid.   **E.**   hypertonic.
           C.   isotonic.

_____   5.   The solution that contains an electrolyte concentration close to that of plasma is a(n):
           A.   colliod.   **D.**   hypotonic.
           B.   crystalloid.   **E.**   hypertonic.
           C.   isotonic.

_____   6.   The solution that contains an electrolyte concentration greater than that of plasma is a(n):
           A.   colliod.   **D.**   hypotonic.
           B.   crystalloid.   **E.**   hypertonic.
           C.   isotonic.

_____   7.   One example of a hypotonic solution is:
           A.   normal saline.   **D.**   5 percent dextrose in water.
           B.   lactated Ringer's solution.   **E.**   dextran.
           C.   plasmanate.

_____   8.   The most desirable replacement for blood lost during trauma is:
           A.   normal saline.   **D.**   5 percent dextrose in water.
           B.   lactated Ringer's solution.   **E.**   none of the above
           C.   plasmanate.

9. Which intravenous fluid bag would you discard?
    A.   one that is cloudy   D.   one that is expired
    B.   one that is discolored   E.   all of the above
    C.   one that is leaking

10. For optimal fluid delivery, the drip chamber should be how full?
    A.   1/4   D.   2/3
    B.   1/3   E.   none of the above
    C.   1/2

11. The administration set most appropriate for administration of intravenous solutions for fluid replacement is the:
    A.   macrodrip administration set.   D.   blood tubing set.
    B.   microdrip administration set.   E.   none of the above
    C.   measured volume administration set.

12. The most common microdrip setting equaling 1 ml is:
    A.   10 gtts.   D.   60 gtts.
    B.   20 gtts.   E.   none of the above
    C.   45 gtts.

13. The administration set most appropriate for administration of a very specific volume of intravenous solution or drug is the:
    A.   macrodrip administration set.
    B.   microdrip administration set.
    C.   measured volume administration set.
    D.   blood tubing set.
    E.   none of the above

14. The most common intravenous cannula used in the prehospital setting is the:
    A.   over-the-needle.   D.   angiocatheter.
    B.   through-the-needle.   E.   A and D
    C.   hollow needle.

15. A venous constricting band should be left in place no longer than:
    A.   1 minute.   D.   5 minutes.
    B.   2 minutes.   E.   10 minutes.
    C.   3 minutes.

16. Leaving the constricting band on for too long is likely to cause:
    A.   collapse of the vein.
    B.   damage to the distal blood vessels.
    C.   damage to the vessels under the band.
    D.   changes in the distal venous blood.
    E.   all of the above

17. The angle of insertion for intravenous cannulation is:
    A.   10 degrees.   D.   60 degrees.
    B.   10 to 30 degrees.   E.   60 to 90 degrees.
    C.   45 degrees.

18. After you feel the "pop" associated with intravenous cannulation, you should:
    A.   advance the catheter.
    B.   advance the needle 0.5 centimeter, then advance the catheter.
    C.   advance the needle 1 centimeter, then advance the catheter.
    D.   advance the needle 2 centimeters, then advance the catheter.
    E.   withdraw the needle, then advance the catheter.

19. During external jugular vein cannulation, the patient's head should be:

A.	moved to the sniffing position.	D.	hyperextended.
B.	turned toward the side of access.	E.	hyperflexed.
C.	turned away from the side of access.		

20. To fill the jugular access site and make the vessel easier to both locate and cannulate, you should:

- **A.** apply a venous constricting band, tightly.
- **B.** apply a venous constricting band, loosely.
- **C.** occlude the vein gently with a finger.
- **D.** perform the procedure without occluding the vein.
- **E.** have the patient take a deep breath and hold it.

21. When establishing an IV with blood tubing, you must be careful to:

- **A.** fill the drip chamber 1/3 full.
- **B.** completely cover the blood filter with blood.
- **C.** fill the set with normal saline first.
- **D.** fill the drip chamber 3/4 full.
- **E.** both A and B above

22. Which of the following is a factor that may affect intravenous flow rates?

- **A.** failure to remove a venous constricting band
- **B.** edema at the access site
- **C.** the cannula tip up against a vein valve
- **D.** a clogged catheter
- **E.** all of the above

23. The complication of peripheral venous access in which a plastic embolus can form is:

A.	pyrogenic reaction.	D.	catheter shear.
B.	pain.	E.	all of the above
C.	thrombophlebitis.		

24. The most common cause of catheter shear is:

- **A.** cannulating thick veins.
- **B.** cannulating underneath the constricting band.
- **C.** withdrawing the needle from within the catheter.
- **D.** withdrawing the catheter from the needle.
- **E.** faulty catheter construction.

25. You should change a large (500- to 1,000-ml) infusion bag when the volume remaining in the bag is:

A.	10 ml.	D.	50 ml.
B.	20 ml.	E.	100 ml.
C.	30 ml.		

26. If air becomes entrained in the administration set when you are changing an IV bag or bottle, you should:

- **A.** continue the infusion, because the volume of air is negligible.
- **B.** discard the set and use a new one.
- **C.** use a syringe placed between the bubbles and patient to withdraw the air.
- **D.** reverse the fluid flow until the bubbles enter the fluid bag or drip chambeR.
- **E.** squeeze the tubing to push them into the drip chamber or bag.

27. Which of the following is NOT true regarding infusion pumps?

- **A.** They deliver fluids under pressure.
- **B.** They are large and difficult to carry.
- **C.** Most pumps contain alarms for occlusion.
- **D.** Most pumps contain alarms for fluid source depletion.
- **E.** They deliver fluids at precise rates.

28. The color of the blood tube container that must be drawn first is:

	A.	blue.	D.	purple.
	B.	red.	E.	gray.
	C.	green.		

_____ 29. Drawing blood and injecting it into the blood tubes in the wrong order may result in:
- A. leaving the wrong volume of blood in a tube.
- B. cross-contamination of the blood with anticoagulants.
- C. depletion of the vacuum in the tubes at too early a stage.
- D. coagulation in the last tubes to be filled.
- E. all but C

_____ 30. The device that accepts the blood tube to permit its filling is:
- A. the leur lock.
- B. the Huber needle.
- C. the vacutainer.
- D. the leur-sampling needle.
- E. either A or C

_____ 31. When using a syringe to fill your blood tubes, you should draw a volume of blood of about:
- A. 5 ml.
- B. 10 ml.
- C. 20 ml.
- D. 35 ml.
- E. 50 ml.

_____ 32. The complication from drawing blood in which red blood cells are destroyed is:
- A. hematocrit.
- B. hemoconcentration.
- C. hemolysis.
- D. hemotypsis.
- E. hematuria.

_____ 33. Hemoconcentration occurs during drawing blood:
- A. when the constricting band is left in place too long.
- B. when blood is drawn back through a needle that is too small.
- C. with premature mixing of the anticoagulant.
- D. with too vigorous a mixing of the blood and anticoagulant.
- E. with too forceful an aspiration of blood into the syringe.

_____ 34. The intraosseous site of infusion is most commonly used for which category of patient?
- A. geriatric patients
- B. cardiac patients
- C. children under 5 years of age
- D. patients with non-skeletal injuries
- E. all of the above

_____ 35. The proper site for intraosseous needle placement in the child is one to two finger widths:
- A. below and medial to the tibial tuberosity.
- B. below and lateral to the tibial tuberosity.
- C. above the medial malleolus.
- D. above the lateral malleolus.
- E. above and lateral to the tibial crest.

_____ 36. Confirmation that you are in the medullary space is achieved by:
- A. feeling the bone "pop."
- B. pushing the needle 2 to 4 mm.
- C. aspirating bone marrow and blood.
- D. feeling resistance to the twisting of insertion.
- E. none of the above

_____ 37. Complications of intraosseous cannulation include all of the following EXCEPT:
- A. pulmonary embolism.
- B. fracture.
- C. growth plate damage.
- D. aspiration of bone marrow.
- E. complete insertion.

_____ **38.** When an intraosseous infusion does not run freely and you note edema at the insertion site, you should suspect:

    A.   pjulmonary embolism.   **D.**   infiltration.
    B.   fracture.   **E.**   thrombus formation.
    C.   growth plate damage.

_____ **39.** Complete insertion is the term that refers to:

    A.   successful cannulation.
    B.   passing the needle through both sides of the tibia.
    C.   advancing the cannula into the medullary canal.
    D.   an improper placement of the cannula into the growth plate.
    E.   none of the above

_____ **40.** Intraosseous placement should not be attempted under which of the following conditions?

    A.   osteoporosis
    B.   osteogenesis imperfecta
    C.   an intravenous line is in place
    D.   there is a fracture of the femur or tibia on the side of access
    E.   all of the above

True/False

_____ **41.** Both central venous and peripheral venous cannulation are common in prehospital care.

    A.   True
    B.   False

_____ **42.** Ringer's Lactate and normal saline are used for fluid replacement because of their immediate ability to expand the circulating volume.

    A.   True
    B.   False

_____ **43.** Hypothermic patients may benefit from administration of warmed colloid solutions.

    A.   True
    B.   False

_____ **44.** The major difference between blood tubing and a standard intravenous administration set is that blood tubing has a filter to remove clots and particulate matter.

    A.   True
    B.   False

_____ **45.** Blood is not administered with fluids like lactated Ringer's solution because such solutions increase blood's potential for coagulation.

    A.   True
    B.   False

_____ **46.** Many patients are prone to develop hypothermia during fluid administration.

    A.   True
    B.   False

_____ **47.** A needle gauge of 18 is smaller than a needle gauge of 22.

    A.   True
    B.   False

_____ **48.** When cleansing the site for intravenous cannulation, you should make one swipe over the intended site with a betadine or alcohol swab.

    A.   True
    B.   False

_____ **49.** You should consider using the external jugular vein as an IV access site only after you have exhausted other means of peripheral access or when the patient needs immediate fluid administration.
- **A.** True
- **B.** False

_____ **50.** If a blood clot appears to stop or slow intravenous fluid flow, forcefully inject a small amount of heparin into the catheter and continue the infusion.
- **A.** True
- **B.** False

_____ **51.** Never administer an intravenous drug infusion as the primary IV line.
- **A.** True
- **B.** False

_____ **52.** The reason venous blood sampling is important in the prehospital setting is that our interventions may alter the blood's composition or erase important information about it.
- **A.** True
- **B.** False

_____ **53.** Do not use a blood tube after its expiration date because the anticoagulant and vacuum may have become ineffective.
- **A.** True
- **B.** False

_____ **54.** You should fill the blood tube to between a third and a half of its volume because the anticoagulant is measured for this amount of blood.
- **A.** True
- **B.** False

_____ **55.** When an IV catheter is withdrawn, place pressure on the venipuncture site with a sterile gauze pad for about 5 minutes.
- **A.** True
- **B.** False

Matching

Write the letter of the appropriate term in the space provided next to the description to which it applies.

Term

A. pyrogen	**F.**	air embolism
B. embolus	**G.**	necrosis
C. circulatory overload	**H.**	anticoagulant
D. thrombophlebitis	**I.**	hemoconcentration
E. thrombus	**J.**	hemolysis

Description

_____ **56.** blood clot

_____ **57.** sloughing off of dead tissue

_____ **58.** foreign protein capable of producing fever

_____ **59.** the destruction of red blood cells

_____ **60.** foreign particle in the blood

_____ **61.** air in the vein

_____ **62.** an excess in intravascular fluid volume

_____ **63.** elevated numbers of red and white blood cells

_____ **64.** inflammation of the vein

_____ **65.** drug that inhibits blood clotting

Chapter 15

Medication Administration

Part 3: Medical Mathematics

Review of Chapter Objectives

After reading this part of the chapter, you should be able to:

1. Review mathematical equivalents.   pp. 835-838

The basic units used for most of medicine are metric: the gram for weight, the liter for volume, and the meter for distance. The metric system is a decimal system that uses suffixes and prefixes to delineate larger and smaller quantities, most commonly kilo (1,000), milli (1/1000), and micro (1/1,000,000). Pharmacology math involves working with addition, subtraction, multiplication, and division as well as working extensively with ratios, fractions, and formulas.

2. Differentiate temperature readings between the centigrade and Fahrenheit scales.   p. 837

The centigrade (officially known as Celsius) scale graduates the temperature between the point at which ice melts and the point at which water boils into 100 degrees. The Fahrenheit scale graduates the range between the lowest temperature at which a salt-water mixture would remain a liquid (0 degrees) and the boiling point of water into 212 degrees. The Celsius scale is used in medicine, and the conversion between the two is demonstrated by the formulas below.

$$°F = 9/5 °C + 32 °C = 5/9 (°F - 32)$$

3. Discuss formulas as a basis for performing drug calculations.   pp. 838-843

The major formula for determining the amount of a drug to be administered is as follows:

Volume to be administered = <u>Volume on hand x Desired dose</u>
Dosage on hand

The formula is mathematically manipulated so that the unknown element can be computed using the known values.
Other elements of drug calculation call for determining the volume flowing through an intravenous administration set by monitoring the number of drops falling in a drip chamber per minute. Conversion is based upon the number of drops that equal one milliliter of fluid.

Drops/Minute = <u>Volume on hand x Drip factor x Desired dose</u>
Dosage on hand

You may also be required to convert pounds to kilograms (if the patient dosing is in weight of drug per kilogram of body weight). To do this you should know that:

1 pound = 2.2 kilograms

In some cases, it is important to administer a volume of medication over time, and the associated formula for such administration is:

Drops/Minute = <u>Volume to be administered x Drip factor</u>
Time in minutes

4. Describe how to perform mathematical conversions from the household system to the metric system.   pp. 836-837

Weight. Weight conversion between household and metric measures is accomplished by dividing a weight in pounds by 2.2 to find the equivalent metric weight in kilograms. Conversely, if you know a weight in kilograms, multiply it by 2.2 to get the weight in pounds

kg = lbs/2.2   lbs = kg 3 2.2

Volume. Volume conversion between household and metric measures is based on the recognition that **1 quart is about equal to 1 liter, 1 cup to 250 milliliters, and so on.**

CONTENT SELF-EVALUATION

_____   1. Grams are a measure of:
        A.   mass.   D.   volume.
        B.   temperature.   E.   area.
        C.   distance.

_____   2. Meters are a measure of:
        A.   mass.   D.   volume.
        B.   temperature.   E.   area.
        C.   distance.

_____   3. Litres are a measure of:
        A.   mass.   D.   volume.
        B.   temperature.   E.   area.
        C.   distance.

_____   4. 7 grams is equivalent to:
        A.   0.007 mg   D.   7,000 mg.
        B.   0.7 mg.   E.   7,000,000 mg
        C.   700 mg.

_____   5. 3.8 micrograms is equivalent to:
        A.   3,800,00 g.   D.   0.0000038 mg.
        B.   0.0038 g.   E.   0.0038mg.
        C.   3,800,000 mg.

_____   6. Your patient weighs 56 lb. This is approximately:
        A.   25 kg.   D.   12.3 kg.
        B.   250 kg.   E.   39 kg.
        C.   123 kg.

_____   7. Your patient weighs 175 lb. This is approximately:

A.	38.5 kg.	**D.**	385 kg.	
B.	70 kg.	**E.**	126 kg.	
C.	12.6 kg.			

_____ **8.** You are ordered to administer 0.4 mg of a medication via IV bolus. The medication comes in a multidose vial containing 1 mg in 1 mL of solution. How much solution must you draw up?

A.	0.4 mL.	**D.**	2.5 mL.
B.	0.1 mL.	**E.**	4 mL.
C.	1 mL.		

_____ **9.** Your patient weighs 45 lb. Your protocol calls for you to administer 0.01 mg/kg of 1:1000 epinephrine SC to a maximum of 0.3 mg. How much epinephrine do you require?

A.	0.02 mg.	**D.**	0.3 mg.
B.	0.1 mg.	**E.**	1.0 mg.
C.	0.2 mg.		

_____ **10.** You are transferring a patient between facilities. You are directed to give 1200 mL of normal saline in the next 90 minutes. Your administration set administers 10 gtts/mL. At what drip rate should you run your infusion?

A.	13.3 gtts/min.	**D.**	72 gtts/min.
B.	133 gtts/min.	**E.**	23.6 gtts/min.
C.	7.2 gtts/min.		

True/False

_____ **11.** A dekagram is larger than a decigram.
- **A.** True
- **B.** False

_____ **12.** A hectogram is smaller than a microgram.
- **A.** True
- **B.** False

_____ **13.** Two cups of fluid is about half a litre.
- **A.** True
- **B.** False

_____ **14.** A degree Fahrenheit is larger than a degree Celsius.
- **A.** True
- **B.** False

_____ **15.** Systems for approximating weights and volumes are adequate for calculating pediatric doses of medications and fluids.
- **A.** True
- **B.** False

Matching

Write the letter of the appropriate metric prefix in the space provided next to the multiplier value to which it applies.

Prefix

A. c		**D.**	h
B. D		**E.**	k
C. d		**F.**	m

Multiplier

_____ **16.** 1000

_____ **17.** 100

_____ **18.** 10

_____ **19.** 1/10 or 0.1

_____ **20.** 1/100 or 0.01

Answer Key

Chapter 1: Introduction to Prehospital Care

Part 1

Multiple Choice

1.	C	*p.* 6
2.	E	*p.* 6
3.	E	*p.* 6
4.	D	*p.* 6
5.	C	*p.* 7
6.	A	*p.* 7
7.	E	*p.* 8
8.	D	*p.* 7

True/False

9.	A	*p.* 6
10.	A	*p.* 7
11.	A	*p.* 7
12.	B	*p.* 7
13.	A	*p.* 7
14.	A	*p.* 7
15.	B	*p.* 8
16.	A	*p.* 8
17.	B	*p.* 8
18.	B	*p.* 8

Matching

19.	E	*p.* 8
20.	A	*p.* 8
21.	C	*p.* 8
22.	F	*p.* 8
23.	D	*p.* 8
24.	B	*p.* 8

Part 2

Multiple Choice

1.	A	*p.* 10
2.	B	*p.* 12
3.	D	*p.* 14
4.	C	*p.* 14
5.	E	*p.* 15
6.	C	*p.* 15
7.	D	*p.* 15
8.	C	*p.* 17
9.	E	*p.* 17
10.	A	*p.* 18
11.	D	*p.* 18
12.	D	*p.* 18
13.	E	*p.* 19
14.	D	*p.* 19
15.	D	*p.* 21
16.	B	*p.* 21
17.	A	*p.* 23
18.	E	*p.* 23
19.	B	*p.* 23
20.	C	*p.* 24
21.	E	*p.* 24
22.	B	*p.* 24
23.	B	*p.* 25
24.	A	*p.* 25
25.	B	*p.* 25

True/False

26.	A	*p.* 8
27.	B	*p.* 9
28.	A	*p.* 12
29.	B	*p.* 14
30.	B	*p.* 15
31.	B	*p.* 17
32.	A	*p.* 18
33.	A	*p.* 19
34.	B	*p.* 23
35.	B	*p.* 25

Matching

36.	B	*p.* 23
37.	C	*p.* 19
38.	A	*p.* 23
39.	H	*p.* 18
40.	F	*p.* 18
41.	D	*p.* 19

Part 3

Multiple Choice

1.	E	*pp. 26–27*
2.	E	*p. 27*
3.	A	*p. 28*
4.	C	*p. 28*
5.	B	*p. 8*
6.	B	*p. 29*
7.	C	*p. 29*
8.	E	*p. 29*
9.	B	*p. 30*
10.	B	*p. 3*
11.	B	*p. 32*
12.	D	*p. 32*
13.	C	*p. 33*
14.	D	*p. 34*
15.	C	*p. 34*

True/False

16.	B	*p. 26*
17.	B	*p. 27*
18.	A	*p. 28*
19.	B	*p. 28*
20.	A	*p. 28*
21.	A	*p. 29*
22.	A	*p. 30*
23.	A	*p. 30*
24.	B	*p. 31*
25.	A	*p. 33*

Matching

26.	G	*p. 29*
27.	C	*p. 28*
28.	D	*p. 28*
29.	C	*p. 28*
30.	F	*p. 29*
31.	A	*p. 27*
32.	C	*p. 28*
33.	C	*p. 28*
34.	E	*p. 29*
35.	B	*p. 27*
36.	E	*p. 29*
37.	A	*p. 27*
38.	G	*p. 29*

39.	D	*p. 28*
40.	S	*p. 28*

Part 4

Multiple Choice

1.	C	*p. 35*
2.	A	*p. 35*
3.	A	*p. 36*
4.	B	*p. 36*
5.	C	*p. 36*
6.	E	*p. 37*
7.	C	*p. 37*
8.	C	*p. 37*
9.	E	*p. 38*
10.	C	*p. 38*
11.	A	*p. 41*
12.	D	*p. 40*
13.	E	*p. 41*
14.	B	*p. 41*
15.	E	*p. 42*
16.	A	*p. 42*
17.	A	*p. 42*
18.	D	*p. 43*
19.	C	*p. 45*
20.	C	*p. 45*
21.	B	*p. 46*
22.	D	*p. 48*
23.	D	*p. 48*
24.	B	*p. 49*
25.	B	*p. 49*
26.	A	*p. 49*
27.	E	*p. 51*
28.	B	*p. 50*
29.	E	*p. 52*
30.	A	*p. 52*
31.	B	*p. 52*
32.	C	*p. 52*
33.	E	*p. 53*
34.	B	*p. 54*
35.	A	*p. 54*

True/False

36.	A	*p. 36*
37.	B	*p. 37*
38.	B	*p. 37*

39.	A	*p. 38*
40.	A	*p. 40*
41.	B	*p. 45*
42.	A	*p. 47*
43.	A	*p. 47*
44.	B	*p. 48*
45.	B	*p. 54*

Matching

46.	A, B	*p. 41*
47.	A, B, D	*p. 41*
48.	A, B	*p. 41*
49.	A, B, C	*p. 41*
50.	A, B	*p. 41*

Part 5

Multiple Choice

1.	D	*p. 55*
2.	C	*p. 55*
3.	B	*p. 56*
4.	C	*p. 56*
5.	A	*p. 58*
6.	B	*p. 58*
7.	E	*p. 59*
8.	E	*p. 61*
9.	B	*p. 61*
10.	E	*p. 62*

True/False

11.	A	*p. 55*
12.	A	*p. 55*
13.	B	*p. 56*
14.	A	*p. 56*
15.	A	*p. 57*
16.	B	*p. 58*
17.	A	*p. 58*
18.	B	*p. 59*
19.	A	*p. 60*
20.	A	*p. 61*

Matching

21.	D	*p. 56*
22.	E	*p. 56*
23.	C	*p. 56*

24.	A	*p. 55*
25.	B	*p. 56*

Part 6

Multiple Choice

1.	B	*p. 63*
2.	A	*p. 63*
3.	E	*p. 63*
4.	A	*p. 64*
5.	D	*p. 64*
6.	A	*p. 65*
7.	D	*p. 65*
8.	B	*p. 67*
9.	A	*p. 69*
10.	E	*p. 73*

True/False

11.	B	*p. 63*
12.	B	*p. 64*
13.	A	*p. 65*
14.	A	*p. 66*
15.	B	*p. 70*

Matching

16.	E	*p. 67*
17.	B	*p. 64*
18.	F	*p. 67*
19.	A	*p. 64*
20.	D	*p. 67*

Part 7

Multiple Choice

1.	E	*p. 74*
2.	D	*p. 74*
3.	A	*p. 75*
4.	B	*p. 75*
5.	A	*p. 76*
6.	B	*p. 77*
7.	E	*p. 79*
8.	C	*p. 79*
9.	A	*p. 84*
10.	D	*p. 85*

True/False

11.	A	*p. 75*
12.	A	*p. 75*
13.	B	*p. 77*
14.	A	*p. 77*
15.	B	*p. 82*

Matching

16.	E	*p. 84*
17.	A	*p. 84*
18.	A	*p. 84*
19.	D	*p. 84*
20.	C	*p. 84*

Chapter 2: Medical-Legal Aspects of Prehospital Care

Multiple Choice

1.	B	*p. 91*
2.	C	*p. 91*
3.	D	*p. 91*
4.	A	*p. 92*
5.	A	*p. 93*
6.	B	*p. 93*
7.	B	*p. 96*
8.	D	*p. 97*
9.	D	*p. 98*
10.	E	*p. 98*
11.	C	*p. 98*
12.	C	*p. 99*
13.	E	*p. 100*
14.	D	*p. 103*
15.	E	*p. 104*
16.	A	*p. 104*
17.	C	*p. 105*
18.	E	*p. 105*
19.	B	*p. 106*
20.	B	*p. 107*
21.	D	*p. 108*
22.	C	*p. 109*
23.	A	*p. 111*
24.	C	*p. 114*
25.	C	*p. 114*

True/False

26.	B	*p. 94*
27.	A	*p. 95*
28.	B	*p. 97*
29.	B	*p. 97*
30.	A	*p. 98*
31.	B	*p. 98*
32.	B	*p. 99*
33.	B	*p. 100*
34.	A	*p. 102*
35.	A	*p. 103*
36.	B	*p. 105*
37.	B	*p. 106*
38.	A	*p. 108*
39.	B	*p. 110*
40.	A	*p. 111*

Matching

41.	I	*p. 100*
42.	L	*p. 104*
43.	E	*p. 99*
44.	C	*p. 98*
45.	K	*p. 104*
46.	H	*p. 99*
47.	B	*p. 98*
48.	N	*p.109*
49.	F	*p. 99*
50.	M	*p.109*

Chapter 3: Operations

Part 1

Multiple Choice

1.	C	*p. 122*
2.	A	*p. 121*
3.	C	*p. 122*
4.	A	*p. 122*
5.	C	*p. 122*
6.	B	*p. 123*
7.	C	*p. 122*
8.	D	*p. 124*
9.	C	*p. 124*
10.	B	*p. 124*

11.	B	*p. 125*
12.	D	*p. 127*
13.	B	*p. 127*
14.	C	*p. 127*
15.	E	*p. 128*
16.	B	*p. 129*
17.	E	*p. 130*
18.	A	*p. 130*
19.	E	*p. 133*
20.	A	*p. 133*

True/False

21.	B	*p. 124*
22.	A	*p. 127*
23.	B	*p. 129*
24.	B	*p. 130*
25.	A	*p. 132*

Matching

26.	D	*p. 124*
27.	F	*p. 124*
28.	I	*p. 122*
29.	A	*p. 124*
30.	E	*p. 125*
31.	B	*p. 124*
32.	C	*p. 124*
33.	J	*p. 125*
34.	H	*p. 125*
35.	G	*p. 126*

Part 2

Multiple Choice

1.	C	*p. 133*
2.	D	*p. 133*
3.	C	*p. 135*
4.	A	*p. 135*
5.	A	*p. 135*
6.	B	*p. 136*
7.	A	*p. 136*
8.	A	*p. 137*
9.	E	*p. 137*
10.	D	*p. 137*
11.	A	*p. 138*
12.	A	*p. 139*

13.	C	*p. 139*
14.	A	*p. 140*
15.	D	*p. 140*
16.	D	*p. 141*
17.	A	*p. 143*
18.	D	*p. 143*
19.	B	*p. 143*
20.	A	*p. 144*
21.	B	*p. 144*
22.	E	*p. 145*
23.	A	*p. 146*
24.	D	*p. 149*
25.	A	*p. 150*

True/False

26.	A	*p. 135*
27.	B	*p. 136*
28.	A	*p. 137*
29.	A	*p. 137*
30.	A	*p. 138*
31.	A	*p. 140*
32.	B	*p. 141*
33.	B	*p. 144*
34.	A	*p. 146*
35.	A	*p. 152*

Matching

36.	D	*p. 135*
37.	J	*p. 139*
38.	I	*p. 140*
39.	H	*p. 135*
40.	A	*p. 140*
41.	B	*p. 137*
42.	G	*p. 139*
43.	C	*p. 150*
44.	F	*p. 140*
45.	E	*p. 136*

Part 3

Multiple Choice

1.	E	*p. 152*
2.	B	*p. 153*
3.	D	*p. 156*
4.	C	*p. 158*

5.	C	_p. 158_
6.	C	_p. 159_
7.	B	_p. 161_
8.	D	_p. 162_
9.	E	_p. 162_
10.	C	_p. 162_
11.	E	_p. 165_
12.	A	_p. 166_
13.	C	_p. 167_
14.	B	_p. 170_
15.	A	_p. 173_
16.	B	_p. 173_
17.	B	_p. 174_
18.	E	_p. 177_
19.	B	_p. 177_
20.	C	_p. 180_

True/False

21.	B	_p. 153_
22.	A	_p. 161_
23.	A	_p. 162_
24.	A	_p. 166_
25.	A	_p. 167_
26.	B	_p. 169_
27.	B	_p. 174_
28.	A	_p. 176_
29.	B	_p. 177_

Matching

30.	B	_p. 180_
31.	H	_p. 160_
32.	C	_p. 159_
33.	F	_p. 162_
34.	A	_p. 162_
35.	J	_p. 173_
36.	I	_p. 178_
37.	D	_p. 164_
38.	E	_p. 165_
39.	G	_p. 173_
40.	B	_p. 166_

Part 4

Multiple Choice

| 1. | A | _p. 181_ |

2.	E	_p. 182_
3.	B	_p. 183_
4.	C	_p. 183_
5.	D	_p. 183_
6.	A	_p. 184_
7.	B	_p. 184_
8.	B	_p. 189_
9.	C	_p. 188_
10.	B	_p. 188_
11.	B	_p. 190_
12.	B	_p. 192_
13.	D	_p. 193_
14.	A	_p. 193_
15.	A	_p. 193_
16.	A	_p. 195_
17.	A	_p. 195_
18.	A	_p. 196_
19.	A	_p. 196_
20.	D	_p. 198_
21.	D	_p. 198_
22.	D	_p. 199_
23.	C	_p. 199_
24.	C	_p. 199_
25.	A	_p. 200_

True/False

26.	A	_p. 181_
27.	B	_p. 188_
28.	A	_p. 183_
29.	A	_p. 185_
30.	B	_p. 188_
31.	B	_p. 189_
32.	B	_p. 191_
33.	B	_p. 192_
34.	A	_p. 195_
35.	A	_p. 200_

Matching

36.	D	_p. 181_
37.	H	_p. 184_
38.	I	_p. 189_
39.	C	_p. 189_
40.	J	_p. 190_
41.	B	_p. 190_
42.	G	_p. 190_
43.	E	_p. 191_

44.	A	*p.* 191
45.	F	*p.* 191

Part 5

Multiple Choice

1.	B	*p.* 201
2.	B	*p.* 201
3.	B	*p.* 202
4.	C	*p.* 202
5.	A	*p.* 202
6.	E	*p.* 202
7.	A	*p.* 204
8.	B	*p.* 203
9.	C	*p.* 205
10.	A	*p.* 205
11.	B	*p.* 205
12.	E	*p.* 206
13.	E	*p.* 206
14.	A	*p.* 206
15.	E	*p.* 206
16.	B	*p.* 207
17.	B	*p.* 208
18.	E	*p.* 207
19.	C	*p.* 209
20.	B	*p.* 209

True/False

21.	B	*p.* 202
22.	A	*p.* 202
23.	B	*p.* 203
24.	B	*p.* 205
25.	B	*p.* 206
26.	B	*p.* 210
27.	B	*p.* 211
28.	A	*p.* 212
29.	A	*p.* 213
30.	A	*p.* 215

Matching

31.	J	*p.* 206
32.	D	*p.* 211
33.	C	*p.* 209
34.	E	*p.* 211
35.	I	*p.* 213

36.	B	*p.* 215
37.	A	*p.* 212
38.	H	*p.* 209
39.	G	*p.* 214
40.	F	*p.* 212

Chapter 4: Therapeutic Communications

Multiple Choice

1.	B	*p.* 219
2.	D	*p.* 219
3.	C	*p.* 219
4.	B	*p.* 220
5.	C	*pp.* 220–221
6.	A	*pp.* 220–221
7.	C	*p.* 222
8.	C	*p.* 222
9.	A	*p.* 222
10.	C	*p.* 222
11.	B	*p.* 222
12.	D	*p.* 222
13.	A	*p.* 222
14.	E	*p.* 222
15.	B	*p.* 223
16.	D	*p.* 224
17.	B	*p.* 224
18.	A	*p.* 224
19.	A	*p.* 225
20.	E	*p.* 226
21.	A	*pp.* 226–227
22.	E	*p.* 227
23.	A	*p.* 228
24.	C	*p.* 230
25.	D	*p.* 232

True/False

26.	A	*p.* 219
27.	B	*p.* 223
28.	A	*p.* 223
29.	B	*p.* 224
30.	B	*p.* 225
31.	B	*p.* 225
32.	A	*p.* 227
33.	A	*p.* 229
34.	A	*p.* 230

35.	B	*p. 232*

Matching

36.	A	*p. 224*
37.	B	*p. 224*
38.	B	*p. 224*
39.	B	*p. 224*
40.	A	*p. 224*
41.	E	*p. 232*
42.	B	*p. 232*
43.	A	*p. 232*
44.	C	*p. 232*
45.	D	*p. 232*

Chapter 5: History Taking

Multiple Choice

1.	D	*p. 235*
2.	C	*p. 235*
3.	B	*p. 235*
4.	D	*p. 236*
5.	A	*p. 236*
6.	E	*p. 237*
7.	E	*p. 238*
8.	B	*p. 238*
9.	A	*p. 239*
10.	B	*p. 239*
11.	C	*p. 241*
12.	E	*p. 242*
13.	C	*p. 242*
14.	D	*p. 242*
15.	B	*p. 242*
16.	A	*p. 243*
17.	D	*p. 244*
18.	B	*pp. 244–245*
19.	A	*p. 246*
20.	C	*p. 247*

True/False

21.	A	*p. 236*
22.	A	*p. 236*
23.	B	*p. 236*
24.	A	*p. 237*
25.	A	*p. 238*

26.	B	*p. 240*
27.	B	*p. 240*
28.	F	*p. 242*
29.	A	*p. 244*
30.	A	*p. 248*

Matching

31.	S	*pp. 239–240*
32.	P	*pp. 239–240*
33.	R	*pp. 239–240*
34.	Q	*pp. 239–240*
35.	P	*pp. 239–240*
36.	O	*pp. 239–240*
37.	R	*pp. 239–240*
38.	T	*pp. 239–240*
39.	Q	*pp. 239–240*
40.	O	*pp. 239–240*
41.	G	*pp. 245*
42.	I	*pp. 245*
43.	F	*pp. 245*
44.	C	*pp. 245*
45.	B	*pp. 245*

Chapter 6: Physical Assessment Techniques

Multiple Choice

1.	A	*p. 254*
2.	B	*p. 257*
3.	A	*p. 255*
4.	C	*p. 255*
5.	B	*p. 255*
6.	C	*p. 256*
7.	C	*p. 256*
8.	A	*p. 256*
9.	C	*p. 257*
10.	B	*p. 258*
11.	C	*p. 258*
12.	A	*p. 258*
13.	E	*p. 260*
14.	A	*p. 260*
15.	D	*p. 260*
16.	C	*p. 260*
17.	A	*p. 260*
18.	E	*p. 260*

19.	B	*p.* 261	65.	E	*p.* 318
20.	C	*p.* 261	66.	A	*p.* 319
21.	E	*p.* 261	67.	E	*p.* 319
22.	C	*p.* 262	68.	B	*p.* 320
23.	D	*p.* 262	69.	C	*p.* 320
24.	D	*p.* 262	70.	D	*p.* 321
25.	B	*p.* 263	71.	D	*p.* 321
26.	B	*p.* 264	72.	B	*p.* 322
27.	D	*p.* 268	73.	A	*p.* 234
28.	B	*p.* 268	74.	C	*p.* 324
29.	D	*p.* 268	75.	D	*p.* 324
30.	E	*p.* 268	76.	D	*p.* 325
31.	C	*p.* 268	77.	E	*p.* 325
32.	A	*p.* 269	78.	B	*p.* 326
33.	E	*p.* 269	79.	B	*p.* 326
34.	D	*p.* 269	80.	D	*p.* 557
35.	B	*p.* 272	81.	C	*p.* 326
36.	D	*p.* 273	82.	E	*p.* 328
37.	E	*p.* 274	83.	C	*p.* 330
38.	A	*p.* 274	84.	E	*p.* 333
39.	B	*p.* 274	85.	A	*p.* 333
40.	D	*p.* 275	86.	C	*p.* 334
41.	A	*p.* 280	87.	E	*p.* 334
42.	A	*p.* 284	88.	E	*p.* 334
43.	B	*p.* 281	89.	A	*p.* 336
44.	E	*p.* 284	90.	A	*p.* 334
45.	A	*p.* 286	91.	B	*p.* 336
46.	D	*p.* 291	92.	A	*p.* 336
47.	B	*p.* 291	93.	D	*p.* 337
48.	E	*p.* 292	94.	E	*p.* 338
49.	B	*p.* 292	95.	A	*p.* 339
50.	A	*p.* 294			

True/False

51.	C	*p.* 294	96.	A	*p.* 256
52.	C	*p.* 294	97.	A	*p.* 256
53.	E	*p.* 296	98.	B	*p.* 257
54.	D	*p.* 300	99.	B	*p.* 259
55.	D	*p.* 300	100.	A	*p.* 259
56.	B	*p.* 305	101.	A	*p.* 261
57.	B	*p.* 305	102.	A	*p.* 268
58.	B	*p.* 314	103.	B	*p.* 269
59.	D	*p.* 314	104.	A	*p.* 261
60.	D	*p.* 316	105.	B	*p.* 262
61.	C	*p.* 316	106.	B	*p.* 269
62.	A	*p.* 316	107.	A	*p.* 272
63.	D	*p.* 318	108.	B	*p.* 295
64.	E	*p.* 316			

109.	B	*p. 292*
110.	A	*p. 295*
111.	B	*p. 297*
112.	A	*p. 300*
113.	B	*p. 316*
114.	A	*p. 325*
115.	A	*p. 326*
116.	A	*p. 329*
117.	B	*p. 330*
118.	B	*p. 333*
119.	B	*p. 334*
120.	B	*p. 336*

Matching

121.	I	*p. 259*
122.	B	*p. 259*
123.	A	*p. 259*
124.	G	*p. 259*
125.	J	*p. 259*
126.	D	*p. 259*
127.	E	*p. 259*
128.	C	*p. 259*
129.	F	*p. 259*
130.	J	*p. 260*
131.	I	*p. 258*
132.	C	*p. 261*
133.	F	*p. 262*
134.	A	*p. 258*
135.	E	*p. 260*
136.	D	*p. 261*
137.	H	*p. 262*
138.	K	*p. 260*
139.	G	*p. 262*
140.	B	*p. 260*

Chapter 7: Patient Assessment in the Field

Multiple Choice

1.	E	*p. 342*
2.	B	*p. 344*
3.	A	*p. 344*
4.	C	*p. 345*
5.	E	*p. 345*
6.	A	*p. 347*

7.	B	*p. 350*
8.	D	*p. 350*
9.	A	*p. 350*
10.	C	*p. 352*
11.	B	*p. 353*
12.	C	*p. 352*
13.	C	*p. 353*
14.	B	*p. 354*
15.	A	*p. 355*
16.	E	*p. 355*
17.	C	*p. 355*
18.	B	*p. 356*
19.	D	*p. 356*
20.	D	*p. 357*
21.	A	*p. 357*
22.	C	*p. 358*
23.	B	*p. 358*
24.	A	*p. 358*
25.	D	*p. 362*
26.	C	*p. 362*
27.	D	*p. 363*
28.	D	*p. 363*
29.	A	*p. 365*
30.	B	*p. 365*
31.	A	*p. 365*
32.	D	*p. 366*
33.	B	*p. 366*
34.	C	*p. 366*
35.	B	*p. 369*
36.	D	*p. 370*
37.	B	*p. 370*
38.	C	*p. 373*
39.	E	*p. 373*
40.	E	*p. 373*
41.	C	*p. 374*
42.	D	*p. 375*
43.	A	*p. 376*
44.	D	*p. 376*
45.	E	*p. 379*
46.	A	*p. 380*
47.	B	*p. 380*
48.	E	*p. 383*
49.	A	*p. 383*
50.	B	*p. 390*

51.	A	*p.* 342
52.	A	*p.* 342
53.	B	*p.* 350
54.	B	*p.* 350
55.	A	*p.* 353
56.	B	*p.* 353
57.	A	*p.* 355
58.	A	*p.* 357
59.	A	*p.* 364
60.	B	*p.* 365
61.	B	*p.* 365
62.	B	*p.* 365
63.	B	*p.* 369
64.	A	*p.* 366
65.	A	*p.* 356
66.	B	*p.* 370
67.	A	*p.* 370
68.	A	*p.* 372
69.	B	*p.* 375
70.	A	*p.* 380

Matching

71.	I	*p.* 370
72.	H	*p.* 370
73.	C	*p.* 369
74.	E	*p.* 369
75.	F	*p.* 369
76.	G	*p.* 369
77.	M	*p.* 377
78.	A, J	*p.* 376
79.	K	*p.* 377
80.	H	*p.* 376
81.	C, D	*p.* 376
82.	I	*p.* 376
83.	A, G	*p.* 377
84.	G	*p.* 377
85.	B	*p.* 376

Chapter 8: Communications

Multiple Choice

1.	E	*p.* 396
2.	A	*p.* 397
3.	D	*p.* 397
4.	C	*p.* 398
5.	A	*p.* 398
6.	D	*p.* 398
7.	C	*p.* 398
8.	E	*p.* 398
9.	D	*p.* 399
10.	B	*p.* 399
11.	B	*p.* 400
12.	A	*p.* 400
13.	E	*pp.* 400–401
14.	B	*pp.* 400–401
15.	D	*p.* 401
16.	E	*p.* 401
17.	A	*p.* 403
18.	B	*p.* 403
19.	D	*p.* 403
20.	D	*p.* 403
21.	B	*p.* 404
22.	C	*p.* 404
23.	A	*p.* 408
24.	A	*p.* 408
25.	A	*p.* 409

True/False

26.	B	*p.* 397
27.	B	*p.* 400
28.	A	*p.* 401
29.	A	*p.* 401
30.	B	*p.* 402
31.	A	*p.* 402
32.	A	*p.* 403
33.	A	*p.* 404
34.	B	*p.* 407
35.	A	*p.* 408

Matching

36.	D	*p.* 399
37.	B	*p.* 399
38.	H	*p.* 399
39.	C	*p.* 399
40.	F	*p.* 399
41.	J	*p.* 399
42.	G	*p.* 399
43.	F	*p.* 399
44.	I	*p.* 399

| 45. | A | *p.* 399 |

Chapter 9: Documentation

Multiple Choice

1.	E	*p.* 412
2.	B	*p.* 412
3.	C	*p.* 414
4.	B	*p.* 414
5.	E	*p.* 415
6.	C	*p.* 420
7.	D	*p.* 421
8.	C	*p.* 421
9.	A	*p.* 422
10.	E	*p.* 424
11.	C	*p.* 424
12.	C	*p.* 424
13.	D	*p.* 425
14.	A	*p.* 425
15.	B	*p.* 426
16.	B	*p.* 427
17.	D	*p.* 428
18.	D	*p.* 427
19.	A	*p.* 429
20.	D	*p.* 429
21.	A	*p.* 428
22.	E	*p.* 429
23.	D	*p.* 430
24.	C	*p.* 431
25.	B	*p.* 434

True/False

26.	A	*p.* 412
27.	A	*p.* 413
28.	B	*p.* 413
29.	A	*p.* 415
30.	A	*p.* 420
31.	B	*p.* 421
32.	B	*p.* 421
33.	A	*p.* 421
34.	A	*p.* 426
35.	B	*p.* 433

Matching

36.	P	*p.* 417
37.	Y	*p.* 417
38.	L	*p.* 417
39.	T	*p.* 417
40.	A	*p.* 417
41.	E	*p.* 417
42.	B	*p.* 417
43.	O	*p.* 417
44.	U	*p.* 417
45.	X	*p.* 417
46.	M	*p.* 417
47.	J	*p.* 418
48.	Q	*p.* 418
49.	G	*p.* 418
50.	R	*p.* 418
51.	V	*p.* 418
52.	I	*p.* 419
53.	N	*p.* 419
54.	F	*p.* 419
55.	C	*p.* 419
56.	W	*p.* 419
57.	K	*p.* 419
58.	S	*p.* 419
59.	D	*p.* 419
60.	H	*p.* 419

Chapter 10: Clinical Decision Making

Multiple Choice

1.	A	*p.* 437
2.	B	*p.* 437
3.	B	*p.* 437
4.	D	*p.* 438
5.	A	*p.* 437
6.	D	*p.* 438
7.	A	*p.* 439
8.	B	*p.* 439
9.	C	*p.* 439
10.	B	*p.* 439
11.	A	*p.* 442
12.	D	*p.* 443
13.	B	*p.* 443
14.	C	*p.* 443
15.	A	*p.* 443

16.	E	*p.* 443
17.	A	*p.* 443
18.	B	*p.* 444
19.	C	*p.* 444
20.	A	*p.* 444
21.	D	*p.* 445
22.	A	*p.* 445
23.	C	*p.* 446
24.	A	*p.* 447
25.	B	*p.* 447

True/False

26.	B	*p.* 437
27.	A	*p.* 438
28.	A	*p.* 438
29.	A	*p.* 439
30.	A	*p.* 439
31.	B	*p.* 441
32.	B	*p.* 441
33.	A	*p.* 442
34.	A	*p.* 444
35.	B	*p.* 448

Matching

36.	B	*p.* 446
37.	D	*p.* 446
38.	A	*p.* 446
39.	A	*p.* 445
40.	C	*p.* 446
41.	B	*p.* 446
42.	A	*p.* 446
43.	C	*p.* 446
44.	D	*p.* 447
45.	E	*p.* 447

Chapter 11: Assessment-Based Management

Multiple Choice

1.	B	*p.* 450
2.	E	*p.* 451
3.	C	*p.* 451
4.	D	*p.* 451
5.	E	*p.* 453

6.	C	*p.* 452
7.	E	*p.* 453
8.	C	*p.* 455
9.	D	*p.* 455
10.	D	*p.* 456
11.	E	*p.* 456
12.	B	*p.* 456
13.	C	*p.* 457
14.	A	*p.* 458
15.	A	*p.* 458
16.	C	*p.* 458
17.	B	*p.* 459
18.	C	*p.* 459
19.	A	*p.* 458
20.	B	*p.* 459
21.	B	*p.* 459
22.	D	*p.* 460
23.	C	*p.* 460
24.	E	*p.* 460
25.	B	*p.* 461

True/False

26.	B	*p.* 451
27.	A	*p.* 451
28.	F	*p.* 452
29.	A	*p.* 452
30.	A	*p.* 453
31.	B	*p.* 454
32.	B	*p.* 455
33.	A	*p.* 460
34.	B	*p.* 460
35.	A	*p.* 461

Matching

36.	A	*p.* 455
37.	B	*p.* 456
38.	A	*p.* 455
39.	B	*p.* 456
40.	B	*p.* 456

Chapter 12: Anatomy and Physiology

Part 1

Multiple Choice

1.	A	*p.* 466
2.	A	*p.* 467
3.	C	*p.* 467
4.	E	*p.* 468
5.	C	*p.* 468
6.	D	*p.* 469
7.	A	*p.* 470
8.	E	*p.* 470
9.	D	*p.* 470
10.	A	*p.* 471
11.	E	*p.* 471
12.	E	*p.* 472
13.	A	*p.* 472
14.	B	*p.* 472
15.	A	*p.* 472
16.	B	*p.* 473
17.	B	*p.* 473
18.	C	*p.* 474
19.	D	*p.* 475
20.	E	*p.* 476
21.	B	*p.* 477
22.	A	*p.* 477
23.	B	*p.* 478
24.	E	*p.* 479
25.	D	*p.* 479
26.	A	*p.* 480
27.	B	*p.* 480
28.	A	*p.* 480
29.	B	*p.* 481
30.	D	*p.* 482
31.	E	*p.* 482
32.	B	*p.* 483
33.	C	*p.* 483
34.	B	*p.* 483
35.	D	*p.* 483

True/False

36.	B	*p.* 469
37.	A	*p.* 469
38.	A	*p.* 472
39.	B	*p.* 473
40.	B	*p.* 474
41.	B	*p.* 475
42.	A	*p.* 483
43.	A	*p.* 483
44.	B	*p.* 483

Matching

45.	B	*p.* 484
46.	J	*p.* 468
47.	C	*p.* 468
48.	E	*p.* 468
49.	B	*p.* 468
50.	D	*p.* 468
51.	A	*p.* 468
52.	H	*p.* 468
53.	G	*p.* 468
54.	I	*p.* 468
55.	F	*p.* 468

Part 2

Multiple Choice

1.	A	*p.* 487
2.	A	*p.* 488
3.	E	*p.* 488
4.	D	*p.* 489
5.	C	*p.* 489
6.	B	*p.* 490
7.	C	*p.* 491
8.	D	*p.* 492
9.	A	*p.* 493
10.	E	*p.* 494
11.	B	*p.* 495
12.	A	*p.* 496
13.	B	*p.* 496
14.	E	*p.* 497
15.	D	*p.* 497
16.	B	*p.* 500
17.	C	*p.* 501
18.	B	*p.* 501
19.	A	*p.* 501
20.	C	*p.* 501
21.	D	*p.* 501
22.	A	*p.* 502
23.	B	*p.* 503
24.	A	*p.* 503

25.	C	*p.* 503		71.	D	*p.* 552
26.	A	*p.* 504		72.	D	*p.* 552
27.	C	*p.* 518		73.	A	*p.* 558
28.	E	*p.* 518		74.	D	*p.* 561
29.	D	*p.* 521		75.	C	*p.* 564
30.	E	*p.* 523		76.	B	*p.* 570
31.	B	*p.* 523		77.	B	*p.* 572
32.	C	*p.* 524		78.	B	*p.* 573
33.	E	*p.* 524		79.	D	*p.* 574
34.	D	*p.* 525		80.	B	*p.* 574
35.	B	*p.* 526		81.	B	*p.* 574
36.	A	*p.* 527		82.	E	*p.* 574
37.	C	*p.* 527		83.	C	*p.* 574
38.	E	*p.* 528		84.	B	*p.* 574
39.	C	*p.* 528		85.	C	*p.* 575
40.	E	*p.* 530		86.	A	*p.* 575
41.	B	*p.* 529		87.	A	*p.* 575
42.	C	*p.* 529		88.	C	*p.* 577
43.	C	*p.* 531		89.	B	*p.* 579
44.	D	*p.* 533		90.	E	*p.* 580
45.	A	*p.* 532		91.	A	*p.* 581
46.	A	*p.* 533		92.	D	*p.* 584
47.	C	*p.* 533		93.	D	*p.* 585
48.	B	*p.* 537		94.	D	*p.* 587
49.	C	*p.* 537		95.	B	*p.* 588
50.	B	*p.* 539		96.	C	*p.* 591
51.	A	*p.* 539		97.	C	*p.* 592
52.	C	*p.* 540		98.	E	*p.* 593
53.	E	*p.* 541		99.	D	*p.* 594
54.	B	*p.* 542		100.	D	*p.* 594
55.	E	*p.* 542		101.	B	*p.* 597
56.	B	*p.* 542		102.	A	*p.* 598
57.	E	*p.* 542		103.	C	*p.* 597
58.	C	*p.* 543		104.	C	*p.* 599
59.	A	*p.* 544		105.	D	*p.* 600
60.	D	*p.* 543		106.	E	*p.* 602
61.	B	*p.* 544		107.	D	*p.* 602
62.	E	*p.* 545		108.	A	*p.* 603
63.	A	*p.* 545		109.	B	*p.* 604
64.	C	*p.* 545		110.	C	*p.* 605
65.	D	*p.* 547		111.	A	*p.* 606
66.	C	*p.* 547		112.	E	*p.* 606
67.	C	*p.* 551		113.	C	*p.* 607
68.	C	*p.* 552		114.	C	*p.* 607
69.	A	*p.* 552		115.	B	*p.* 608
70.	E	*p.* 552		116.	A	*p.* 608

117.	E	*p. 609*
118.	C	*p. 609*
119.	C	*p. 609*
120.	A	*p. 610*
121.	C	*p. 611*
122.	E	*p. 611*
123.	E	*p. 585*
124.	B	*p. 585*
125.	A	*p. 585*
126.	E	*p. 585*
127.	A	*p. 616*
128.	B	*p. 619*
129.	D	*p. 622*
130.	B	*p. 623*
131.	C	*p. 624*
132.	E	*p. 625*
133.	A	*p. 627*
134.	B	*p. 627*
135.	A	*p. 627*
136.	C	*p. 627*
137.	D	*p. 627*
138.	C	*p. 628*
139.	D	*p. 629*
140.	C	*p. 629*

True/False

141.	A	*p. 488*
142.	A	*p. 492*
143.	A	*p. 522*
144.	B	*p. 527*
145.	A	*p. 527*
146.	A	*p. 528*
147.	A	*p. 541*
148.	B	*p. 545*
149.	A	*p. 571*
150.	A	*p. 575*
151.	A	*p. 582*
152.	A	*p. 584*
153.	A	*p. 597*
154.	A	*p. 600*
155.	A	*p. 621*
156.	B	*p. 622*

Matching

157.	J	*p. 468*
158.	C	*p. 468*

159.	E	*p. 468*
160.	B	*p. 468*
161.	D	*p. 468*
162.	A	*p. 468*
163.	H	*p. 468*
164.	G	*p. 468*
165.	I	*p. 468*
166.	F	*p. 468*
167.	B or H	*p. 505*
168.	H or B	*p. 505*
169.	C	*p. 505*
170.	E	*p. 505*
171.	G	*p. 505*
172.	A	*p. 505*
173.	D	*p. 505*
174.	F	*p. 505*
175.	C	*p. 587*
176.	F	*p. 587*
177.	A	*p. 585*
178.	G	*p. 582*
179.	B	*p. 587*
180.	D	*p. 582*

Chapter 13: General Principles of Pathophysiology

Part 1

Multiple Choice

1.	B	*p. 633*
2.	B	*p. 633*
3.	E	*p. 635*
4.	A	*p. 634*
5.	C	*p. 634*
6.	A	*p. 635*
7.	D	*p. 635*
8.	E	*p. 635*
9.	A	*p. 636*
10.	E	*p. 636*
11.	E	*p. 637*
12.	D	*p. 638*
13.	A	*p. 639*
14.	C	*p. 639*
15.	A	*p. 640*
16.	B	*p. 640*

17.	B	*p.* 641
18.	A	*p.* 641
19.	D	*p.* 643
20.	C	*p.* 643
21.	B	*p.* 643
22.	C	*p.* 643
23.	D	*p.* 645
24.	E	*p.* 646
25.	D	*p.* 647
26.	B	*p.* 647
27.	C	*p.* 648
28.	A	*p.* 650
29.	E	*p.* 650
30.	C	*p.* 649
31.	A	*p.* 651
32.	C	*p.* 649
33.	E	*p.* 652
34.	C	*p.* 653
35.	C	*p.* 654
36.	A	*p.* 654
37.	C	*p.* 655
38.	C	*p.* 656
39.	D	*p.* 656
40.	A	*p.* 656
41.	C	*p.* 656
42.	D	*p.* 656
43.	D	*p.* 656
44.	B	*p.* 649
45.	E	*p.* 660
46.	D	*p.* 661
47.	C	*p.* 659
48.	C	*p.* 659
49.	B	*p.* 662
50.	E	*p.* 664

True/False

51.	B	*p.* 634
52.	A	*p.* 634
53.	B	*p.* 635
54.	B	*p.* 641
55.	B	*p.* 643
56.	A	*p.* 645
57.	B	*p.* 645
58.	A	*p.* 645
59.	B	*p.* 647
60.	A	*p.* 648

61.	B	*p.* 648
62.	A	*p.* 649
63.	A	*p.* 653
64.	B	*p.* 654
65.	A	*p.* 662

Matching

66.	A	*p.* 657
67.	C	*p.* 659
68.	E	*p.* 660
69.	D	*p.* 661
70.	E	*p.* 660
71.	D	*p.* 661
72.	E	*p.* 660
73.	E	*p.* 660
74.	C	*p.* 659
75.	B	*p.* 658

Part 2

Multiple Choice

1.	B	*p.* 664
2.	C	*p.* 665
3.	B	*p.* 667
4.	C	*p.* 667
5.	A	*p.* 668
6.	B	*p.* 668
7.	B	*p.* 669
8.	E	*p.* 669
9.	E	*p.* 670
10.	C	*p.* 670
11.	E	*p.* 670
12.	B	*p.* 671
13.	E	*p.* 671
14.	D	*p.* 674
15.	B	*p.* 674
16.	E	*p.* 674
17.	C	*p.* 676
18.	C	*p.* 677
19.	D	*p.* 677
20.	D	*p.* 677
21.	E	*p.* 679
22.	C	*p.* 681
23.	D	*p.* 681
24.	B	*p.* 681
25.	A	*p.* 681

26.	B	*p.* 681
27.	E	*p.* 682
28.	B	*p.* 682
29.	E	*p.* 682
30.	C	*p.* 683
31.	D	*p.* 684

True/False

32.	B	*p.* 666
33.	B	*p.* 667
34.	A	*p.* 667
35.	B	*p.* 672
36.	A	*p.* 675
37.	B	*p.* 676
38.	A	*p.* 677
39.	B	*p.* 679
40.	B	*p.* 683

Matching

41.	B	*p.* 686
42.	B	*p.* 674
43.	D	*p.* 674
44.	E	*p.* 674
45.	C	*p.* 675

Chapter 14: General Principles of Pharmacology

Part 1

Multiple Choice

1.	D	*p.* 690
2.	A	*p.* 691
3.	B	*p.* 691
4.	A	*p.* 691
5.	B	*p.* 691
6.	B	*p.* 691
7.	C	*p.* 692
8.	C	*p.* 692
9.	B	*p.* 693
10.	B	*p.* 694
11.	E	*p.* 694
12.	E	*p.* 695

13.	D	*p.* 693
14.	E	*p.* 693
15.	D	*p.* 696
16.	E	*p.* 697
17.	D	*p.* 698
18.	A	*p.* 698
19.	C	*p.* 698
20.	B	*p.* 698
21.	D	*p.* 699
22.	A	*p.* 700
23.	D	*p.* 702
24.	B	*p.* 703
25.	D	*p.* 703
26.	A	*p.* 704
27.	C	*p.* 704
28.	C	*p.* 704
29.	E	*p.* 704
30.	C	*p.* 705
31.	C	*p.* 705
32.	B	*p.* 705
33.	D	*p.* 706
34.	B	*p.* 706
35.	C	*p.* 706
36.	A	*p.* 706
37.	A	*p.* 707
38.	D	*p.* 708
39.	E	*p.* 708
40.	C	*p.* 708

True/False

41.	B	*p.* 691
42.	A	*p.* 693
43.	B	*p.* 693
44.	A	*p.* 695
45.	A	*p.* 695
46.	B	*p.* 696
47.	B	*p.* 696
48.	A	*p.* 696
49.	B	*p.* 698
50.	A	*p.* 698
51.	A	*p.* 698
52.	B	*p.* 699
53.	B	*p.* 700
54.	A	*p.* 703
55.	B	*p.* 705

Matching

56.	D	*p. 699*
57.	F	*p. 696*
58.	A	*p. 698*
59.	E	*p. 699*
60.	H	*p. 699*
61.	B	*p. 700*
62.	C	*p. 694*
63.	G	*p. 699*
64.	J	*p. 699*
65.	I	*p. 705*
66.	E	*p. 706*
67.	B	*p. 706*
68.	A	*p. 706*
69.	D	*p. 706*
70.	C	*p. 706*

Part 2

Multiple Choice

1.	E	*p. 710*
2.	B	*p. 711*
3.	E	*p. 711*
4.	A	*p. 711*
5.	D	*p. 711*
6.	C	*p. 712*
7.	B	*p. 712*
8.	C	*p. 712*
9.	C	*p. 713*
10.	A	*p. 712*
11.	D	*p. 713*
12.	A	*p. 714*
13.	B	*p. 714*
14.	B	*p. 716*
15.	A	*p. 716*
16.	B	*p. 716*
17.	A	*p. 715*
18.	C	*p. 717*
19.	D	*p. 717*
20.	D	*p. 718*
21.	D	*p. 718*
22.	B	*p. 718*
23.	B	*p. 719*
24.	B	*p. 719*
25.	A	*p. 719*
26.	B	*p. 720*

27.	B	*p. 721*
28.	B	*p. 721*
29.	A	*p. 722*
30.	A	*p. 722*
31.	D	*p. 722*
32.	D	*p. 722*
33.	C	*p. 722*
34.	B	*p. 722*
35.	D	*p. 723*
36.	A	*p. 723*
37.	D	*p. 723*
38.	A	*p. 725*
39.	E	*p. 725*
40.	B	*p. 725*
41.	D	*p. 728*
42.	D	*p. 727*
43.	A	*p. 726*
44.	A	*p. 725*
45.	B	*p. 730*
46.	C	*p. 731*
47.	D	*p. 732*
48.	C	*p. 734*
49.	C	*p. 735*
50.	C	*p. 736*
51.	A	*p. 737*
52.	D	*p. 738*
53.	B	*p. 738*
54.	B	*p. 738*
55.	B	*p. 739*
56.	D	*p. 739*
57.	C	*p. 739*
58.	E	*p. 740*
59.	C	*p. 741*
60.	A	*p. 741*
61.	C	*p. 743*
62.	B	*p. 743*
63.	A	*p. 743*
64.	C	*p. 744*
65.	E	*p. 745*
66.	E	*p. 746*
67.	A	*p. 748*
68.	E	*p. 748*
69.	A	*p. 749*
70.	C	*p. 749*
71.	C	*p. 749*
72.	B	*p. 750*

73.	B	*p. 750*
74.	A	*p. 751*
75.	D	*p. 751*
76.	A	*p. 753*
77.	B	*p. 755*
78.	E	*p. 756*
79.	B	*p. 758*
80.	A	*p. 759*

True/False

81.	A	*p. 713*
82.	A	*p. 717*
83.	B	*p. 718*
84.	A	*p. 719*
85.	B	*p. 720*
86.	B	*p. 723*
87.	A	*p. 725*
88.	A	*p. 728*
89.	B	*p. 743*
90.	A	*p. 743*

Matching

91.	B	*p. 712*
92.	F	*p. 714*
93.	C	*p. 712*
94.	D	*p. 713*
95.	E	*p. 713*
96.	D	*p. 719*
97.	B	*p. 736*
98.	C	*p. 729*
99.	F	*p. 739*
100.	A	*p. 729*
101.	C	*p. 725*
102.	A	*p. 725*
103.	D	*p. 725*
104.	A	*p. 725*
105.	C	*p. 725*

Chapter 15: Medication Administration

Part 1

Multiple Choice

1.	B	*p. 763*

2.	D	*p. 763*
3.	E	*p. 764*
4.	A	*p. 764*
5.	A	*p. 764*
6.	C	*p. 764*
7.	D	*p. 765*
8.	A	*p. 765*
9.	C	*p. 766*
10.	E	*p. 766*
11.	E	*p. 767*
12.	D	*p. 767*
13.	C	*p. 767*
14.	C	*p. 767*
15.	E	*p. 768*
16.	D	*p. 768*
17.	B	*p. 770*
18.	C	*p. 772*
19.	E	*p. 773*
20.	A	*p. 773*
21.	B	*p. 773*
22.	B	*p. 775*
23.	C	*p. 775*
24.	B	*p. 778*
25.	C	*p. 779*
26.	B	*p. 782*
27.	A	*p. 782*
28.	C	*p. 785*
29.	D	*p. 787*
30.	D	*p. 787*
31.	E	*p. 785*
32.	A	*p. 788*
33.	C	*p. 790*
34.	D	*p. 789*
35.	A	*p. 792*
36.	D	*p. 794*
37.	C	*p. 794*
38.	D	*p. 794*
39.	D	*p. 794*
40.	B	*p. 796*

True/False

41.	B	*p. 763*
42.	A	*p. 764*
43.	A	*p. 765*
44.	B	*p. 772*
45.	A	*p. 773*

46.	A	*p. 774*
47.	B	*p. 781*
48.	A	*p. 789*
49.	A	*p. 790*
50.	B	*p. 796*

Matching

51.	D	*p. 764*
52.	B	*p. 765*
53.	C	*p. 764*
54.	F	*p. 764*
55.	A	*p. 765*
56.	I	*p. 796*
57.	M	*p. 789*
58.	C	*p. 773*
59.	N	*p. 767*
60.	A	*p. 769*
61.	B	*p. 767*
62.	H	*p. 828*
63.	O	*p. 766*
64.	J	*p. 768*
65.	K	*p. 780*

Part 2

Multiple Choice

1.	E	*p. 796*
2.	E	*p. 797*
3.	D	*p. 797*
4.	A	*p. 798*
5.	C	*p. 799*
6.	E	*p. 799*
7.	D	*p. 799*
8.	E	*p. 800*
9.	E	*p. 800*
10.	B	*p. 800*
11.	A	*p. 800*
12.	D	*p. 800*
13.	C	*p. 802*
14.	E	*p. 804*
15.	B	*p. 805*
16.	D	*p. 806*
17.	B	*p. 806*
18.	B	*p. 806*
19.	C	*p. 808*
20.	C	*p. 810*

21.	E	*p. 812*
22.	E	*p. 812*
23.	D	*p. 814*
24.	D	*p. 814*
25.	D	*p. 814*
26.	D	*p. 815*
27.	B	*p. 823*
28.	B	*p. 825*
29.	B	*p. 825*
30.	C	*p. 826*
31.	C	*p. 826*
32.	C	*p. 828*
33.	A	*p. 828*
34.	C	*p. 828*
35.	A	*p. 830*
36.	C	*p. 834*
37.	E	*p. 834*
38.	D	*p. 834*
39.	B	*p. 834*
40.	E	*p. 835*

True/False

41.	B	*p. 797*
42.	A	*p. 799*
43.	B	*p. 799*
44.	A	*p. 803*
45.	A	*p. 803*
46.	A	*p. 803*
47.	B	*p. 804*
48.	B	*p. 806*
49.	A	*p. 808*
50.	B	*p. 814*
51.	A	*p. 817*
52.	A	*p. 824*
53.	A	*p. 825*
54.	A	*p. 826*
55.	A	*p. 828*

Matching

56.	E	*p. 814*
57.	G	*p. 814*
58.	A	*p. 813*
59.	J	*p. 828*
60.	B	*p. 814*
61.	F	*p. 814*
62.	C	*p. 814*

63.	I	*p. 828*
64.	D	*p. 814*
65.	H	*p. 814*

Part 3

Multiple Choice

1.	A	*p. 835*
2.	C	*p. 835*
3.	D	*p. 835*
4.	D	*p. 835*
5.	E	*p. 835*
6.	A	*p. 837*
7.	B	*p. 837*
8.	A	*p. 839*
9.	C	*p. 840*
10.	B	*p. 844*

True/False

11.	A	*p. 835*
12.	B	*p. 835*
13.	A	*p. 837*
14.	B	*p. 837*
15.	B	*p. 843*

Matching

16.	E	*p. 835*
17.	D	*p. 835*
18.	B	*p. 835*
19.	C	*p. 835*
20.	A	*p. 835*